Comprehensive Atlas of 3D Echocardiography

Edited by:

Roberto M. Lang, MD, FASE, FACC, FESC, FAHA, FRCP
Professor of Medicine and Radiolog, Director of Cardiac Imaging
Department of Medicine/Section of Cardiology
University of Chicago Medical Center
Chicago, Illinois

Stanton K. Shernan, MD, FAHA, FASE
Professor of Anesthesia
Department of Anesthesiology, Perioperative and Pain Medicine
Brigham and Women's Hospital
Harvard Medical School
Boston, Massachusetts

Girish S. Shirali, MBBS, FACC, FASE
Melva and Randall L. O'Donnell Family Chair in Cardiology
Section Chief, Cardiology
Medical Co-Director, The Ward Family Center For Congenital Heart Disease
Children's Mercy Hospital
University of Missouri—Kansas City School of Medicine
Kansas City, Missouri

Victor Mor-Avi, PhD, FASE
Professor, Director of Cardiac Imaging Research
Department of Medicine/Section of Cardiology
University of Chicago
Chicago, Illinois

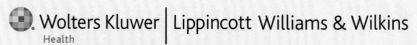

Wolters Kluwer | Lippincott Williams & Wilkins
Health

Philadelphia • Baltimore • New York • London
Buenos Aires • Hong Kong • Sydney • Tokyo

Acquisitions Editor: Brian Brown
Product Manager: Nicole Dernoski
Vendor Manager: Alicia Jackson
Senior Manufacturing Manager: Benjamin Rivera
Marketing Manager: Lisa Lawrence
Design Coordinator: Teresa Mallon
Production Service: SPi Global

Copyright © 2013 by LIPPINCOTT WILLIAMS & WILKINS, a WOLTERS KLUWER business
Two Commerce Square
2001 Market Street
Philadelphia, PA 19103 USA
LWW.com

Cover image has been reused with permission from Lang RM, Tsang W, Weinert L, et al. Valvular heart disease: The value of 3-dimensional echocardiography. *J Am Coll Cardiol.* 2011;58(19):1933–1944.

Printed in China

Library of Congress Cataloging-in-Publication Data
Comprehensive atlas of 3D echocardiography / edited by Roberto Lang ... [et al.].
   p. ; cm.
  Includes bibliographical references and index.
  ISBN 978-1-4511-4322-5
 I. Lang, Roberto M.
  [DNLM: 1. Echocardiography, Three-Dimensional—Atlases. 2. Heart Diseases—ultrasonography—Atlases. WG 17]
  616.1'207543—dc23

                                         2012018559

To purchase additional copies of this book, call our customer service department at (800) 638-3030 or fax orders to (301) 223-2320. International customers should call (301) 223-2300.

Visit Lippincott Williams & Wilkins on the Internet: at LWW.com. Lippincott Williams & Wilkins customer service representatives are available from 8:30 am to 6 pm, EST.

10 9 8 7 6 5 4 3 2 1

I would like to acknowledge the hard work of our cardiac sonographers and cardiology fellows at the University of Chicago Medical Center. Special thanks are due to Lynn Weinert for her unwavering support of our 3D ultrasound imaging program. On a personal level, I would like to acknowledge the support of my family: Lili, Gabriel, Daniella, and Lindsey during the preparation of this book.

—*Roberto M. Lang*

I would like to dedicate this book to my wife, Audrey, and children, Ethan and Mina, for their precious support, patience, and love; to my parents Sidney and Phyllis for their guidance and encouragement to pursue a passion for learning and excellence; and finally to my mentors, colleagues, and students over the years who have generously given me their extraordinary wisdom.

—*Stanton K. Shernan*

I would like to acknowledge the guidance of Drs. Tal Geva, Scott Bradley, Stella and Richard van Praagh, and Professor Robert Anderson. The assistance of our sonographers, especially Karen Chessa, is appreciated. I appreciate the support and understanding shown by Shefali, Raena, and Rohan Shirali over the course of the development of this work.

—*Girish S. Shirali*

I would like to thank all those who have contributed directly and indirectly to my ability to be part of this unique project. This includes my colleagues whose hard work resulted in the beautiful images on almost every page of this book. This also includes my family whose support makes a world of a difference. Special thanks to my life partner, Andy, for being there for me day in and day out. And finally, I want to thank my son Yarden and my daughter Eden for being the sunshine of my life, and for teaching me so many things about this world, which I could have never learned without them.

—*Victor Mor-Avi*

CONTRIBUTORS

Luigi P. Badano, MD, FESC, FACC
Medical Department of Cardiac, Thoracic and
    Vascular Sciences
University of Padua
Padua, Italy

Enrico G. Caiani, MS, PhD
Department of Biomedical Engineering
Politecnico di Milano
Milano, Italy

Sonal Chandra, MD
Department of Medicine/Section of Cardiology
University of Chicago Medical Center
Chicago, Illinois

Carlo Dal Lin, MD
Department of Cardiac, Thoracic and
    Vascular Sciences
University of Padua
Padua, Italy

Jeanne M. DeCara, MD
Department of Medicine/Section of Cardiology
University of Chicago Medical Center
Chicago, Illinois

Benjamin H. Freed, MD
Department of Medicine/Section of Cardiology
University of Chicago Medicine
Chicago, Illinois

Swaminatha Gurudevan, MD
Cedars Sinai Heart Institute
Cedars Sinai Medical Center
Los Angeles, California

Mark S. Hynes, MD, FRCPC
Division of Cardiac Anesthesia and
    Critical Care Medicine
University of Ottawa Heart Institute
Ottawa, Canada

Sabino Iliceto, MD, FESC, FAHA
Department of Cardiac, Thoracic and
    Vascular Sciences
University of Padua
University Hospital
Padua, Italy

Itzhak Kronzon, MD
Department of Cardiovascular Medicine
North Shore—LIJ/Lenox Hill Hospital
New York, New York

Stephane Lambert, MD, FRCPC
Division of Cardiac Anesthesiology
University of Ottawa Heart Institute
Cardiac Anesthesia, Ottawa Heart Institute
Ottawa, Ontario
Canada

Roberto M. Lang, MD
Department of Medicine/Section of Cardiology
University of Chicago Medical Center
Chicago, Illinois

Huai Luo, MD
Cedars Sinai Heart Institute
Cedars Sinai Medical Center
Los Angeles, California

Victor Mor-Avi, PhD
Department of Medicine/Section of Cardiology
University of Chicago
Chicago, Illinois

Denisa Muraru, MD
Department of Cardiac, Thoracic and Vascular Sciences
University of Padua
Padua, Italy

Gila Perk, MD, FACC, FASE
Echocardiography Laboratory
Lenox Hill Hospital
North Shore LIJ Health System
New York, New York

David A. Roberson, MD
The Heart Institute for Children
Hope Children's Hospital
Oak Lawn, Illinois

Carlos Ruiz, MD
Department of Interventional Cardiology
Lenox Hill Hospital
New York, New York

Muhamed Saric, MD, PhD, FACC, FASE
New York University Langone Medical Center
New York, New York

Stanton K. Shernan, MD, FAHA, FASE
Department of Anesthesiology, Perioperative and Pain
  Medicine
Brigham and Women's Hospital
Harvard Medical School
Boston, Massachusetts

Takahiro Shiota, MD
Cedars-Sinai Heart Institute
Cedars-Sinai Medical Center and UCLA
Los Angeles, California

Girish S. Shirali, MBBS, FACC, FASE
Children's Mercy Hospital
University of Missouri—Kansas City School of Medicine
Kansas City, Missouri

Robert J. Siegel, MD
Cedars-Sinai Heart Institute
Cedars-Sinai Medical Center and Geffen School of
  Medicine at UCLA
Los Angeles, California

John M. Simpson, MD, FRCP, FESC
Department of Congenital Heart Disease
Evelina Children's Hospital
Guy's and St. Thomas' NHS Foundation Trust
London, United Kingdom

Nirmal Singh, MBBS
Cedars Sinai Heart Institute
Cedars Sinai Medical Center
Los Angeles, California

Masaaki Takeuchi, MD, PhD
Second Department of Internal Medicine
University of Occupational and Environmental Health
School of Medicine
Kitakyushu, Japan

Kirsten Tolstrup, MD
Cedars Sinai Heart Institute
Cedars Sinai Medical Center
Los Angeles, California

Wendy Tsang, MD, FRCP(C)
Non-Invasive Cardiac Imaging Laboratory
University of Chicago Medical Center
Chicago, Illinois

Vivian Wei Cui, MD
The Heart Institute for Children
Hope Children's Hospital
Oak Lawn, Illinois

Lynn Weinert, BS
Department of Medicine/Section of Cardiology
University of Chicago Medical Center
Chicago, Illinois

PREFACE

Over the past several decades, technological advances have significantly contributed to the development of echocardiography as an invaluable diagnostic tool, which is also used to monitor cardiac performance. Although the concept of three-dimensional (3D) echocardiography was first introduced in the 1970s, it was only recently that it gained widespread clinical use and appropriate recognition with the development of real-time 3D imaging. Today, echocardiography provides more than just pretty pictures. Its advantages in improving the diagnostic confidence of the echocardiographic examination are well established and rapidly broadening as these techniques are being incorporated into mainstream clinical imaging protocols.

The advantages of 3D echocardiography stem from the fact that with the preservation of spatial and temporal resolution, the addition of the third dimension of depth contributes to our understanding of and ability to accurately quantify complex anatomy and functional geometry of cardiac chambers, valves, and great vessels. Consequently, 3D echocardiography greatly enhances diagnosis, while facilitating interpretation, communication, education, and clinical decision making.

The *Comprehensive Atlas of 3D Echocardiography* uses the advantages of a multimedia format to address the unique dynamic nature of this imaging modality. The use of a combination of figures and videos provides examples of unique imaging windows, along with novel displays using dedicated cropping tools, in order to appreciate how a comprehensive 3D echocardiographic examination can be performed in patients with normal anatomy and physiology, as well as those with complex heart disease and congenital heart defects. The significant number and variety of case studies in this Atlas demonstrate the advantages of 3D echocardiography in terms of unique quantitative and qualitative analyses that far exceed what can be accomplished using standard two-dimensional techniques. We hope that this Atlas will be of use to all echocardiography professionals, including sonographers, anesthesiologists, intensivists, cardiac surgeons, and cardiologists.

ACKNOWLEDGMENTS

The photographic images of cardiac specimens in this volume are from the Archiving Working Group (AWG) (http://ipccc-awg.net), of the International Society for Nomenclature of Paediatric and Congenital Heart Disease (ISNPCHD). Diane E. Spicer BS, PA (ASCP) of the Congenital Heart Institute of Florida (CHIF) is the Senior Archivist for the AWG. (The AWG is supported in part by a grant from The Children's Heart Foundation.) The editors are grateful to Diane Spicer for her invaluable contributions to this work.

CONTENTS

TRANSTHORACIC AND TRANSESOPHAGEAL MATRIX TRANSDUCERS AND IMAGE FORMATION

1

Enrico G. Caiani

Three-dimensional echocardiography (3DE) is a relatively young ultrasound imaging modality that was developed in the 1980s, when off-line 3D reconstruction from serial multiplane 2D acquisitions was reported for the first time.[1,2] In the early 1990s, technologic improvements in the field of transducer design and electronic circuitry led to the development of a probe with piezoelectric crystals arranged as a sparse matrix of about 300 elements, instead of linear vectors, capable of scanning pyramidal volumes, rather than single-plane sectors.[3] Despite the relatively low spatial and temporal resolution, this system allowed fast acquisition of pyramidal datasets during a single breath-hold without the need for off-line reconstruction.

In the last 10 years, impressive progress has been attained by the development of a full matrix array probe technology of about 3,000 piezoelectric elements, based on advanced digital processing and improved image formation algorithms, capable of providing higher spatial and temporal resolution for real-time volumetric imaging (Fig. 1-1). This second-generation transducers, the first to become commercially available, overcame many of the limitations that had precluded 3DE from being used in the clinical setting,[4,5] despite the fact that for wider-angle acquisition to be possible, multiple ECG-gated narrow-angle images had to be acquired.

Further advances in miniaturization of the electronics and in element interconnection technology resulted in the ability to insert a full matrix array into the tip of a transesophageal probe[6] as well as the possibility of full-volume imaging to include the entire left ventricular (LV) cavity in a single beat.[7] Also, the continuous technologic improvements in circuitry miniaturization recently resulted in the development of new probes capable of both 2D and 3D imaging, thus preserving image quality, in the attempt to improve the workflow of the echocardiographic examination.

A conventional phased array probe utilizes multiple piezoelectric elements, electrically isolated from each other, oriented in a single row (Fig. 1-2). Individual wave fronts are generated by firing elements in a specific sequence, with a delay in phase with respect to the transmit initiation time. Each element constructively and destructively adds and subtracts pulses to generate an overall wave with a specific direction that constitutes a radially propagating scan line. The one-dimensional array can be steered in two dimensions: radial and azimuthal (lateral), while resolution in elevation is fixed by the slice thickness, which is related to the piezoelectric element vertical dimension. In the full matrix array probe, about 3,000 independent piezoelectric elements are arranged in a checkerboard fashion and used to steer the beam electronically. This checkerboard pattern allows phasic firing of all elements to generate a radially propagating scan line that can be steered in both depth, azimuth, and elevation directions in order to scan a true 3D volume.

The major technologic advances that allowed the manufacturing of the fully sampled matrix array transducer were (1) the ability to develop electrical interconnections for every piezoelectric element, which enables each element to be independently controlled, both with respect to transmitting and receiving[8] (Fig. 1-3) as well as (2) microbeamforming that allows the same transducer cable size of conventional 2D imaging to be used with 3D imaging despite the 3,000 elements, thus keeping the transducer head and cable sizes practical for routine scanning.[9,10]

Beamforming is a signal processing technique used to create directional or spatial selectivity of signals sent to or received from an array of sensors (Fig. 1-4). In 2D echocardiography, all the components of the beamforming electronics (high-voltage transmitters, low-noise receivers, analog-to-digital converters, digital delay lines, delay controllers) are in the system and usually consume about 100 W using 1,500 cm^2 of personal computer's electronic board area. The extension of the classical beamforming approach for full matrix array probe would be impractical, since it would require a 3,000 channel system and cable, 4-kW power consumption, and a huge PC board area to contain all the needed circuitry. Therefore, the adopted solution was to move part

1

of the beamforming circuitry directly into the transducer (Figs. 1-5 and 1-6). This single circuit design that results in an active probe allows microbeamforming of the signal with very low power consumption (<1 W). However, the engineering of active transducers involves thermal management, since the electronics inside the transducer generate heat, which increases during imaging with the mechanical index (Fig. 1-7). Improved crystal technology obtained using new manufacturing processes (PureWave, Philips) allows the acquisition of single crystal materials with homogeneous solid-state domains and piezoelectric properties (Fig. 1-8). These new transducers result in reduced heating production by increasing the efficiency in the transduction process. In this manner, a better conversion of transmit power into ultrasound energy, and of received ultrasound into electrical energy, is achieved, together with a wider bandwidth, resulting in increased echo penetration and resolution, with the additional benefits of improved image quality, less artifacts, lower power consumption, and higher Doppler sensitivity (Fig. 1-9).

When considering the ideal performance of the 3D system, in terms of frame rate, volume size and resolution, the main limiting factor is nowadays represented by the speed of sound, equal to approximately 1,540 m/s in myocardial tissue and blood. This value, divided by the distance a single pulse has to propagate back and forth (determined by the imaging depth), results in the maximum number of pulses that can be fired per second without getting interference. Based on the pyramid angular width and the desired beam spacing in each dimension, this number is related to the volumes per second that can be imaged. Possible solutions to cope with this limitation include parallel receive beamforming that allows true real-time full-volume acquisition, ECG-gated stitching for subvolumes, or real-time zoom feature by reducing the field of view.

Parallel beamforming or multiline acquisition ("explososcan") is a technique where the system transmits one wide beam and receives multiple narrow beams in parallel.[11] In this way, frame (volume) rate is increased by a factor equal to the number of the receiving beams. Each beamformer focuses along a slightly different direction that was insonified by the broad transmit pulse. This parallel processing of the received data permits multiple scan lines to be sampled in the amount of time a conventional scanner would take for a single line, at the expense of reduced signal strength and resolution, as the receive beams are steered farther and farther away from the center of the transmit beam, thus receiving lower energy signals (Fig. 1-10).

The relation between frame rate, receive beams, sector width, depth, and line density can be described by the following equation[12,13]:

$$\text{Frame rate} = \frac{1,540 \times \text{Number of parallel receive beams}}{2 \times (\text{Volume width / lateral resolution})^2 \times \text{Volume depth}}$$

By either changing volume widths or depth, frame rate can be adjusted to the specific needs. Also, the 3D system could allow the user to modify the lateral resolution, by changing the density of the scan lines in the pyramidal sector (Fig. 1-11). However, a decrease in spatial resolution also affects the contrast resolution of the image. By increasing the number of parallel receive beams, the frame rate increases but at the expense of a lower signal-to-noise ratio and thus image quality (Fig. 1-12).[14]

In multibeat acquisition, ECG-gated stitching of subvolumes acquired from different cardiac cycles allows increasing the volume size, while maintaining the frame rate, and vice versa (Fig. 1-13). ECG-gated stitching is of course prone to motion artifacts caused by transducer movement, respiration, and varying heart rate.[15] It is important that the 3D system is able to display the stitched data in real time so that the sonographer, while imaging, can verify that the data are acquired without artifacts. Matrix array probes can also provide real-time multiple 2D images, at high frame rates, oriented in predefined or user-selected plane orientations. This concept has been further developed in the last generation of 2D/3D matrix array probes, where the 2D imaging plane is obtained by electronically rotating the beam, keeping the transducer in the same position, to avoid foreshortening (Fig. 1-14). During acquisition, or once the 3D dataset has been stored, different visualization strategies are available: (1) visualize one or multiple cross sections as standard 2D images, manually or automatically selected[16]; (2) simulate the 3D appearance by volume rendering[17]; or (3) detect off-line the cardiac structures and visualize them as surface rendered models in 3D.

In summary, improvements in probe technology achieved by circuitry miniaturization and crystal technology have enabled impressive performances in the field of real-time 3D echocardiography, which is now limited only by the laws of physics.

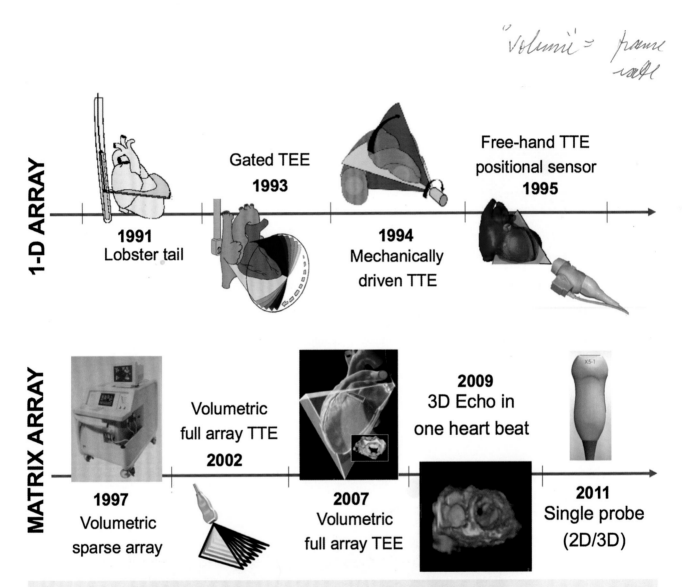

Figure 1-1. Evolution of 3DE over time. Top. Acquisition techniques of multiple ECG- and respiration-gated 2D acquisitions, resulting in off-line 3D reconstruction. Bottom. Major advances relevant to matrix array technology.

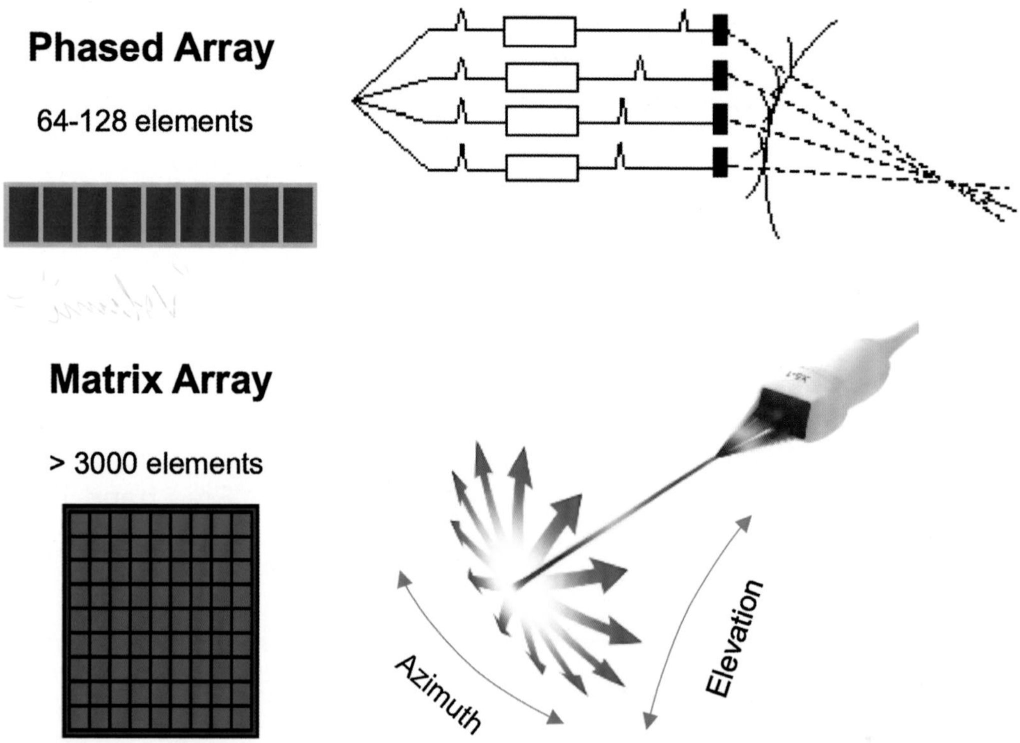

Phased Array

64-128 elements

Matrix Array

> 3000 elements

Azimuth

Elevation

Figure 1-2. **Steering capabilities of transducers.** Schematic of the phased array (top) and the matrix array (bottom) transducer, with their respective steering capabilities. The phased array can only steer in two dimensions (radial and azimuthal), by firing elements in a specific sequence, with a delay in phase with respect to a transmit initiation time and with resolution in elevation related to the piezoelectric element vertical dimension. In contrast, the checkerboard pattern of the matrix array allows phasic firing of all the elements to generate a radially propagated scanline that can be steered in both depth, azimuth, and elevation in order to scan a true 3D volume.

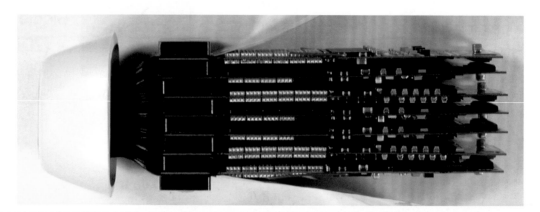

Figure 1-3. **Interconnection technology.** 3D transducer with fully sampled 2D matrix array, interconnection technology, and custom-made transmit and receive electronics. (With kind permission from Springer Science + Business Media: *Textbook of real-time three dimensional echocardiography,* Badano L, Lang RM, Zamorano JL, eds. Technical principles of transthoracic three-dimensional echocardiography, 2011, Stain I Rabben, Figure 2.1.b, and any original (first) copyright notice displayed with material.)

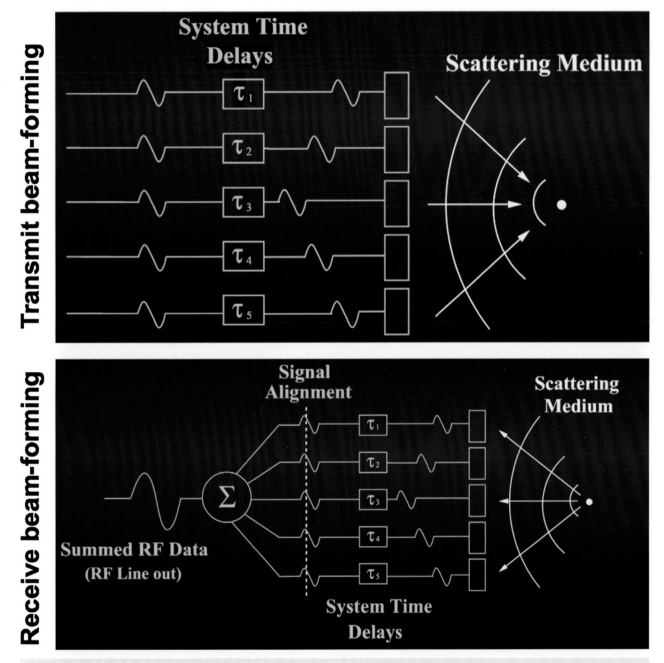

Figure 1-4. **Schematic of beamforming.** On the transmit side (**top**), focused beams of ultrasound are created using a phased array, thus introducing delays in each element line. In the receive beamforming (**bottom**), focusing is achieved by appropriately delaying echo signals arriving at different elements to align them in a way that creates an isophase plane. These aligned echoes are then all summed coherently.

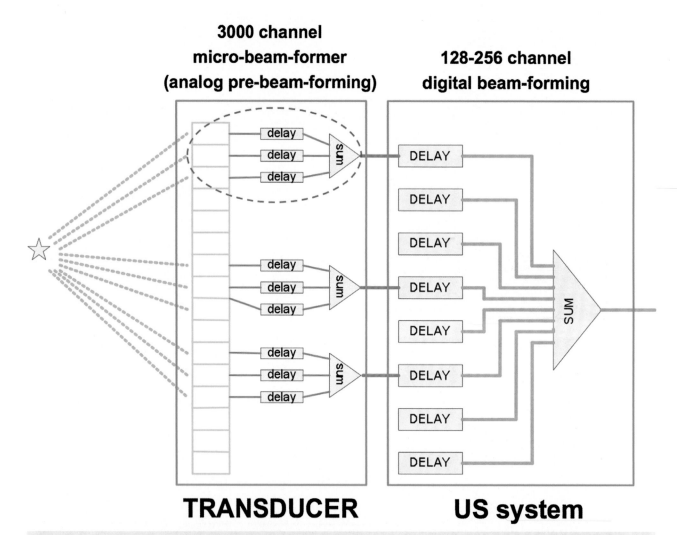

Figure 1-5. Schematic of the cascaded beamformer approach for full matrix probe. In this two level approach, the steering process is split into two pieces: coarse and fine steering. Fine steering is performed by the 3,000 channel analog microbeam-former, implemented by placing fine analog delay circuitry into application of specific integrated circuits (or ASIC) placed into the transducer head, and connected to the 3,000 piezoelectric elements. Fine steering is performed in the transducer using different subsections of the element matrix known as patches (evidenced by the *dashed red line*), by delaying and summing signals within each patch. This allows the number of control lines to be put into the transducer coaxial cable that links the transducer to the ultrasound system to the downsized from 3,000 to the conventional size of 128 to 256 channels. Coarse steering is digitally performed within the system, where the analog-to-digital conversion takes place, using digital delay lines. (Courtesy from Philips Medical System.)

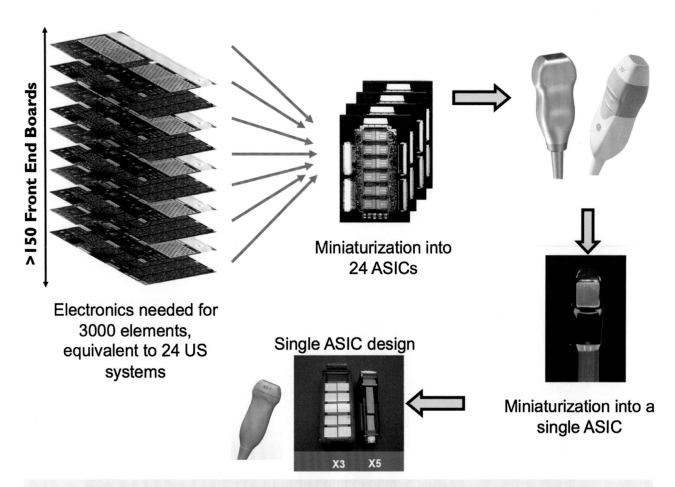

Figure 1-6. Evolution of the miniaturization of the electronic circuitry. From the 150 front-end boards potentially needed to control beamforming in a full matrix array probe, their miniaturization led to 24 application specific integrated circuits (ASICs) that were fitted into the ergonomic housing of the transducer. Further technologic improvements led to the miniaturization into a single ASIC to be contained in the transesophageal tip. This concept was then transferred to the design of new transthoracic probes, based on single ASIC.

Active cooling

Passive cooling

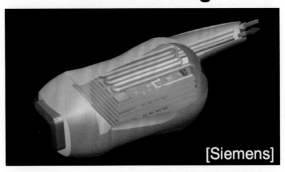 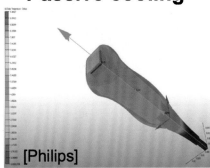

Figure 1-7. **3D probe thermal management solutions.** Two different strategies are shown: active cooling (left), where the heat is actively transported through the transducer cable, or active cooling, or passive cooling (right), where cooling is obtained by a reduction in heating production by improved crystal technology, low power-specific integrated circuit, and efficient acoustic design.

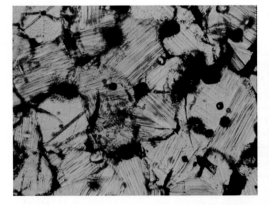 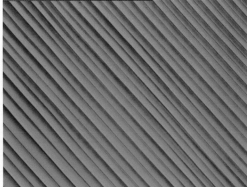

800 x Magnification

Figure 1-8. **Improvements in crystal technology.** Comparison of conventional PZT (lead–zirconate–tungsten) ceramic (left) versus novel single crystal materials (right) obtained with PureWave (Philips) technology. While the ceramic material appears imperfect, multicrystalline with randomly oriented grains, the single crystal shows a perfect atomic level arrangements, uniform, and without grain boundaries, thus resulting in a more efficient transduction process. (Courtesy from Philips Medical System.)

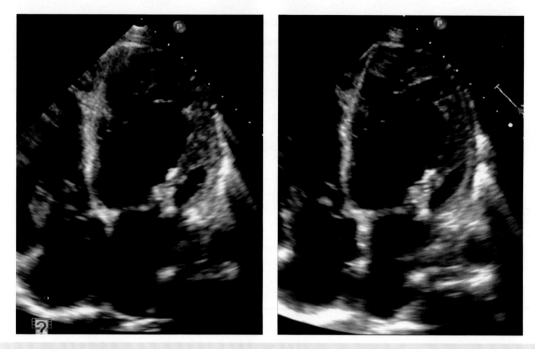

Figure 1-9. Performance of 3D probe with novel crystal technology. Example of the same patient in an apical four-chamber view using conventional 2D probe (S5-1, left) and the novel full matrix probe (X5-1, right) with PureWave crystal technology. One of the advantages related to the use of this improved crystal technology consists in the possibility of utilizing the same transducer for both 2D and 3D imaging, without losing 2D image quality. This results in improved workflow during the echo-cardiographic examination.

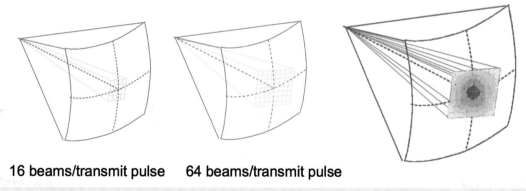

16 beams/transmit pulse   64 beams/transmit pulse

Figure 1-10. Parallel beamforming. Schematic of the process, receiving in parallel 16 (left) or 64 (center) beams for each transmit pulse. For example, to obtain a 90×90 16-cm depth volume at a rate of 25 Hz, 200,000 lines/s need to be received. Since the capability of emission is about 5,000 pulses/s, there is a need to receive 42 beams in parallel for each transmit pulse. But increasing the number of parallel beams to improve frame rate leads to an increase in size, cost, and power consumption of the beamforming electronics, broader width of the transmit beam, and deterioration in the signal-to-noise ratio and contrast resolution. On the right, a schematic of the amplitude (from *red* as max to *yellow* as min) of the broad transmit pulse, centered in the transmitted scan line, resulting in received lower energy signals from the parallel receiving beams steered farther away from the center of the transmit beam, is shown.

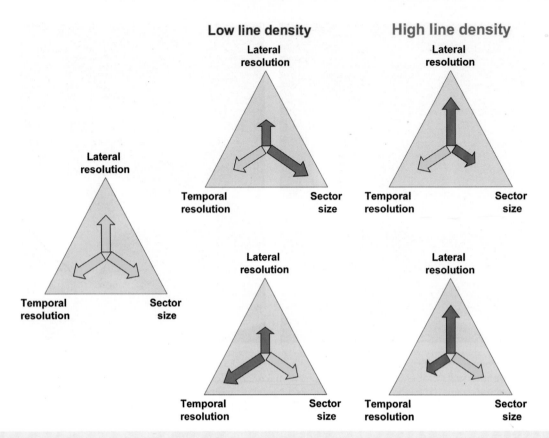

Figure 1-11. Spatial and temporal resolution. Schematic of the relation between temporal resolution (frame rate), sector size (width and depth), and lateral resolution (line density). For a constant frame rate, lines widely spaced can increase the volume size at the cost of lowering resolution (**top center**), or at the price of a smaller volume, tight line spacing can be used (as in zoom mode) to increase lateral resolution (**top right**). In a similar manner, with a constant sector size, lower line density increases the frame rate reducing lateral resolution (**bottom center**), while higher line density results in the opposite (**bottom right**).

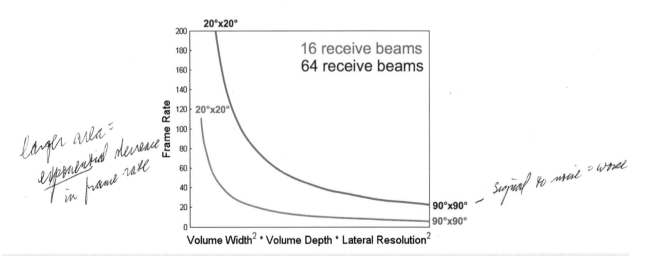

Figure 1-12. Parallel beamforming and frame rate. Visualization of the relationship between frame rate and the other variables described by the formula in the text, using 16 or 64 receive beams. For each number of receive beams, by increasing the scan volume from 20×20 to 90×90 (moving from left to right along the curve), the frame rate is exponentially decreased. By increasing the number of receive beams from 16 to 64, the curve is upper translated, with an improvement in frame rate due to the fixed value of the denominator in the formula. However, the signal-to-noise ratio of the acquired data is worse, as seen in this figure, due to the receiving lower energy signals. (With kind permission from Springer Science + Business Media: *Textbook of real-time three dimensional echocardiography*, Badano L, Lang RM, Zamorano JL, eds. Technical principles of transthoracic three-dimensional echocardiography, 2011, Stain I Rabben, Figure 2.4, and any original (first) copyright notice displayed with material.)

Live 3D   **Full volume: 1 beat**

Full volume: 4 beats   **Full volume: 8 beat**

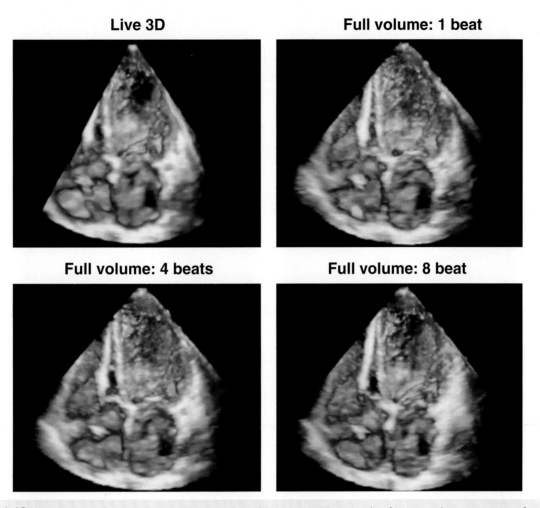

Figure 1-13. Parallel beamforming versus ECG-gated stitching. (MOVIES) Example of imaging the same patient from transthoracic apical view using live 3D mode (**top left**), full volume in one heartbeat (**top right**), and ECG-gated full volume in four (**bottom left**) and eight (**bottom right**) consecutive beats.

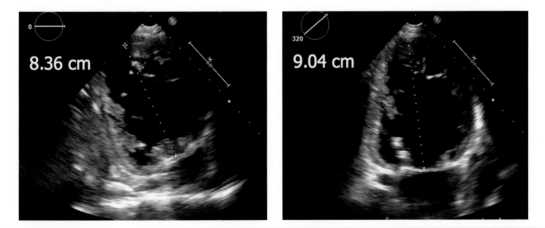

Figure 1-14. Novel 2D electronic steering advantages. Example of the electronic correction of the imaging plane to avoid foreshortening, by electronically rotating the beam, keeping the transducer in the same imaging position. The increase in the long-axis measurement corresponding to the nonforeshortened view is visible (**right panel**).

References

1. Matsumoto M, Inoue M, Tamura S, et al. Three-dimensional echocardiography for spatial visualization and volume calculation of cardiac structures. *J Clin Ultrasound*. 1981;9:157–165.

2. Stickels KR, Wann LS. An analysis of three-dimensional reconstructive echocardiography. *Ultrasound Med Biol*. 1984;10:575–580.

3. von Ramm OT, Smith SW. Real time volumetric ultrasound imaging system. *J Digit Imaging*. 1990;3:261–266.

4. Sugeng L, Weinert L, Lang RM. Left ventricular assessment using real time three-dimensional echocardiography. *Heart*. 2003;89:29–36.

5. Sugeng L, Weinert L, Thiele K, et al. Real-time three-dimensional echocardiography using a novel matrix array transducer. *Echocardiography*. 2003;20:623–635.

6. Sugeng L, Shernan SK, Salgo IS, et al. Live three-dimensional transesophageal echocardiography: initial experience using the fully-sampled matrix array probe. *J Am Coll Cardiol*. 2008;52:446–449.

7. Gonçalves A, Zamorano JL. Valve anatomy and function with transthoracic three-dimensional echocardiography: advantages and limitations of instantaneous full-volume color Doppler imaging. *Ther Adv Cardiovasc Dis*. 2010;4:385–394.

8. Savord B, Solomon R. Fully sampled matrix transducer for real time 3D ultrasonic imaging. *Proc IEEE Ultrason Symp*. 2003:945–953.

9. Zhang F, Bilas A, Dhanantwari A, et al. Parallelization and performance of 3D ultrasound imaging beamforming algorithms on modern clusters. *Proc ICS*. 2002.

10. Dhanantwari AC, Stergiopoulos S, Song L, et al. An efficient 3D beamformer implementation for real-time 4D ultrasound systems deploying planar array probes. *Proc IEEE Ultrason Symp*. 2004;1421–1424.

11. Bredthauer G, von Ramm OT. Array design for ultrasound imaging with simultaneous beams. *Proc IEEE International Symposium on Biomedical Imaging*. 2002:981–984.

12. Rabben SI. Technical principles of transthoracic three-dimensional echocardiography. In: Badano L, Lang RM, Zamorano JL, eds. *Textbook of real-time three dimensional echocardiography*. London: Springer, 2011.

13. Angelini E, Gerard O. Imagerie cardiaque ultrasonore dynamique. In: Clarysse P, ed. *Imagerie dynamique cardiaque et thoracique (Traité Information et Science du Vivant, IC2)*. France: Hermes Science Publications - Lavoisier, 2011: Chapter 5.

14. Salgo IS. Three-dimensional echocardiographic technology. *Cardiol Clin*. 2007;25:231–239.

15. Brekke S, Rabben SI, Støylen A, et al. Volume stitching in three-dimensional echocardiography: distortion analysis and extension to real time. *Ultrasound Med Biol*. 2007;33:782–796.

16. Nucifora G, Badano LP, Dall'Armellina E, et al. Fast data acquisition and analysis with real time triplane echocardiography for the assessment of left ventricular size and function: a validation study. *Echocardiography*. 2009;26:66–75.

17. Steen E, Olstad B. Volume rendering of 3D medical ultrasound data using direct feature mapping. *IEEE Trans Med Imaging* 1994;13:517–525.

2

INSTRUMENTATION AND DATA ACQUISITION

Luigi P. Badano, Denisa Muraru, Carlo Dal Lin, Sabino Iliceto

FULLY SAMPLED MATRIX ARRAY TRANSDUCERS

An important milestone in the history of real-time three-dimensional echocardiography (3DE) has been the development of fully sampled matrix array transthoracic transducers, which allowed the operators to acquire within a short time good-quality volume-rendered images.

Currently, 3DE matrix array transducers are composed of nearly 3,000 piezoelectric elements with operating frequencies ranging from 2 to 4 MHz for transthoracic echocardiography (TTE) and 5 to 7 MHz for transesophageal echocardiography (TEE). These piezoelectric elements are arranged in a matrix configuration within the transducer and require a large number of digital channels for these elements to be connected. To reduce both power consumption and the size of the connecting cable, several miniaturized circuit boards are incorporated into the transducer, allowing partial beamforming to be performed in the probe. A fully sampled matrix array transducer allows the ultrasound beam to be steered along the usual two-dimensional (2D) x-axis (lateral or azimuthal: left and right), y-axis (vertical or axial: up and down), and the z-axis (elevation: front and back) (Fig. 2-1).

Additionally, developments in transducer technology have resulted in a reduced transducer footprint, improved side-lobe suppression, increased sensitivity and penetration, and harmonic capabilities that can be used for both gray-scale and contrast imaging. The most recent generation of matrix transducers are significantly smaller than the previous ones; they allow both the 2D and 3DE imaging; the quality of the 2D and 3D imaging has improved significantly, compared to the previous generations.

DATA ACQUISITION

With current 3DE technology, there are two data acquisition methods: electrocardiogram (ECG)-triggered multibeat 3DE reconstruction and real-time or live 3DE imaging. Multibeat 3DE provides images of higher spatial and temporal resolution. This is achieved through consecutive acquisitions of narrow volumes of data over several heartbeats (ranging from two to seven cardiac cycles) that are subsequently stitched together to create a single volumetric dataset (Fig. 2-2). However, gated imaging of the heart is inherently prone to imaging artifacts created by the patient's body or respiratory motion or irregular cardiac rhythm (Fig. 2-3).

In contrast, real-time or live 3DE imaging refers to acquisition of a pyramidal dataset in a single heartbeat. Most ultrasound systems have real-time 3DE volume imaging available in the following modes: live 3D narrow volume, live 3D zoomed, live 3D wide-angled (full volume), and live 3D color Doppler. While this methodology overcomes the limitations imposed by rhythm disturbances or respiratory motion, it is limited by relatively poor temporal and spatial resolution.

The main trade-off in 3DE imaging is between volume rate (i.e., temporal resolution) and spatial resolution. In order to improve spatial resolution, an increase in the number of scan lines per volume (scan line density) is required, which takes longer to acquire and process and thereby limits the overall volume rate. Fortunately, imaging volumes can be adjusted in size (i.e., by reducing volume size), in order to increase volume rate while maintaining spatial resolution. Due to the frequent artifacts associated with multibeat 3DE acquisition, ultrasound manufacturers are pursuing improvements in processing power needed to provide full-volume (90 degrees × 90 degrees) real-time 3DE datasets with adequate spatial and temporal resolution. *saw this - GE @ BHR 3/14/14*

Multibeat datasets can be challenging in patients with arrhythmias and/or respiratory difficulties. Figure 2-3 shows an example of a 2D depiction of an artifact caused by ECG-gated multibeat 3DE acquisition.

Prior to 3DE acquisition, the 2D image should be optimized, since suboptimal 2D images result in suboptimal 3DE datasets. Then the number of heartbeats to acquire and the size of the dataset volume should be tailored to the clinical question to be addressed, taking into account that with more beats the volume would be wider and the temporal resolution higher. In contrast, to improve spatial resolution (i.e., the number of scan lines per volume), the pyramidal volume should be optimized to acquire the smallest volume that can encompass the cardiac structure of interest.

One of the most critical controls to set properly in order to acquire optimal 3DE datasets is the gain setting (Fig. 2-4). As a general rule, both gain and compression settings should be set in the mid range (50 units) and optimized with slightly higher time gain controls (TGCs) rather than using the power-output gain in order to enable greatest flexibility with postprocessing gain and compression. Another issue to consider while optimizing the 3DE dataset is the image resolution (Figs. 2-5–2-7).

DATA DISPLAY

The ability to acquire 3DE datasets brought about the question as to how to display moving structures contained within the volumetric dataset on a flat, 2D monitor. This can be obtained by using the three basic functions of 3D analysis: rotating, cropping, and thresholding. Rotating is a basic function that allows manual freehand rotation of the dataset to provide the best perspective to visualize the structure of interest. Cropping the volumetric dataset means to remove volumetric proximal data in order to visualize the more distal structure of interest (Fig. 2-8). Usually, there are two cropping modalities: the cropping box and the single arbitrary cropping plane (Fig. 2-9). After cropping the 3D dataset, in order to display a specific cardiac structure, one should rotate it to reorient the dataset until the desired structure is in the front of the display. Since the volume-rendered 3D dataset of the heart can be cropped to display intracardiac structures by choosing a cutting plane and the image beyond this plane reconstructed as if the heart is cut by a surgeon, we will no longer use the word "view" (referring to heart's orientation to the body axis), which will be replaced by the term "anatomical planes" or simply "planes" (referring to the heart itself), to describe the orientation of the images. The use of anatomical planes to display the cardiac structures allows easy comparisons between anatomic specimens and 3DE images and facilitates the communication with surgeons and pathologists (Figs. 2-10–2-12).

After having removed the undesired volumetric data, the adequate display of cardiac structures requires some thresholding. Thresholding allows the echocardiographer to determine how much of the volumetric data is part of the cardiac structure of interest, deemed noise or part of the blood pool (Fig. 2-4). This is mainly controlled using the gain settings.

The last action to perform is to decide from which point of view one needs/wants to look at the desired structure (e.g., mitral valve can be viewed from the atrial side, the so-called surgical view, or from the ventricular side) (Fig. 2-11).

Once the cardiac structure of interest has been identified within the volumetric dataset, there are several ways to display it on a 2D monitor. There are three broad classes of techniques for displaying 3D images: volume rendering, surface rendering, and 2D tomographic slices (Fig. 2-13). The choice of the display technique is generally determined by the clinical application and is controlled by the user. Volume rendering (Figs. 2-13A and 2-14) is a technique used to display 3D images in a 2D plane to closely resemble the true anatomy of the heart. Surface rendering technique (Figs. 2-13B and 2-15) is based on visualization of the surfaces of structures or organs as solid casts. Finally, the last way to visualize the content of the dataset is by creating parallel slices to obtain tomographic views.

CONCLUSIONS

Over the last two decades, echocardiography has witnessed significant technologic developments and breakthroughs that have transformed 3DE into a clinically useful imaging modality. Transducer miniaturization and multitasking (simultaneous 2D and 3D imaging), improved spatial and temporal resolution of single-beat datasets, and new automated software packages for quantitative analysis make the 3DE platforms simpler and faster to use and further extend the application of 3DE to provide effective solutions for clinical problems.

ACKNOWLEDGMENTS

Dr. Denisa Muraru was supported by a research grant program awarded by the European Association of Echocardiography.

CONFLICTS OF INTEREST

Dr. Denisa Muraru has received equipment and research funding from GE Healthcare. Dr. Luigi P. Badano has received equipment grants from GE Healthcare and is on the Speakers' Bureau of this company. Dr. Carlo Dal Lin and Prof. Sabino Iliceto have no conflicts of interest to disclose.

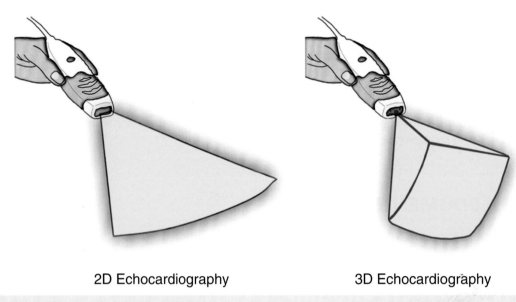

2D Echocardiography   3D Echocardiography

Figure 2-1. **The probe.** Two-dimensional echocardiography is based on phased array transducers, which consist of a series of rectangular piezoelectric elements sequentially fired in order to obtain ultrasound beam steering (**left**). Three-dimensional echocardiography is based on real-time volumetric imaging that allows acquisition of pyramid datasets (**right**) using 3,000 to 4,000 piezoelectric elements arranged in a matrix array inside the transducer head.

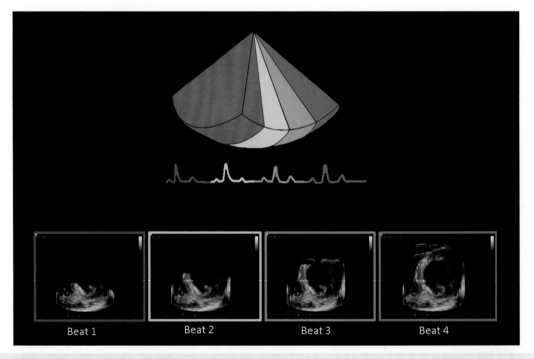

Beat 1   Beat 2   Beat 3   Beat 4

Figure 2-2. **ECG-gated multibeat acquisition of pyramidal datasets.** Creation of a full-volume 3D dataset from multibeat acquisitions involves acquisition of narrow volumes of information over several consecutive heartbeats (ranging from two to seven cardiac cycles) that are then stitched together to create a larger volumetric dataset. This acquisition mode compensates for the poor temporal resolution of single-beat full-volume real-time 3DE acquisition but is prone to stitch artifacts.

Interference = motion
cant hold breath (??)
irregular rhythm

transverse cut plane ~~cut~~ vs longitudinal cut plane

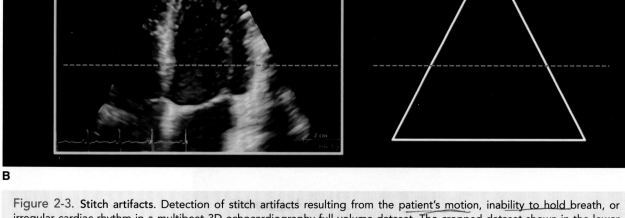

A

longitudinal ~~plane cut~~ cut plane

B

Figure 2-3. **Stitch artifacts.** Detection of stitch artifacts resulting from the patient's motion, inability to hold breath, or irregular cardiac rhythm in a multibeat 3D echocardiography full-volume dataset. The cropped dataset shown in the lower panel appears to be free of artifacts, whereas the one in the upper panel has distinct stitching artifacts. The *yellow and blue dashed lines* show the respective transversal and longitudinal cut planes. If the gated acquisition acquires sector slices in a sweeping motion parallel to the reference image, then every image parallel to the reference image would appear normal. Stitching artifacts where the individual components constitute the 3DE image are most prominent when the volumetric dataset is viewed from a cut plane perpendicular to the sweep plane (i.e., the transversal cut plane for datasets acquired from the apical approach). Accompanying Videos 2.3A and 2.3B correspond to panels A and B, respectively.

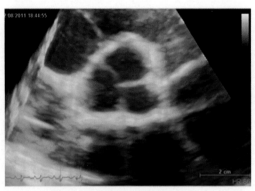

A **Too much gain** = *lose 3D perspective*

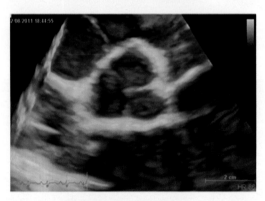

B **Optimal gain**

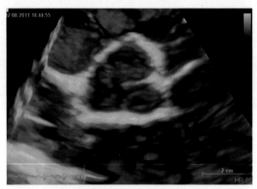

C **Too low gain** = *Echo drop out*

Figure 2-4. **The importance of gain settings.** Excess gain settings will decrease resolution and result in a loss of the 3D perspective or depth within the dataset (A). Conversely, low gain settings will result in echo dropout with the potential for loss of anatomic structures in the dataset that cannot be recovered during postprocessing (C). Optimal gain settings (B) allow clear detection of anatomic details of the aortic valve from the aorta perspective without dropout artifacts.

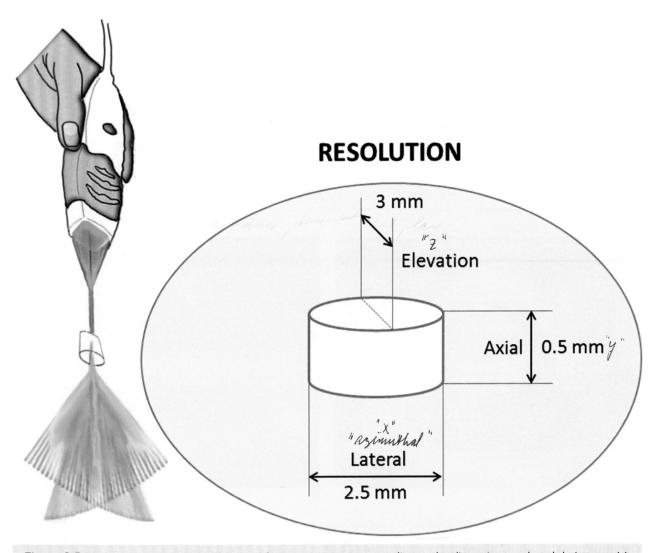

RESOLUTION

3 mm

Elevation "z"

Axial | 0.5 mm "y"

"x"
"azimuthal"
Lateral

2.5 mm

Figure 2-5. Spatial resolution. The resolution of 3DE images varies according to the dimension employed during acquisition. For current 3D transducers, spatial resolution is approximately 0.5 to 1 mm in the axial (y) dimension, 1.5 to 2.0 mm in the azimuthal (x) dimension, and around 2.5 to 3 mm in the elevation (z) dimension.

∴ cant get too much depth
but can get OK width
but think - AV ~ 25 mm diameter

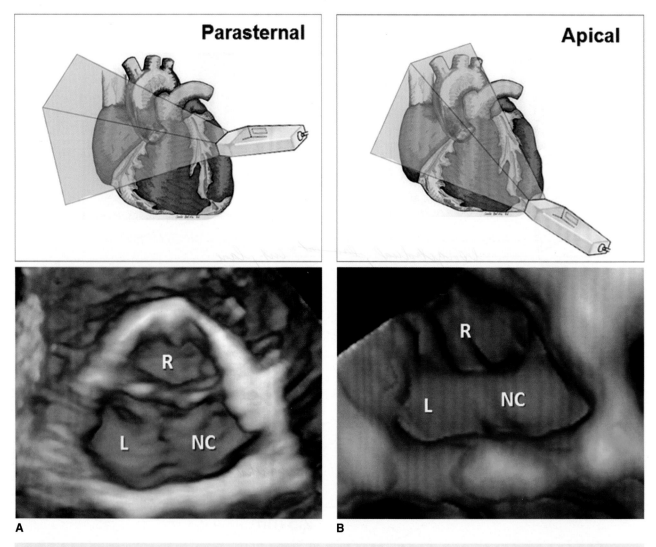

A

B

Figure 2-6. Dependence of spatial resolution of volume rendering on acquisition approach. When the goal is to obtain an en-face view of the aortic valve from the aortic root (the so called surgical view), the best results can be obtained by using the parasternal short-axis approach, because structures are imaged using the axial and azimuthal dimensions (A). Conversely, the worst result is expected to be obtained using the apical approach, which uses the azimuthal and elevation dimensions (B). Accompanying Videos 2.6A and 2.6B correspond to panels A and B, respectively.

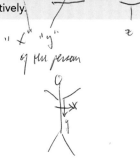

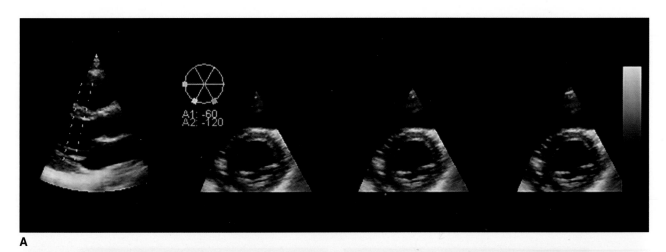

A

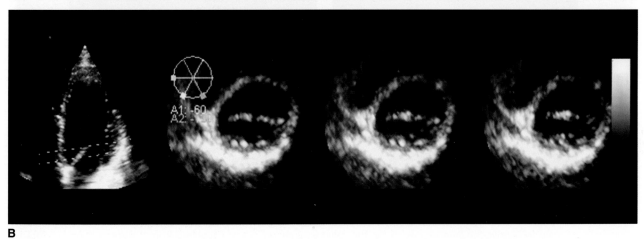

B

Figure 2-7. Dependence of spatial resolution of slicing according to acquisition approach. Multislice display of the basal part of the left ventricle. Better spatial resolution is obtained by imaging from the parasternal approach (A) than from the apical approach (B). Accompanying Videos 2.7A and 2.7B correspond to panels A and B, respectively.

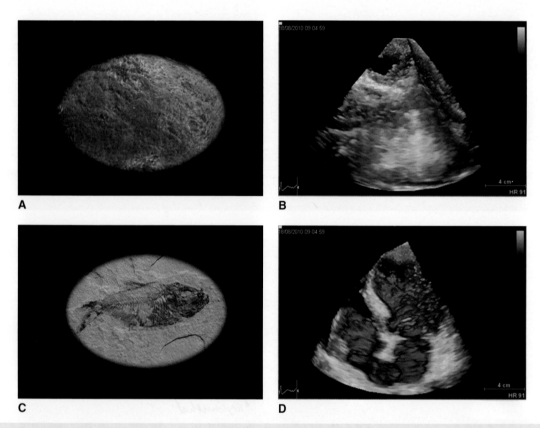

Figure 2-8. The concept of cropping. Once having cropped away part of the dataset, one is able to see inside the heart. This is similar to a rock that contains a fossil (A). One needs to break the stone and remove part of it to see the fossil inside (C). Similarly, we need to remove the anterior part of this full-volume pyramidal dataset acquired from the apical approach (B) to visualize the heart chambers (D). Accompanying Videos 2.8A and 2.8B correspond to panels B and D, respectively.

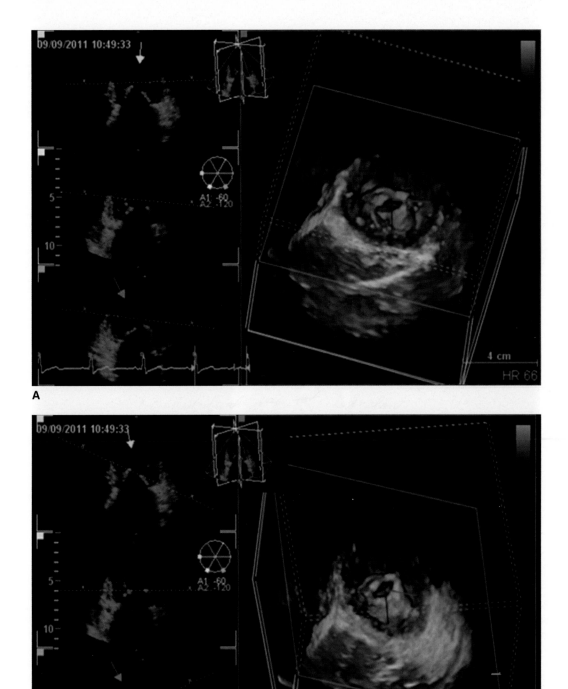

Figure 2-9. The cropping box tool. The cropping function can be performed in two ways using a cropping box. The cropping box is a transparent reference box, which contains the 3D dataset. The three pairs of planes, frontal, lateral, and horizontal, are displayed in three different colors: blue, red, and yellow. By moving one plane at a time, cropping of the dataset is performed (A). In addition, the freehand cropping plane is used to align the cut plane in any direction for the best visualization of the cardiac structure of interest (B). Accompanying Videos 2.9A and 2.9B correspond to panels A and B, respectively.

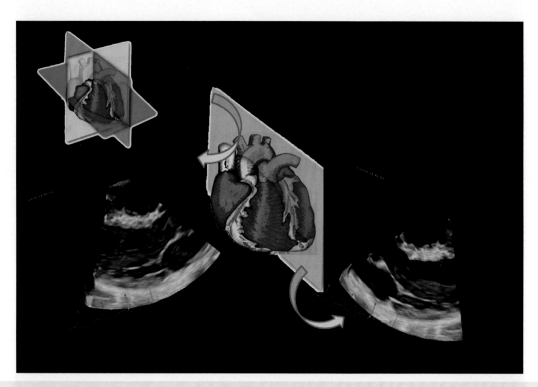

Figure 2-10. The sagittal cutting plane. The most frequently used planes in dissection are (1) the <u>sagittal plane</u>, a vertical plane that divides the heart into right and left portions (the *blue plane* in the drawing); (2) the coronal plane, a vertical plane, which divides the heart into anterior and posterior portions (*shown in yellow*); and (3) the transverse plane, a horizontal plane that runs parallel to the ground and divides the heart into superior and inferior portions (*shown in green*). The figure shows the two parts of the heart (left and right) when cutting along the sagittal plane a dataset of the left ventricle and the atrium with the aortic root acquired from the parasternal approach. Accompanying Videos 2.10A and 2.10B correspond to images on the left and the right, respectively.

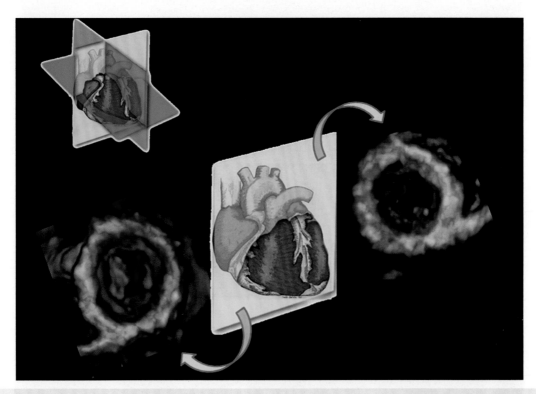

Figure 2-11. **The transversal cutting plane.** The figure shows the two parts of the heart (anterior and posterior) when cutting along the coronal or transversal plane a dataset of the left ventricle and the atrium with the aortic root acquired from the parasternal approach. Accompanying Videos 2.11A and 2.11B correspond to images on the left and the right, respectively.

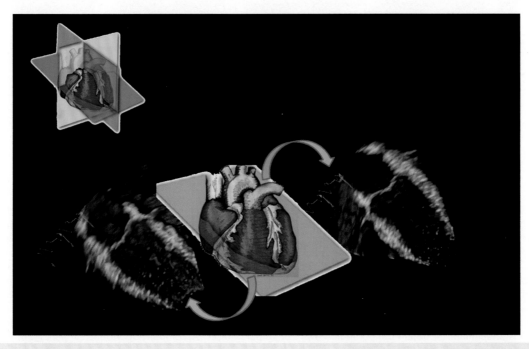

Figure 2-12. **The horizontal cutting plane.** The figure shows the two parts of the heart (superior and inferior) when cutting along the horizontal plane a dataset of the heart acquired from the apical approach. Accompanying Videos 2.12A and 2.12B correspond to images on the left and the right, respectively.

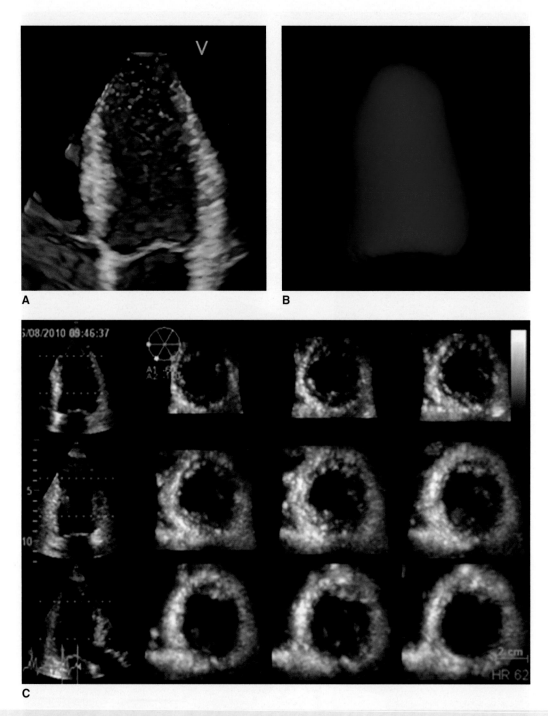

Figure 2-13. **Techniques for displaying 3D images on 2D monitors.** Volume rendering (A) is a technique used to display 3D images in a 2D plane to closely resemble the true anatomy of the heart. The techniques commonly used to obtain this display mode cast a light beam through the collected voxels. Then, the voxels along each light beam are weighted to obtain a gradient of voxel values intensity that integrated with levels of opacity, shading, and lighting allows a structure to appear either solid (e.g., tissue) or transparent (e.g., blood pool). Finally, shading and/or depth encoded colorization techniques are used to generate a 3D display of the depths and textures of the cardiac structures. This kind of display mode enables the assessment of the cardiac anatomy and the complex spatial relationships between the structures. Surface rendering technique (B) is based on the visualization of the surfaces of structures or organs as a solid cast. Once the organ boundaries are identified, shadowing algorithms can be used to create a 3D perspective. Information of the tissue beneath the surface is not visible. Slicing (C) is a technique to obtain tomographic views from a 3D dataset. Accompanying Videos 2.13A, 2.13B, and 2.13C correspond to panels A, B, and C, respectively.

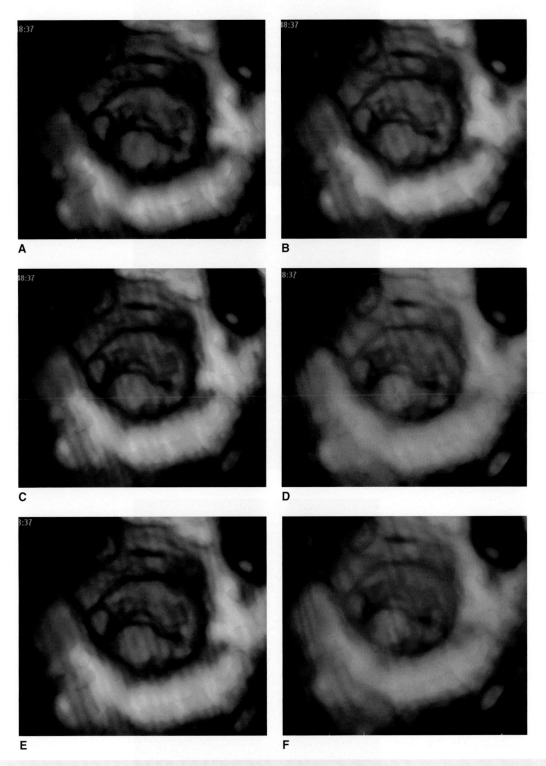

Figure 2-14. Use of colorization maps to appreciate depth. A large prolapsed P2 scallop of a mitral valve is shown from the atrial perspective ("surgical view") using the volume rendering technique with different colorization maps to enhance the perception of depth: gray (A), bronze (B), bronze-blue (C), gray-red (D), bronze-gray (E), bronze-red (F). See accompanying Videos 2.14A, 2.14B, 2.14C, and 2.14E.

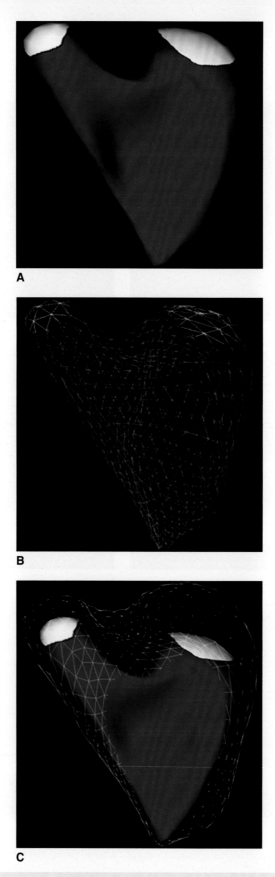

Figure 2-15. Wire frame display technique. The right ventricular cavity is shown using different surface rendering techniques to assess the size and function of the ventricle: solid surface rendering (A); wire frame is another way to display a 3D surface while allowing the visualization of its distal portion (B). The combination of the two techniques (wire frame for end-diastolic volume and solid surface for the volume changes throughout the cardiac cycle) is an effective way to depict ventricular function (C). Accompanying Videos 2.15A, 2.15B, and 2.15C correspond to panels A, B, and C, respectively.

Victor Mor-Avi, Lynn Weinert, Roberto M. Lang

The main characteristics of the left ventricle (LV) are volume, mass, shape, and global as well as regional function. The goal of this chapter is to focus on each of these entities and the 3D echocardiographic (3DE) techniques used to measure them and to highlight their intrinsic strengths and weaknesses.

The main limitations of 2D echocardiography (2DE) from the point of view of cardiac chamber quantification are the fact that single-plane apical views are frequently foreshortened[1] and the need for geometric modeling, which can be inaccurate in the presence of pathology. This is because it is impossible to expect that imaging plane obtained through the intercostal window would always cut through the true LV apex. Three-dimensional echocardiography allows us to overcome the first limitation, because one can select from the 3D dataset anatomically correct, nonforeshortened apical views and use them for volume measurements (Figs. 3-1 and 3-2).[1,2] The feasibility of this 3D-guided biplane approach was initially tested in the context of LV mass measurements, which were compared to MRI reference values, side-by-side with the biplane 2D measurements.[1] While LV mass was underestimated by 2DE, this underestimation was significantly reduced by using the 3D-guided biplane technique,[3–7] paving the way for clinical use of 3DE measurements of LV mass (Fig. 3-3).

The more recently developed direct volumetric measurement using automated detection of the 3D endocardial surface (Figs. 3-4 and 3-5)[8,9] has an additional important advantage over the 3D-guided biplane technique: volume measurements do not rely on any geometric modeling, as volume can be obtained by directly counting voxels inside the endocardial surface, thus eliminating the second well-known confounding factor from ventricular volume measurements. Also, endocardial surface can be automatically detected throughout the cardiac cycle, allowing accurate identification of the timing of end of ejection, without the need to guess the end-systolic frame in order to measure end-systolic volume and eventually the ejection fraction (EF). In addition, this approach provides useful information on the timing of systolic and diastolic function and allows accurate calculation of the rates of ejection and filling.[8]

The fact that repeated measurements can be performed on nonforeshortened views, rather than views that are randomly foreshortened during consecutive acquisitions, brings about another important advantage of 3D chamber quantification: its improved reproducibility.[2,10,11] Both intra- and interobserver variability of LV volume measurements using the standard 2D biplane technique were in most studies several times higher than those of the 3D-based measurements (Fig. 3-6). Importantly, this translates into smaller patient groups necessary to test a hypothesis and thus into potential cost savings in clinical trials, making 3DE imaging an attractive alternative to other costly and cumbersome imaging modalities in such trials.

Of course, the question is how accurate the 3DE-based LV volume measurements are. Several groups compared RT3DE-derived volumes and EFs with MRI and found excellent agreement, reflected by correlation coefficients >0.85 as well as small biases and tight limits of agreement.[10,12–16] However, several studies reported that despite the high correlation with MRI, 3D echocardiography consistently underestimated LV volumes.[17–19] In order to find out how much foreshortening contributed to this underestimation versus geometric modeling, the 2D biplane technique, 3D-guided biplane technique, and the volumetric approach were compared side-by-side against MRI in the same group of patients.[2] Not surprisingly, a stepwise improvement in accuracy was noted, with the 2D technique being the least accurate (Fig. 3-7).

A multicenter study designed to validate endocardial surface analysis of LV volumes against MRI reference and to identify the potential sources of underestimation[20] reported that 3DE-derived volumes correlated highly with MRI, in agreement with previous studies, but the underestimation was even bigger than previously reported in single-center studies. After ruling out every possible source of error, endocardial tracing, which in human ventricles is further complicated by the presence of endocardial trabeculae, was found to be the primary source of error leading to volume underestimation in humans (Figs. 3-8 and 3-9). Importantly, this error can be minimized by learning how to identify the true endocardial boundaries in the 3DE images beyond what appears to be the blood–trabeculae interface. Moreover, several more recent studies have demonstrated the value of contrast enhancement in accurate delineation of LV endocardial boundaries, resulting in improved quantification of ventricular volumes.[21,22]

Lately, in addition to MRI and 3D echocardiography, cardiac computed tomography (CCT) has become increasingly popular. CCT has exceptionally high spatial resolution and has the potential to provide highly accurate ventricular volume measurements.[23] It is important to determine to what extent volume measurements obtained using these three imaging modalities are interchangeable.[17] Studies comparing MRI, 3DE, and CCT measurements showed that LV volumes obtained using different imaging modalities are not necessarily identical. The main implication of these findings is that serial evaluation of ventricular volumes should preferably be performed using the same imaging modality or that measurements should be adjusted accordingly in order to correctly evaluate LV remodeling (Fig. 3-10).

Of course, LV volume, EF, and mass do not always accurately characterize the ventricle. Another important determinant is LV shape and there is a variety of ways to describe shape, among which probably the most well known is the sphericity index (Fig. 3-11). It has been demonstrated that patients with dilated cardiomyopathy (DCM) and more spherical ventricles have worse outcomes than those with less spherical ventricles.[24] Also, a recent study reported age-related changes in LV sphericity index.[25] Nevertheless, this is a rather crude index of shape, as it does not reflect regional changes in shape. Alternative approaches to characterize LV shape in a more detailed manner are warranted (Figs. 3-12 and 3-13).[26,27]

The value of 3D echocardiography with respect to the assessment of regional LV function lies in that we can not only visualize wall motion (Fig. 3-14) but also quantify it using commonly available tools (Fig. 3-15), resulting in a variety of parameters of regional systolic and diastolic function. Importantly, regional volumes derived from 3DE datasets are accurate when compared to MRI reference,[8] indicating that quantitative analysis of RT3DE datasets may become the new clinical standard for the evaluation of regional LV wall motion as an alternative to subjective and experience-dependent visual interpretation of multiple 2D planes.

This is particularly advantageous in the context of stress testing, where 3DE imaging reduces the time between the peak stress and image acquisition, from which any view can be extracted for review at a later time (Fig. 3-16). Another interesting and potential useful application of 3DE-based analysis of regional wall motion is the evaluation of LV dyssynchrony[28–33] and the evaluation of the success of resynchronization therapy (Figs. 3-17 and 3-18).

One of the latest developments in 3D echocardiography is 3D speckle tracking. This is a 3D extension of the 2D speckle tracking echocardiography (STE), which has established itself as a way to quantify myocardial deformation. One potentially clinically useful application of 3D STE is its ability to automatically measure LV volume continuously throughout the cardiac cycle. LV volumes obtained using this methodology were found to correlate better with MRI with smaller biases and tighter limits of agreement compared to 2D STE.[34–36] However, the main advantage of the 3D approach over 2D STE is that the latter may easily misdiagnose abnormal function simply because it is "blind" to out-of-plane myocardial motion (Figs. 3-19 and 3-20).[34,37] In contrast, 3D STE–derived radial, longitudinal, and rotational components of myocardial displacement and the corresponding strains measured at three different levels of the LV were found to not only accurately characterize the known normal patterns of regional LV function but also differentiate normal from hypokinetic myocardium (Figs. 3-21 and 3-22).[37]

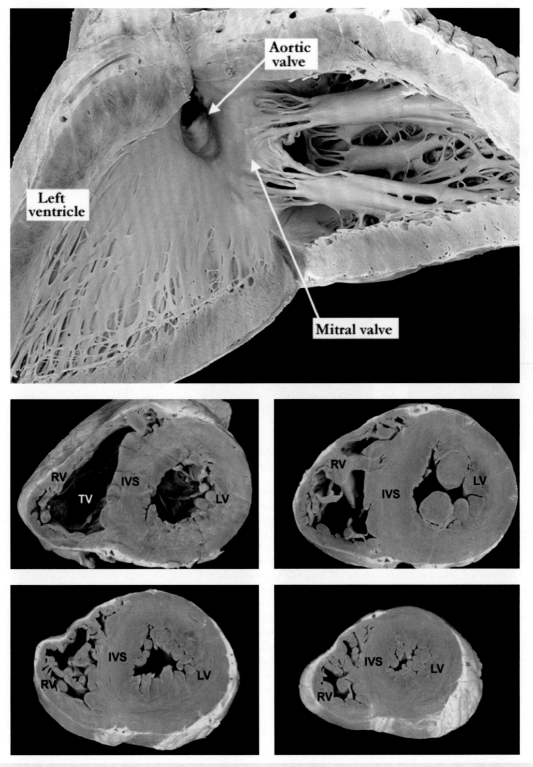

Figure 3-1. Anatomical views of the normal heart. Top. Longitudinal section of the left ventricle (LV) depicting both mitral and aortic valves. Bottom panels. Short-axis slices at four different levels from base to apex, depicting the LV, right ventricle (RV), interventricular septum (IVS), and tricuspid valve (TV).

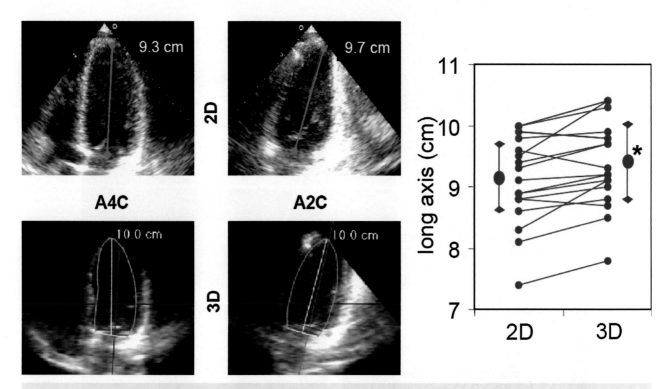

Figure 3-2. **The effect of foreshortening on 2DE volume determinations. Left. The top panels** represent 2DE apical four-chamber (A4C) and two-chamber (A2C) images with their respective long axes indicated by the *green lines*. The bottom panels show the anatomically correct four- and two-chamber images that were extracted from the RT3DE dataset obtained in the same subject. When these nonforeshortened images are used to measure the long axis of the ventricle, it is clear that the 2DE images are foreshortened, which explains the underestimation of the ventricular volume obtained by the biplane technique. By performing a biplane measurements on the nonforeshortened images extracted from the RT3DE datasets, a more accurate result is obtained. (Modified from Jacobs LD, Salgo IS, Goonewardena S, et al. Rapid online quantification of left ventricular volume from real-time three-dimensional echocardiographic data. *Eur Heart J* 2006;27:460–468.) Accompanying Video 3.2 corresponds to the bottom panels. **Right.** Left ventricular long-axis dimension measured in 19 patients from conventional 2D images and from anatomically correct apical views extracted from RT3DE datasets. Note the increase in LV length, as assessed by the 3D technique in most patients (*large circles* and *error bars* represent mean ± SD, *$p < 0.05$). (Modified from Mor-Avi V, Sugeng L, Weinert L, et al. Fast measurement of left ventricular mass with real-time three-dimensional echocardiography: comparison with magnetic resonance imaging. *Circulation* 2004;110:1814–1818.)

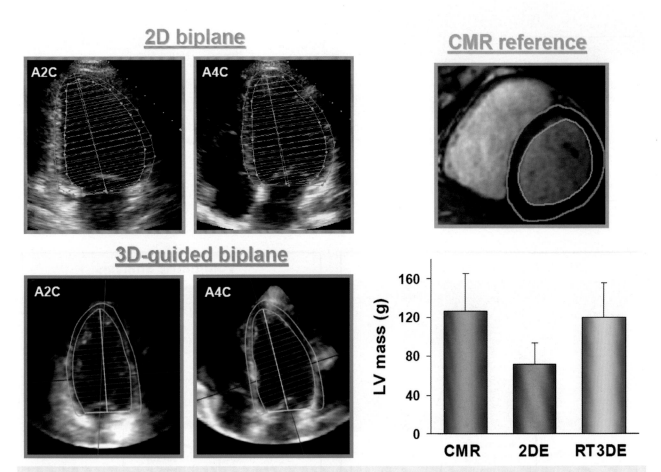

Figure 3-3. Advantage of 3D-guided biplane for LV mass measurements. Left. Example of end-diastolic apical four- and two-chamber views of the LV (A2C and A4C, respectively) obtained using conventional 2D imaging. Below. end-diastolic, anatomically correct A4C and A2C views extracted from the RT3DE dataset obtained in the same subject for 3D-guided biplane measurement of LV mass. Right. LV mass measurements were compared to MRI reference values, showing that the underestimation by the 2D technique was eliminated by using RT3DE-derived nonforeshortened views. (Modified from Mor-Avi V, Sugeng L, Weinert L, et al. Fast measurement of left ventricular mass with real-time three-dimensional echocardiography: comparison with magnetic resonance imaging. *Circulation* 2004;110:1814–1818.)

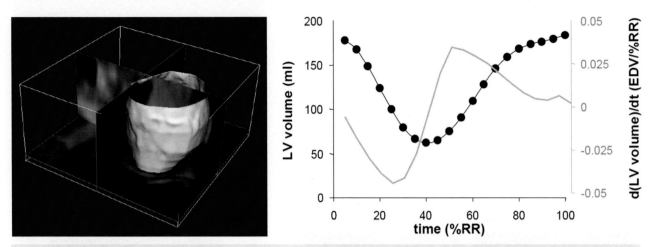

Figure 3-4. Volumetric analysis of the LV. Left. Example of LV endocardial surface detected from a RT3DE dataset obtained in a normal subject, shown superimposed on cross-sectional long-axis planes of the original data. This image was created before this idea was implemented in commercial software. Accompanying Video 3.4 corresponds to the right panel. Right. LV volume time curve shown with the time derivative (*solid lines* without symbols, secondary *y*-axis). (Modified from Corsi C, Lang RM, Veronesi F, et al. Volumetric quantification of global and regional left ventricular function from real-time three-dimensional echocardiographic images. *Circulation* 2005;112:1161–1170.)

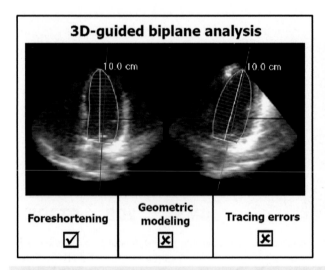

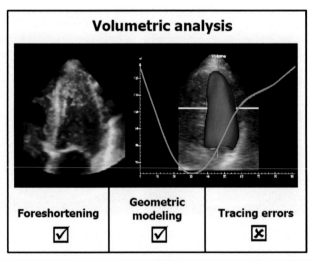

Figure 3-5. 3D-guided biplane versus volumetric analyses: sources of error. Two approaches to measure LV volume from RT3DE datasets: (Left) 3D-guided biplane analysis based on selecting from the entire 3D dataset anatomically correct, non-foreshortened apical three- and four-chamber views and then using the biplane calculation identical to that used with 2D imaging, and (Right) direct phase-by-phase volumetric analysis based on counting pixels contained inside the 3D endocardial surface, which results in a volume over time curve (*green curve*). Accompanying Video 3.5 corresponds to the right panel. Key:☑, resolved;☒, remains unresolved.

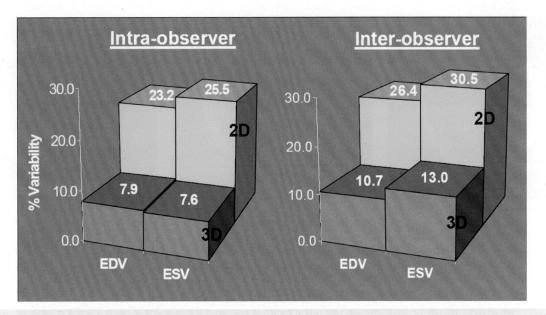

Figure 3-6. Reproducibility: 3D-guided biplane versus volumetric analyses. Intra- and interobserver variability in end-systolic and end-diastolic LV volumes (ESV, EDV) calculated using the 2D biplane technique and the direct volume calculation from reconstructed 3D endocardial surface. (Based on data reported in Jacobs LD, Salgo IS, Goonewardena S, et al. Rapid online quantification of left ventricular volume from real-time three-dimensional echocardiographic data. *Eur Heart J* 2006;27:460–468.)

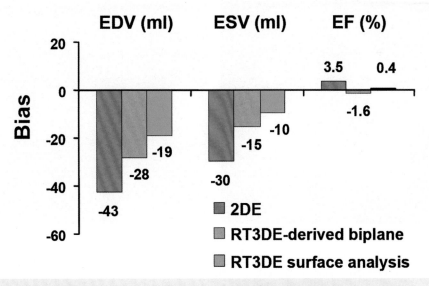

Figure 3-7. Accuracy against MRI: 3D-guided biplane versus volumetric analyses. Biases compared to MRI reference values noted in end-diastolic and end-systolic volumes (EDV, ESV) and ejection fraction (EF) in a group of 20 patients. (Reproduced from Jacobs LD, Salgo IS, Goonewardena S, et al. Rapid online quantification of left ventricular volume from real-time three-dimensional echocardiographic data. *Eur Heart J* 2006;27:460–468, with permission.)

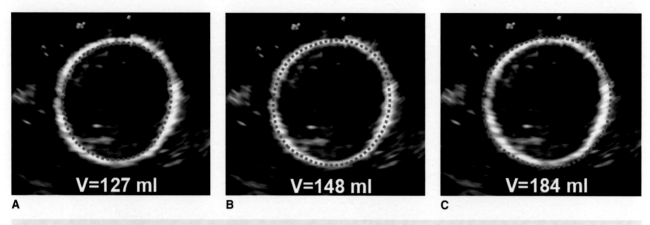

Figure 3-8. Effects of tracing: volume measurements in vitro. Cross-sectional views of a water-filled latex balloon with three alternative manually traced boundaries: along the inner interface (A), along the outer interface (B), and in the center of the latex layer (C). Volumes resulting from each tracing session in this balloon are shown to be compared with the true volume of 150 mL. When this image was traced along what appeared to be the water–latex interface, the measured volume was 14% below the true volume. Surprisingly, most accurate measurements (<1% error) were obtained by tracing through what appeared to be the center of the latex layer. (Modified from Mor-Avi V, Jenkins C, Kuhl HP, et al. Real-time 3-dimensional echocardiographic quantification of left ventricular volumes: multicenter study for validation with magnetic resonance imaging and investigation of sources of error. *J Am Coll Cardiol Img* 2008;1:413–423, with permission.)

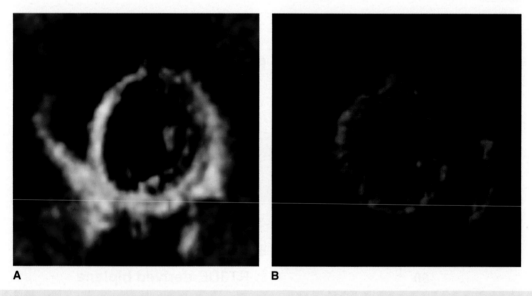

Figure 3-9. Effects of endocardial tracing in humans. Example of short-axis cut planes extracted from RT3DE datasets. In some patients (A), endocardial trabeculae can be well visualized and clearly differentiated from the myocardium, so that one would be able to trace the endocardium, while including the trabeculae in the LV cavity according to the standard convention. In contrast, in other patients (B), the spatial resolution of the RT3DE image is not sufficient to provide this kind of detail, and as a result, it can be extremely difficult to accurately identify the endocardial boundary. (Modified from Mor-Avi V, Jenkins C, Kuhl HP, et al. Real-time 3-dimensional echocardiographic quantification of left ventricular volumes: multicenter study for validation with magnetic resonance imaging and investigation of sources of error. *J Am Coll Cardiol Img* 2008;1:413–423, with permission.)

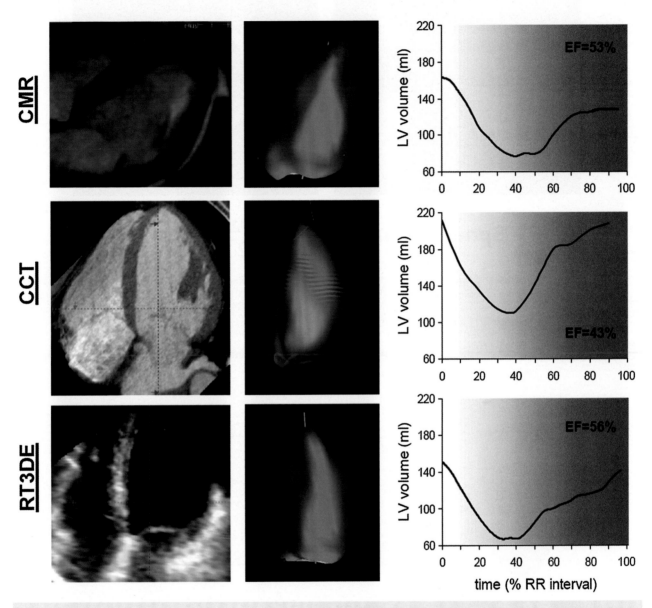

Figure 3-10. Multimodality comparison of volumetric analysis of the LV. Example of long-axis views of the LV obtained at end-diastole in one patient from cardiac magnetic resonance (CMR) images (top), CCT images (center), and 3DE images (bottom), with the corresponding reconstructed LV endocardial surfaces (*middle column*) and volume over time curves (*right column*). To avoid analysis-related differences, all three types of images were analyzed using the same software. One expected finding of this study was that reproducibility of volume measurements was directly related to spatial resolution of the three imaging modalities, with 3DE being the worst, CCT the best, and MRI in between. In other words, as expected, the best image resulted in the highest reproducibility. As far as accuracy, when MRI was used as a reference, the correlations were very high, as reflected by r^2 values between 0.93 and 0.96. While 3D echo measurements showed only minimal volume underestimation, CCT-derived volumes were significantly higher than MRI reference values for reasons that are not fully understood. (Reproduced from Sugeng L, Mor-Avi V, Weinert L, et al. Quantitative assessment of left ventricular size and function: side-by-side comparison of real-time three-dimensional echocardiography and computed tomography with magnetic resonance reference. *Circulation* 2006;114:654–661, with permission.)

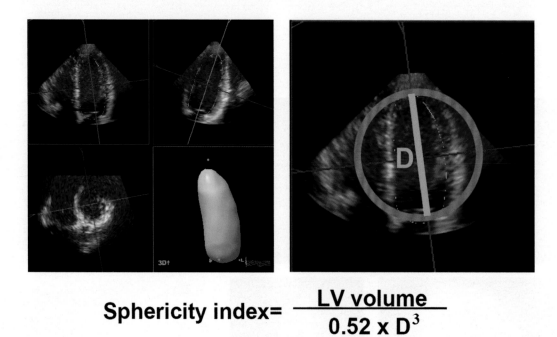

$$\text{Sphericity index} = \frac{\text{LV volume}}{0.52 \times D^3}$$

Figure 3-11. Left ventricular shape: sphericity index. LV sphericity index is defined the ratio between the actual LV volume and the volume of a sphere of a diameter equal to the length of the LV long axis. Three-dimensional echocardiographic imaging offers an opportunity for easy evaluation of ventricular sphericity, which was shown to be affected by a variety of disease states. Accompanying Video 3.11 corresponds to the left panel.

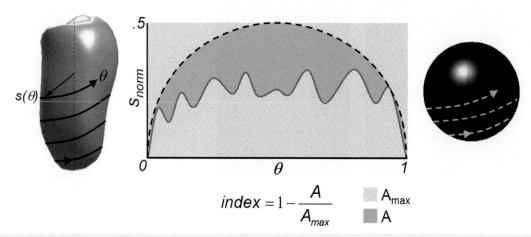

$$index = 1 - \frac{A}{A_{max}}$$

Figure 3-12. Left ventricular shape: beyond sphericity. One mathematical approach provides quantitative shape indices that compare the shape of the ventricle to different predetermined 3D objects, such as a sphere, a cone, an ellipsoid, etc. Changes in LV shape were noted throughout the cardiac cycle in the normal heart, for example, the ventricle becomes less spherical and more conical at end systole. (Reproduced from Maffessanti F, Lang RM, Corsi C, et al. Feasibility of left ventricular shape analysis from transthoracic real-time 3-D echocardiographic images. *Ultrasound Med Biol* 2009;35:1953–1962.)

Pre-operative   6 months

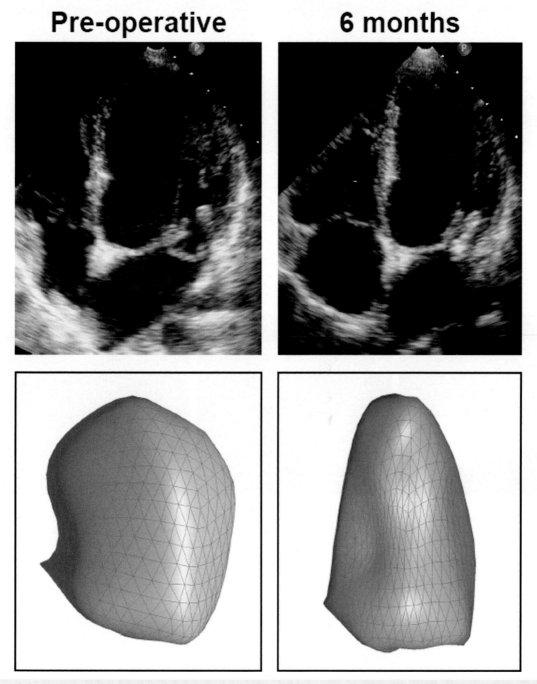

Figure 3-13. Left ventricular shape: assessment of remodeling. Apical four-chamber views obtained in a patient with normal LV EF undergoing mitral valve repair before and 6 months after surgery (top) and the corresponding RT3DE-derived endocardial surfaces. Note that preoperatively, LV has a *spherical shape* that remodels into a more *conical shape* after surgery. (Modified from Maffessanti F, Caiani EG, Tamborini G, et al. Serial changes in left ventricular shape following early mitral valve repair. *Am J Cardiol* 2010;106:836–842.)

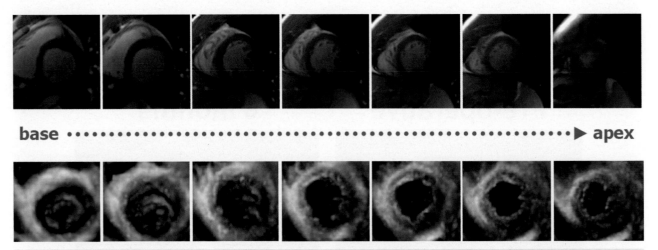

base ••• ▶ **apex**

Figure 3-14. **Multislice assessment of LV function.** Parallel short-axis views of the LV from base to apex obtained using CMR (top) and 3DE imaging (bottom). While CMR acquisition time needed to generate 10 slices is approximately 5 minutes and requires multiple breath-holds, 3DE dataset from which multiple parallel slices can be extracted from a pyramidal dataset acquired within a single breath-hold. Accompanying Video 3.14 depicts this in a dynamic format.

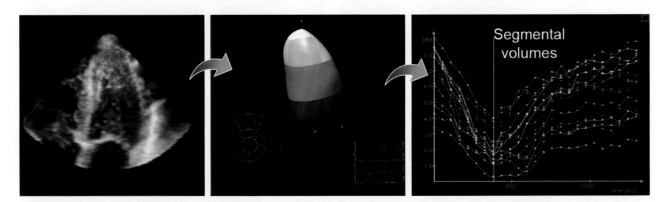

Figure 3-15. Quantification of regional LV function. Endocardial surface extracted from a RT3DE dataset (left) can be divided into segments corresponding to specific LV walls (middle). Accompanying Videos 3.5 and 3.15 correspond to the left and middle panels. For each wall, a segmental volume can be obtained over time throughout the cardiac cycle (right). From these curves, a variety of quantitative indices of regional LV systolic and diastolic function, including segmental EF, can be calculated.

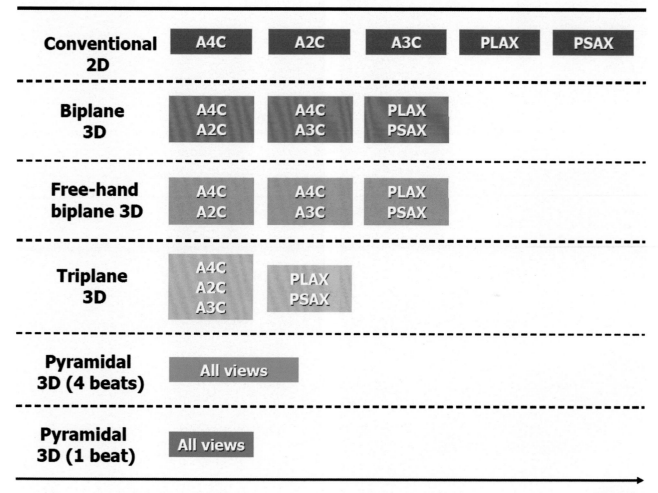

Figure 3-16. **Time-saving implications for stress testing.** Gradual decrease in the time required for different acquisition modes currently used with stress testing, beyond the conventional 2D protocol that images one plane at a time and involves changes of transducer position from plane to plane. Time is saved by imaging more than one plane at a time and also by reducing the number of transducer positions.

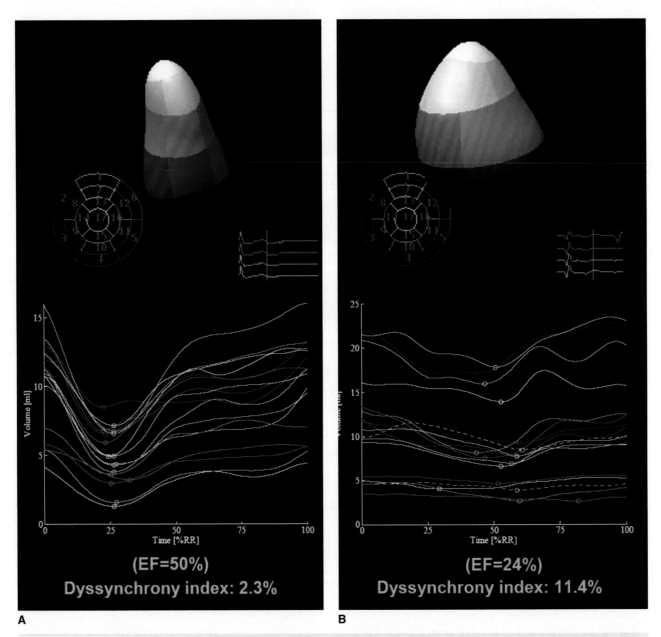

Figure 3-17. **Quantification of LV dyssynchrony.** Two LV casts shown here were obtained in a normal subject (**A**) and in a patient with DCM (**B**). Accompanying Videos 3.17A and 3.17B correspond to the top panels. The individual regional ejection time intervals are used to calculate the dyssynchrony index, calculated as the standard deviation of the mean of these time intervals. In this example, in the normal subject, the end of ejection occurs almost simultaneously in all segments, indicating synchronous contraction, and consequently, the calculated index of systolic dyssynchrony is considerably shorter (**A**, **bottom**), compared to the disorganized contraction pattern in the patient with the dilated ventricle, resulting in an index of dyssynchrony that is five times higher (**B**, **bottom**).

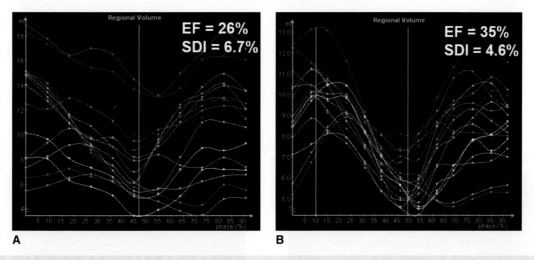

Figure 3-18. Quantification of response to cardiac resynchronization. Segmental volume time curves obtained in a patient with LV dyssynchrony without (A) and with (B) biventricular pacing. Note the change from disorganized to more organized pattern of segmental volume curves with pacing reflecting the effects of resynchronization therapy, which in this case resulted in a more uniform contraction reflected by a decrease in the dyssynchrony index and an increase in EF.

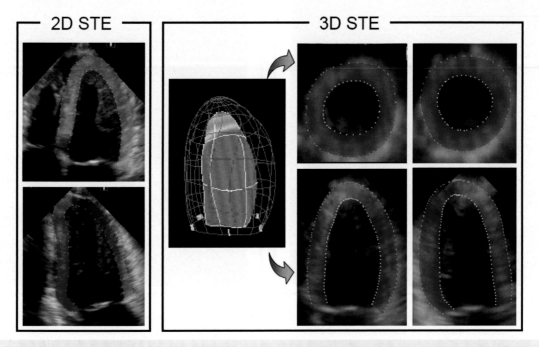

Figure 3-19. Two-dimensional versus three-dimensional speckle tracking: effects of out-of-plane motion. In this patient with normal LV wall motion, 2D speckle tracking (STE) showed uneven color distribution, indicating nonuniform deformation (left panels). Accompanying Videos 3.19A and 3.19B correspond to the left panel. In contrast, cut planes extracted from the 3D STE data showed very even color distribution, indicating uniform contraction with a gradual decrease toward the apex (right panels). This can likely be explained by the fact that 2D STE misinterprets regional differences noted in the imaging plane simply because it is "blinded" to the out-of-plane motion of the heart. Accompanying Video 3.19C depicts this in a dynamic format. (Modified from Nesser HJ, Mor-Avi V, Gorissen W, et al. Quantification of left ventricular volumes using three-dimensional echocardiographic speckle tracking: comparison with MRI. *Eur Heart J* 2009;30:1565–1573.)

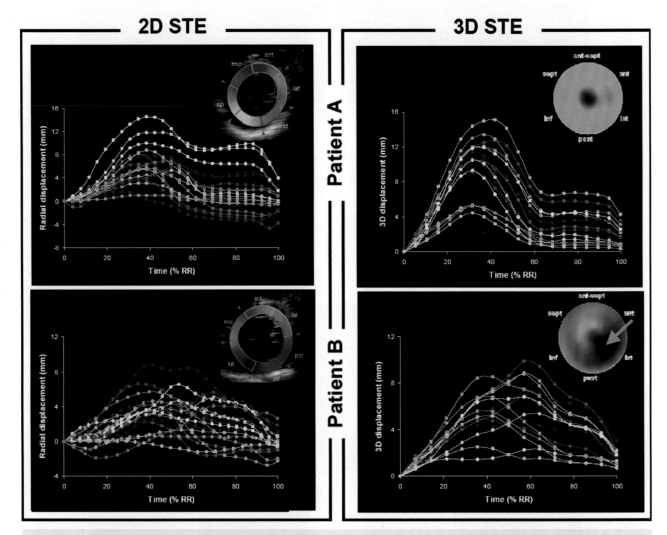

Figure 3-20. Two-dimensional versus three-dimensional speckle tracking: pathology or artifact? Segmental endocardial displacement curves obtained by 2D (left) and 3D (right) speckle tracking (STE) in two patients: patient A (top) with normal wall motion and patient B (bottom) with a hypokinetic apex and inferolateral wall due to ischemic heart disease. While 2D STE shows uneven color distribution and disorganized regional curves, potentially indicating wall motion abnormalities in both patients, 3D STE showed a normal pattern of contraction with synchronized curves in patient A but clearly depicted the area of hypokinesis and dyssynchronized curves in patient B (*green arrow*). Importantly, patient A had normal LV function, while patient B had prior myocardial infarction in the lateral wall. (Modified from Maffessanti F, Nesser HJ, Weinert L, et al. Quantitative evaluation of regional left ventricular function using three-dimensional speckle tracking echocardiography in patients with and without heart disease. *Am J Cardiol* 2009;104:1755–1762, with permission.)

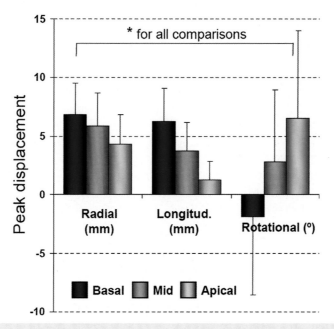

Figure 3-21. Three-dimensional speckle tracking: normal contraction patterns. Three-dimensional STE–derived radial and longitudinal displacement and rotation measured in normal myocardial segments at three different LV levels: base, midventricle, and apex. While radial and longitudinal displacement gradually decrease from base to apex, the rotation increases in magnitude and reverses its direction, which is consistent with the well-known wringing motion of the heart during systole. (Modified from Maffessanti F, Nesser HJ, Weinert L, et al. Quantitative evaluation of regional left ventricular function using three-dimensional speckle tracking echocardiography in patients with and without heart disease. *Am J Cardiol* 2009;104:1755–1762, with permission.)

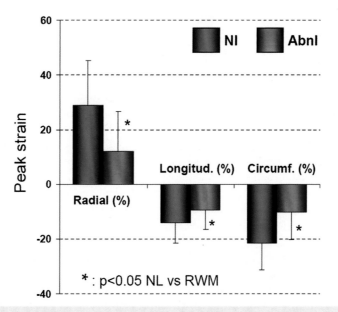

Figure 3-22. Three-dimensional speckle tracking: detection of regional hypokinesis. Radial, longitudinal, and circumferential peak strain compared between normal segments and segments judged by an expert reader as hypokinetic. All three strain components were significantly reduced in the abnormal segments. (Modified from Maffessanti F, Nesser HJ, Weinert L, et al. Quantitative evaluation of regional left ventricular function using three-dimensional speckle tracking echocardiography in patients with and without heart disease. *Am J Cardiol* 2009;104:1755–1762, with permission.)

References

1. Mor-Avi V, Sugeng L, Weinert L, et al. Fast measurement of left ventricular mass with real-time three-dimensional echocardiography: comparison with magnetic resonance imaging. *Circulation* 2004;110:1814–1818.

2. Jacobs LD, Salgo IS, Goonewardena S, et al. Rapid online quantification of left ventricular volume from real-time three-dimensional echocardiographic data. *Eur Heart J* 2006;27:460–468.

3. van den Bosch AE, Robbers-Visser D, Krenning BJ, et al. Comparison of real-time three-dimensional echocardiography to magnetic resonance imaging for assessment of left ventricular mass. *Am J Cardiol* 2006;97:113–117.

4. Poutanen T, Jokinen E. Left ventricular mass in 169 healthy children and young adults assessed by three-dimensional echocardiography. *Pediatr Cardiol* 2007;28:201–207.

5. Singh A, Pothineni KR, Panwar SR. Left ventricular mass assessment by real-time three-dimensional echocardiography. *Am J Cardiol* 2007;99:1180–1181.

6. Takeuchi M, Nishikage T, Mor-Avi V, et al. Measurement of left ventricular mass by real-time three-dimensional echocardiography: validation against magnetic resonance and comparison with two-dimensional and m-mode measurements. *J Am Soc Echocardiogr* 2008;21:1001–1005.

7. Pouleur AC, le Polain de Waroux JB, Pasquet A, et al. Assessment of left ventricular mass and volumes by three-dimensional echocardiography in patients with or without wall motion abnormalities: comparison against cine magnetic resonance imaging. *Heart* 2008;94:1050–1057.

8. Corsi C, Lang RM, Veronesi F, et al. Volumetric quantification of global and regional left ventricular function from real-time three-dimensional echocardiographic images. *Circulation* 2005;112:1161–1170.

9. Caiani EG, Corsi C, Sugeng L, et al. Improved quantification of left ventricular mass based on endocardial and epicardial surface detection with real time three dimensional echocardiography. *Heart* 2006;92:213–219.

10. Jenkins C, Bricknell K, Hanekom L, et al. Reproducibility and accuracy of echocardiographic measurements of left ventricular parameters using real-time three-dimensional echocardiography. *J Am Coll Cardiol* 2004;44:878–886.

11. Soliman OI, Kirschbaum SW, van Dalen BM, et al. Accuracy and reproducibility of quantitation of left ventricular function by real-time three-dimensional echocardiography versus cardiac magnetic resonance. *Am J Cardiol* 2008;102:778–783.

12. Qin JX, Jones M, Shiota T, et al. Validation of real-time three-dimensional echocardiography for quantifying left ventricular volumes in the presence of a left ventricular aneurysm: in vitro and in vivo studies. *J Am Coll Cardiol* 2000;36:900–907.

13. Ahmad M, Xie T, McCulloch M, et al. Real-time three-dimensional dobutamine stress echocardiography in assessment of ischemia: comparison with two-dimensional dobutamine stress echocardiography. *J Am Coll Cardiol* 2001;37:1303–1309.

14. Arai K, Hozumi T, Matsumura Y, et al. Accuracy of measurement of left ventricular volume and ejection fraction by new real-time three-dimensional echocardiography in patients with wall motion abnormalities secondary to myocardial infarction. *Am J Cardiol* 2004;94:552–558.

15. Kuhl HP, Schreckenberg M, Rulands D, et al. High-resolution transthoracic real-time three-dimensional echocardiography: quantitation of cardiac volumes and function using semi-automatic border detection and comparison with cardiac magnetic resonance imaging. *J Am Coll Cardiol* 2004;43:2083–2090.

16. Gutierrez-Chico JL, Zamorano JL, Perez de Isla L, et al. Comparison of left ventricular volumes and ejection fractions measured by three-dimensional echocardiography versus by two-dimensional echocardiography and cardiac magnetic resonance in patients with various cardiomyopathies. *Am J Cardiol* 2005;95:809–813.

17. Sugeng L, Mor-Avi V, Weinert L, et al. Quantitative assessment of left ventricular size and function: side-by-side comparison of real-time three-dimensional echocardiography and computed tomography with magnetic resonance reference. *Circulation* 2006;114:654–661.

18. Jenkins C, Leano R, Chan J, et al. Reconstructed versus real-time 3-dimensional echocardiography: comparison with magnetic resonance imaging. *J Am Soc Echocardiogr* 2007;20:862–868.

19. Soliman OI, Krenning BJ, Geleijnse ML, et al. Quantification of left ventricular volumes and function in patients with cardiomyopathies by real-time three-dimensional echocardiography: a head-to-head comparison between two different semiautomated endocardial border detection algorithms. *J Am Soc Echocardiogr* 2007;20:1042–1049.

20. Mor-Avi V, Jenkins C, Kuhl HP, et al. Real-time 3-dimensional echocardiographic quantification of left ventricular volumes: multicenter study for validation with magnetic resonance imaging and investigation of sources of error. *J Am Coll Cardiol Img* 2008;1:413–423.

21. Jenkins C, Moir S, Chan J, et al. Left ventricular volume measurement with echocardiography: a comparison of left ventricular opacification, three-dimensional echocardiography, or both with magnetic resonance imaging. *Eur Heart J* 2009;30:98–106.

22. van der Heide JA, Mannaerts HF, Yang L, et al. Contrast-enhanced versus non-enhanced three-dimensional echocardiography of left ventricular volumes. *Neth Heart J* 2008;16:47–52.

23. Bardo DM, Kachenoura N, Newby B, et al. Multidetector computed tomography evaluation of left ventricular volumes: sources of error and guidelines for their minimization. *J Cardiovasc Comput Tomogr* 2008;2:222–230.

24. Opie LH, Commerford PJ, Gersh BJ, et al. Controversies in ventricular remodelling. *Lancet* 2006;367:356–367.

25. Kaku K, Takeuchi M, Otani K, et al. Age- and gender-dependency of left ventricular geometry assessed with real-time three-dimensional transthoracic echocardiography. *J Am Soc Echocardiogr* 2011;24:541–547.

26. Maffessanti F, Lang RM, Corsi C, et al. Feasibility of left ventricular shape analysis from transthoracic real-time 3-D echocardiographic images. *Ultrasound Med Biol* 2009;35:1953–1962.

27. Maffessanti F, Caiani EG, Tamborini G, et al. Serial changes in left ventricular shape following early mitral valve repair. *Am J Cardiol* 2010;106:836–842.

28. Kapetanakis S, Kearney MT, Siva A, et al. Real-time three-dimensional echocardiography: a novel technique to quantify global left ventricular mechanical dyssynchrony. *Circulation* 2005;112:992–1000.

29. Burgess MI, Jenkins C, Chan J, et al. Measurement of left ventricular dyssynchrony in patients with ischaemic cardiomyopathy: a comparison of real-time three-dimensional and tissue Doppler echocardiography. *Heart* 2007;93:1191–1196.

30. Takeuchi M, Jacobs A, Sugeng L, et al. Assessment of left ventricular dyssynchrony with real-time 3-dimensional echocardiography: comparison with Doppler tissue imaging. *J Am Soc Echocardiogr* 2007;20:1321–1329.

31. Marsan NA, Henneman MM, Chen J, et al. Real-time 3-dimensional echocardiography as a novel approach to quantify left ventricular dyssynchrony: a comparison study with phase analysis of gated myocardial perfusion single photon emission computed tomography. *J Am Soc Echocardiogr* 2008;21:801–807.

32. van Dijk J, Dijkmans PA, Gotte MJ, et al. Evaluation of global left ventricular function and mechanical dys-synchrony in patients with an asymptomatic left bundle branch block: a real-time 3D echocardiography study. *Eur J Echocardiogr* 2008;9:40–46.

33. Soliman OI, van Dalen BM, Nemes A, et al. Quantification of left ventricular systolic dyssynchrony by real-time three-dimensional echocardiography. *J Am Soc Echocardiogr* 2009;22:232–239.

34. Nesser HJ, Mor-Avi V, Gorissen W, et al. Quantification of left ventricular volumes using three-dimensional echocardiographic speckle tracking: comparison with MRI. *Eur Heart J* 2009;30:1565–1573.

35. Flu WJ, van Kuijk JP, Bax JJ, et al. Three-dimensional speckle tracking echocardiography: a novel approach in the assessment of left ventricular volume and function? *Eur Heart J* 2009;30:2304–2307.

36. Muraru D, Badano LP, Piccoli G, et al. Validation of a novel automated border-detection algorithm for rapid and accurate quantitation of left ventricular volumes based on three-dimensional echocardiography. *Eur J Echocardiogr* 2010;11:359–368.

37. Maffessanti F, Nesser HJ, Weinert L, et al. Quantitative evaluation of regional left ventricular function using three-dimensional speckle tracking echocardiography in patients with and without heart disease. *Am J Cardiol* 2009;104:1755–1762.

4

CHAMBER QUANTIFICATION: BEYOND THE LEFT VENTRICLE

Lynn Weinert, Victor Mor-Avi, Roberto M. Lang

RIGHT VENTRICLE

The right ventricle (Fig. 4-1) is composed of three anatomical and functional subunits, which extend from (1) the tricuspid valve (TV) annulus to the proximal os infundibulum, (2) the right ventricular (RV) body to the apex, and (3) the RV outflow tract to the pulmonary valve. This divides the RV cavity into three sections: inlet, apical trabecular, and outlet. The musculature of the RV extends from the atrioventricular to the ventriculoarterial junctions. The RV is highly trabeculated, with several muscle bands including the septoparietal trabeculations and the moderator band. From a functional point of view and due to the orientation of the RV fibers, global assessment of the RV is difficult with the two main sections contracting in directions perpendicular to each other: the proximal (RV inflow) longitudinally and the distal (RV outflow) circumferentially.

Due to the complex RV shape and function, functional assessment of the right ventricle by two-dimensional echocardiography (2DE) remains a conundrum due to the unique geometry of this chamber and limitations of the current methods of quantification (Figs. 4-2 through 4-4). Since the evaluation of the right ventricle using three-dimensional echocardiography (3DE) does not require geometric modeling, it has the potential of improved accuracy (Figs. 4-4 and 4-5).[1,2]

Full-volume datasets of the entire right ventricle acquired from the four-chamber apical view can be cropped to depict in any desired RV cut plane (Figs. 4-6 through 4-9). The anatomy and pathology of the TV and the RV are best visualized using volume-rendered images, which can depict the valve from either the atrial or ventricular perspectives (Fig. 4-10). To allow RV volume measurements, RV endocardial boundary can be semiautomatically detected frame by frame, from which RV volume can be directly obtained throughout the cardiac cycle (Figs. 4-11 and 4-12), including separate analysis of the different RV sections (inlet, apex, and outflow). This technique uses a combination of views that allow the visualization of the TV, RV outflow tract, and apex in order to reconstruct RV endocardial surface and directly calculate RV volumes without using geometrical modeling.[3,4] This analysis relies on manual initialization of RV boundaries in a number of planes and adjustments of the automatically detected 3D surface.

This analysis was validated using in vitro models as well as in vivo using cardiac magnetic resonance as the gold standard (Figs. 4-13, 4-14, and 4-15).[5] This multimodality study showed that this analysis overcomes many of the known hurdles that impeded accurate assessment of this geometrically complex chamber in the past and can be used with either cardiac magnetic resonance (CMR), cardiac computed tomography (CCT), or 3DE. However, the results of this study also showed that RV volume measurements are not interchangeable between modalities, and therefore, serial evaluations should preferably be performed using the same modality.

Data on RV volumes and function are of diagnostic and prognostic importance in a variety of cardiac disease including valve disease, congenital heart disease, pulmonary hypertension, and heart failure. With the above analysis tools, 3DE allows the quantification of volumes and function, thereby allowing identification of patients with different severity of RV dilatation and dysfunction.[4,6] Several clinical studies have shown good agreement between cardiac magnetic resonance and 3DE volumes and ejection fraction of the RV in selected populations with the majority of studies showing a slight underestimation of volumes compared to the reference technique.[3,5,7,8] Differences in RV volumes have been demonstrated between men (129 ± 25 mL) and women (102 ± 33 mL); however, by adjusting to lean body mass (but not to body surface area or height), these differences can be eliminated.[8–10] The use of 3D TTE has been validated in patients with pulmonic valve regurgitation, secundum atrial septal defect, tetralogy of Fallot repair, Ebstein's anomaly, and RV cardiomyopathy.[11–13] The feasibility and utility of 3D TTE for guidance of RV endomyocardial biopsies in children has also been demonstrated.[14]

Assessment of RV function is of great interest in cardiovascular surgery because right-sided heart failure is one of the most frequent causes of morbidity and mortality post valvular and congenital surgery, coronary artery bypass, and heart transplantation (Fig. 4-16). This highlights the importance of an accurate preoperative assessment of the right ventricle to improve risk stratification and an early postoperative follow-up to optimize treatment. In this regard, 2DE and Doppler parameters (TAPSE, Doppler tissue imaging of the annulus) have several limitations, particularly in the postoperative follow-up. The evaluation of RV volumes and ejection fraction using 3DE overcomes many of the limitations of 2DE methods.[15]

Currently, 3DE assessment of RV volumes and ejection fraction shows great promise. Although routine clinical use is currently limited by the need for excellent quality of transthoracic images, 3DE imaging in combination with dedicated analysis software will undoubtedly provide more accurate assessment of the right ventricle than 2DE and will have significant impact on diagnosis and management of disease states that involve this geometrically and physiologically complex chamber.

LEFT ATRIUM

It is well established that increased left atrial (LA) volume is associated with adverse cardiovascular outcomes and is among the first criteria used to diagnose LV diastolic dysfunction according to the current recommendations of the American Society of Echocardiography (ASE).[16] Accordingly, techniques for accurate LA volume (LAV) measurement are highly sought after.

The left atrium consists of three parts: the appendage, the vestibule, and the venous component. The LA appendage is a multilobar structure located between the left upper pulmonary vein and the left ventricle. The vestibule is the part of the left atrium that surrounds the mitral valve (MV) orifice and has no distinctive anatomical characteristics. The pulmonary veins drain oxygenated blood from the lung into the left atrium through oval-shaped ostia. While there is significant variability in dimensions, shape, and branching patterns of the pulmonary veins, the most common pattern of entry is two veins from the hilum of each lung. The superior pulmonary vein ostia tend to be larger and have longer distances from the ostium to the first-order branches than the inferior veins. The right superior pulmonary vein lies just behind the superior vena cava. The left pulmonary veins are separated from the LA appendage by the ligament of Marshall.

Today, LAV measurements are routinely performed using 2DE (Fig. 4-17). Most commonly, LAV is estimated using either the single- or biplane area-length technique or method of disks.[17] The accuracy of these approximations is limited because of their view dependency and their reliance on geometrical assumptions regarding LA shape (Fig. 4-18). In addition, LA remodeling as a result of disease processes is frequently asymmetric, rendering the standard geometrical assumptions even more inadequate. Not surprisingly, several studies have shown that 2DE underestimates LAV compared to imaging techniques that are free of these limitations, such as CCT[18,19] and CMR.[20]

Since real-time 3DE can also overcome these limitations by allowing direct detection of LA boundaries in 3D space, it is attractive as a potentially more accurate and more reproducible alternative for the LAV measurements.[21–23] To date, only few studies have prospectively validated 3DE-derived LAV measurements in large groups of patients against an accepted independent reference standard[24,25] because of the lack of appropriate tools for volumetric analysis of LAV from 3DE datasets, the high cost of CMR or CCT studies, and the radiation concerns associated with the latter.

Three-dimensional echocardiography imaging of the left atrium for volume and function measurements should be performed from TTE views or TEE transgastric views. With midesophageal TEE views, the entire left atrium cannot be seen within the imaging pyramid and precluding the measurements of LA volumes. Also, 3D TEE cannot visualize the entire atrial posterior wall with all four pulmonary veins. However, it can provide high-quality images of one or two of the pulmonary vein ostia and surrounding LA tissue. Three-dimensional TEE is ideal for visualization of the interatrial septum and its adjacent structures.

Once a wide-angled acquisition 3D dataset of the septum is obtained, the cropping plane can be used to optimize views of the septum demonstrating its relationship to structures such as the MV, right upper pulmonary vein, and aorta. As well, the cropping planes can be aligned perpendicular to the pulmonary vein orifices to obtain ostial dimensions.

A new dedicated software for volumetric measurement of LAV, based on semiautomated detection of LA boundaries (Figs. 4-19, 4-20 and 4-21), was recently tested in a large group of patients with a wide range of LA sizes.[26–28] When compared to CMR reference, 3DE-derived LAV measurements were found to be more accurate than 2DE-based analysis with similar reproducibility. Importantly, the improved accuracy resulted in fewer patients with undetected atrial enragement, which has important implications for echocardiographic evaluation of LV diastolic function (Figs. 4-22 and 4-23).[26–28]

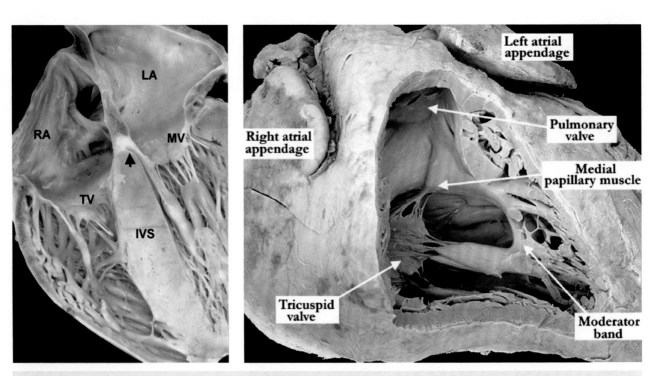

Figure 4-1. Anatomical views of a normal right ventricle. Left. Longitudinal midventricular section also depicting the right atrium (RA) and tricuspid valve (TV), as well as the interventricular septum (IVS), left atrium (LA), and mitral valve (MV). Right. A different longitudinal section depicting additional anatomical structures.

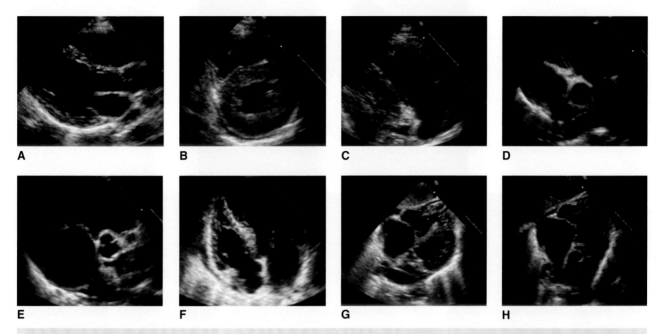

Figure 4-2. The complex shape of the right ventricle depicted in different cross-sectional planes. Because of the 3D geometry of the right ventricle, its echocardiographic assessment involves imaging in multiple planes designed to visualize different aspects of this complex chamber: (A) parasternal long-axis, (B) parasternal short-axis, (C) parasternal RV inflow, (D) parasternal short-axis RV outflow, (E) parasternal long-axis RV outflow, (F) apical four-chamber, (G) subcostal RV inflow, and (H) subcostal RV outflow.

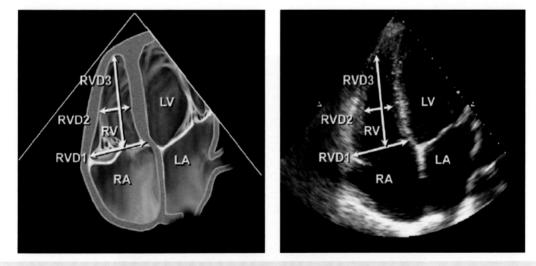

Figure 4-3. Two-dimensional evaluation of RV dilatation. Current guidelines define a dilated RV chamber by diameter >42 mm at the base and a longitudinal dimension >86 mm, measured at end diastole in the apical four-chamber view, as shown on a model (left) and an actual 2D image (right).

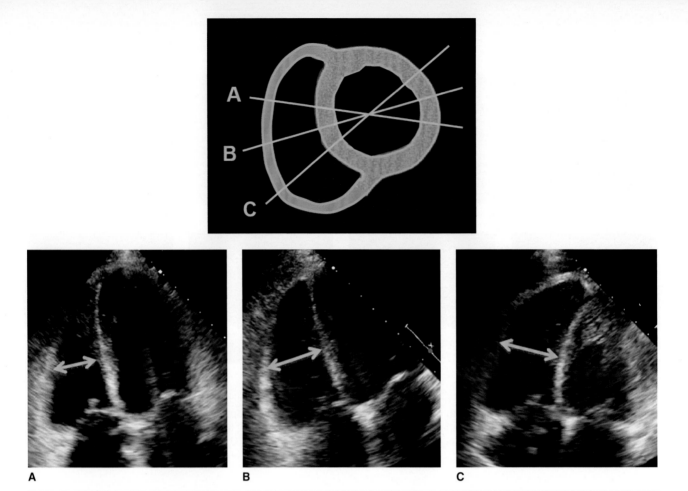

Figure 4-4. Angle dependency of 2D measurements of RV dimensions. Since the apical four-chamber view is not uniquely defined (planes A, B, and C are all apical four-chamber views), as one can see, the measurements used to define a dilated right ventricle (Fig. 4-3) can vary depending on the specific plane (**bottom panels**), resulting in divergent classifications of the ventricle as normal or dilated.

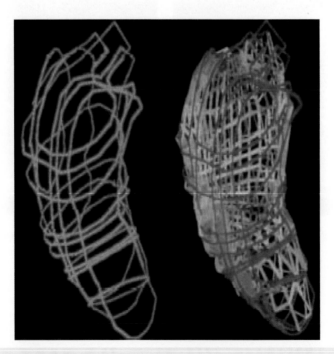

Figure 4-5. Early 3D reconstruction of the right ventricle. The geometrical complexity of the right ventricle has driven the development of 3D reconstruction techniques to allow accurate quantification of the dimensions of this chamber and its function. This wireframe representation of the RV cavity was obtained by 3D reconstruction from multiple 2D planes. (Reproduced from Jiang L, Siu SC, Handschumacher MD, et al. Three-dimensional echocardiography. In vivo validation for right ventricular volume and function. *Circulation* 1994;89:2342–2350, with permission.)

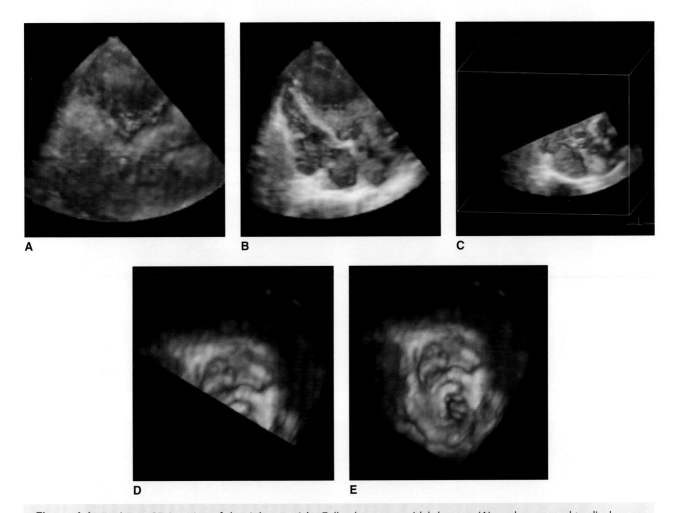

Figure 4-6. **Real-time 3D imaging of the right ventricle.** Full-volume pyramidal datasets (A) can be cropped to display any desired view. (B, accompanying Video 4.6B) Apical four-chamber view obtained by cropping the pyramid in the middle. Cropping the half-pyramid from the apex (C) to the level of the TV and rotating the dataset result in an en-face view of the valve (D). Further uncropping in the lateral direction results in a view of the valve that includes the RV inflow and outflow tracts (E, accompanying Video 4.6E).

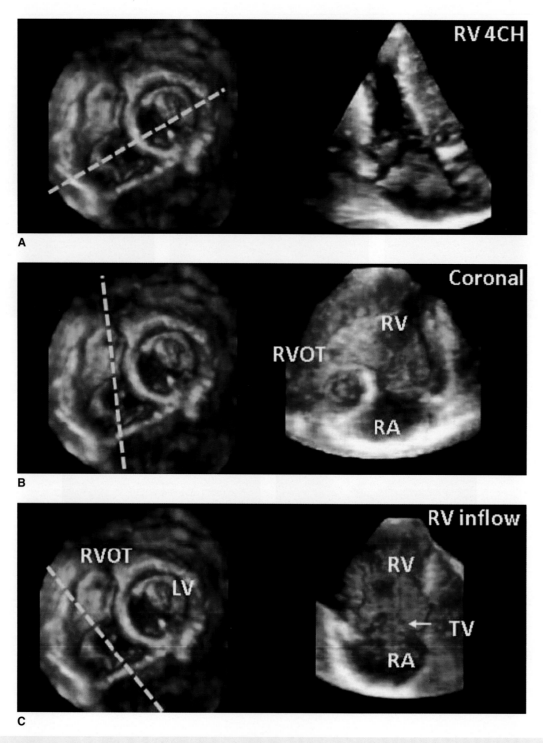

Figure 4-7. Views of the right ventricle obtained from the 3D dataset. Examples depicting: (A) the four-chamber view, (B) the coronal view, and (C) the RV inflow view. RA, right atrium; RV, right ventricle; RVOT, right ventricular outflow tract; TV, tricuspid valve.

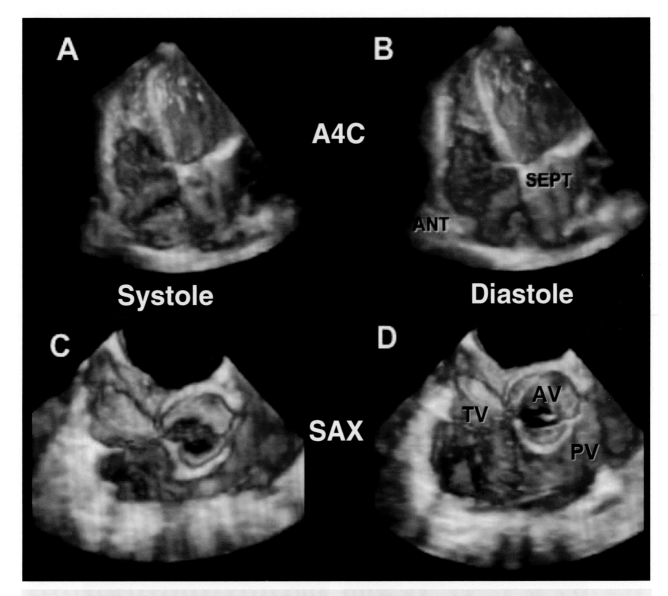

Figure 4-8. Examples of 3D images of the right ventricle in different phases of the cardiac cycle. Apical four-chamber view in systole (A) and diastole (B) (accompanying Video 4.8AB) and the RV inflow and outflow tracts in systole (C) and diastole (D) (accompanying Video 4.8CD) with the aortic valve in the center, the TV to the left, and the pulmonic valve to the right. A4C, apical four-chamber view; SAX, short-axis view; Ant, anterior; Sept, septum; TV, tricuspid valve; AV, aortic valve; PV, pulmonic valve.

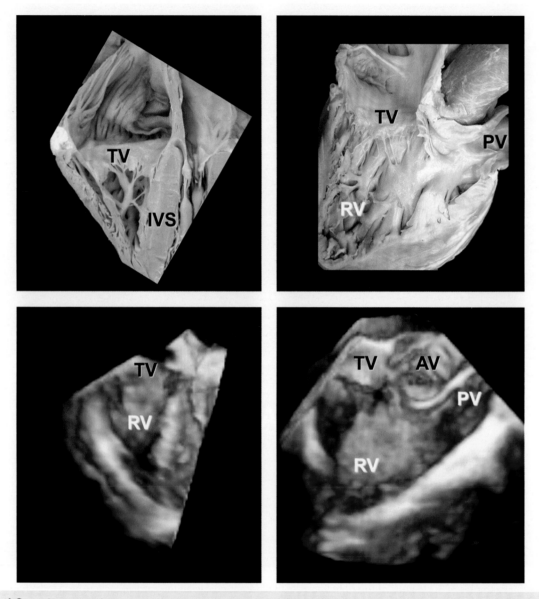

Figure 4-9. Right ventricular views: anatomy versus 3D echocardiography. Anatomical specimens (top) and 3D transesophageal images (bottom) depicting the right ventricle: four-chamber (left, accompanying Video 4.9A) and coronal (right, accompanying Video 4.9B) views. TV, tricuspid valve; AV, aortic valve; PV, pulmonic valve.

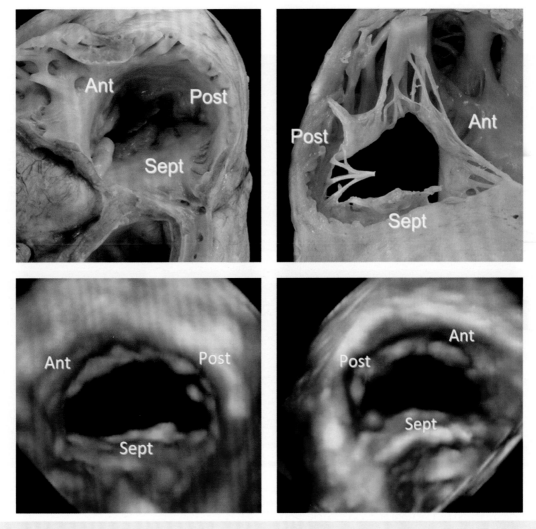

Figure 4-10. **Tricuspid valve: anatomy versus 3D echocardiography.** Anatomical specimens (top) and 3D transesophageal images (bottom) depicting the valve as viewed from the right atrium (left) and the right ventricle (right). Ant, anterior; Post, posterior; Sept, septum.

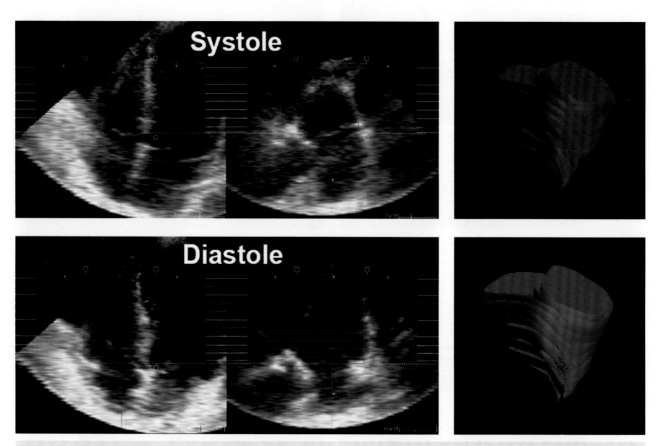

Figure 4-11. Volumetric quantification of RV volume. Chamber volume can be calculated from the 3DE datasets using the disk approximation by summation of slices of the RV cavity. Example in this figure depicts RV cavity casts reconstructed using this methodology at end systole (top) and end diastole (bottom).

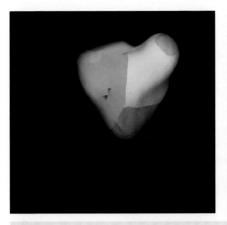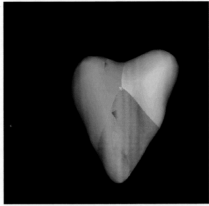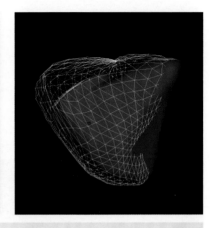

Figure 4-12. Dynamic reconstruction of RV endocardial surface. Three-dimensional reconstruction of the RV endocardial surface can be performed on every consecutive frame throughout the cardiac cycle, resulting in a dynamic display of a "beating" RV cast. Left and middle panels display the RV cast at end systole and end diastole. The "beating cast" can also be displayed with its end-diastolic silhouette in a transparent wireframe representation to facilitate the visualization of RV regional function. Accompanying Video 4.13 corresponds to the right panel and depicts this in a dynamic format.

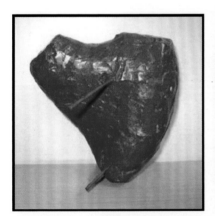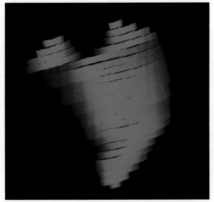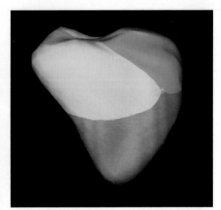

Figure 4-13. Validation of RV reconstruction and volume measurements in a phantom. RV-shaped phantom of known volume (left) was initially used to validate volume measurements by disk approximation (middle) and direct volumetric measurements from reconstructed RV endocardial surface (right). Comparing these measurements side by side against the true volume demonstrated the superior accuracy of the latter approach. (Modified from Sugeng L, Mor-Avi V, Weinert L, et al. Multimodality comparison of quantitative volumetric analysis of the right ventricle. *JACC Cardiovasc Imaging* 2010;3:10–18, with permission.)

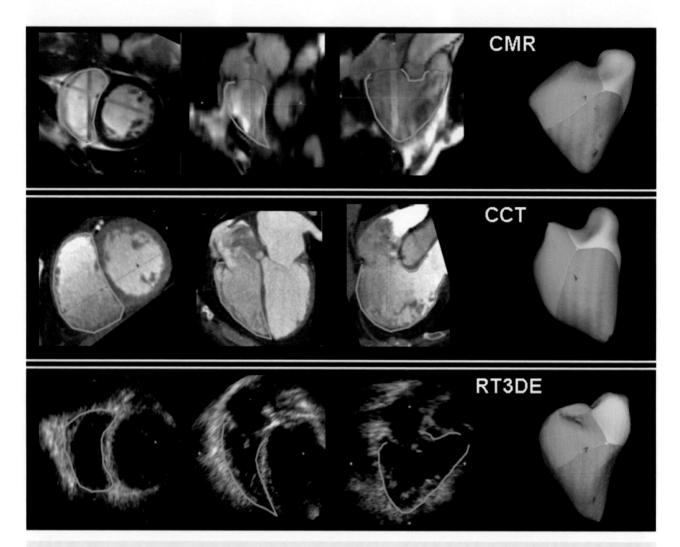

Figure 4-14. Multimodality comparisons of RV volume measurements in humans. Example of RV volumetric analysis across three imaging modalities: cardiac MRI (top), cardiac CT (middle), and 3DE (bottom) images obtained in one patient. From left to right: RV boundaries initialized in a midventricular short-axis view, apical four-chamber view, and coronal view, shown along with the calculated RV endocardial 3D surfaces (right), with the cast representing end systole and the wireframe representing end diastole. CMR, cardiac magnetic resonance; CCT, cardiac computed tomography; RT3DE, real-time 3DE. (Modified from Sugeng L, Mor-Avi V, Weinert L, et al. Multimodality comparison of quantitative volumetric analysis of the right ventricle. *JACC Cardiovasc Imaging* 2010;3:10–18, with permission.)

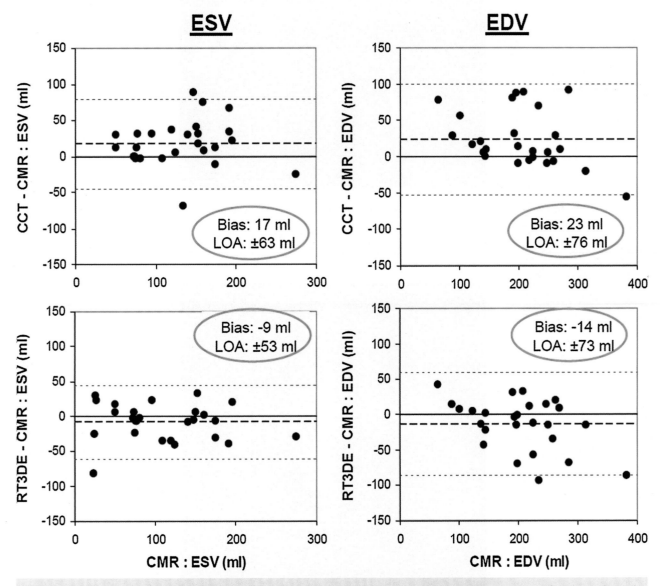

Figure 4-15. **Intermodality differences in RV volume measurements.** Results of Bland-Altman analysis of end-systolic and end-diastolic RV volumes (ESV—left, EDV—right), calculated using volumetric analysis of cardiac CT (top) and 3DE (bottom) images against CMR reference values obtained in 28 patients. While CCT overestimated both volumes, RT3DE underestimated them. *Dashed horizontal lines* show the bias, while the *dotted lines* show the 95% limits of agreement (LOA). CMR, cardiac magnetic resonance; CCT, cardiac computed tomography. (Modified from Sugeng L, Mor-Avi V, Weinert L, et al. Multimodality comparison of quantitative volumetric analysis of the right ventricle. *JACC Cardiovasc Imaging* 2010;3:10–18, with permission.)

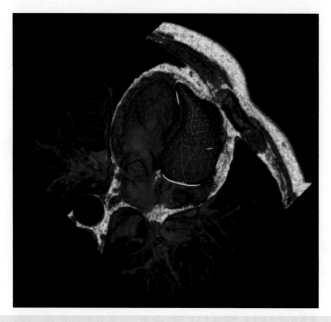

Figure 4-16. Multimodality fusion imaging of the right ventricle. A new intriguing application is multimodality fusion imaging. This image is a result of fusion of cardiac CT and 3DE.

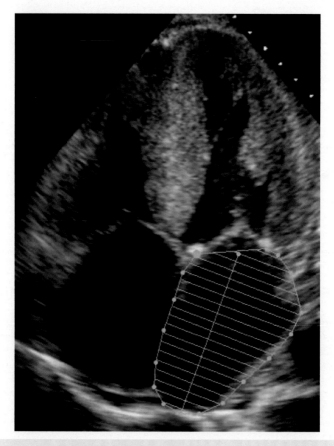

Figure 4-17. Two-dimensional echocardiographic measurement of left atrial volume. Two-dimensional echocardiography is routinely used to measure LAV using the disk summation method. To improve the accuracy of the measurements, biplane disk approximation is frequently used by averaging measurements from the apical four- and two-chamber views.

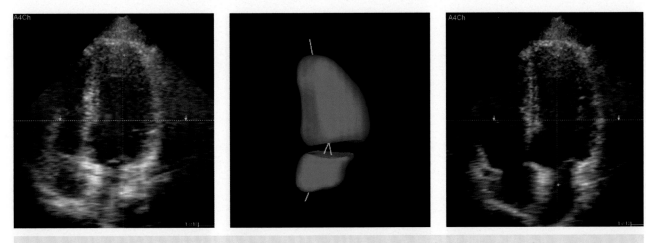

Figure 4-18. Limitations of 2D echocardiographic measurements of left atrial volume. The accuracy of 2DE measurements of LAV is limited because these measurements are view dependent and rely on geometrical assumptions regarding LA shape. This is especially problematic because LAV is frequently measured in apical views optimized for the left ventricle (left), in which the left atrium may be foreshortened, compared to views specifically optimized to visualize the left atrium (right). This is because the long axes of the ventricle and the atrium do not necessarily coincide, as depicted in this 3D reconstruction of both left heart chambers (center). Accompanying Videos 4.18A and 4.18B depict this in a dynamic format.

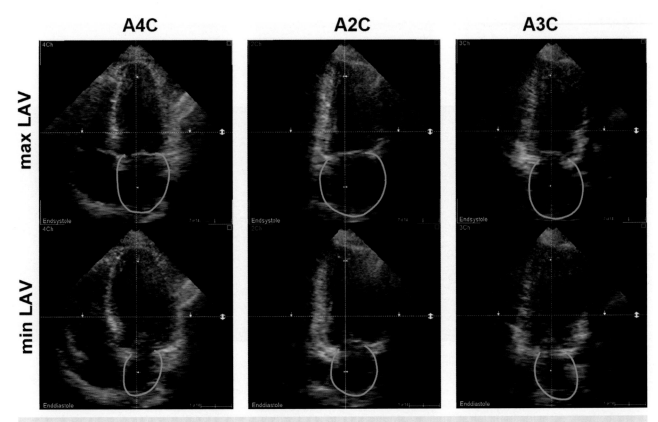

Figure 4-19. Three-dimensional measurement of LAV. To improve the accuracy of the evaluation of LA size, atrial volume can be measured directly by reconstructing the LA cavity in three dimensions. This reconstruction requires manual initialization of the atrial boundaries in three apical views (four-, two-, and three-chamber) extracted from the 3DE datasets at the end of ventricular systole, just before MV opening, when atrial volume reaches its peak value (top), and at end diastole, just before MV closing, when the volume is minimal (bottom). (Reprinted from Mor-Avi V, Yodwut C, Jenkins C, et al. Real-time 3D echocardiographic quantification of left atrial volume: Multicenter study for validation with magnetic resonance imaging. *J Am Coll Cardiol Img* 2012;5:769–777, with permission.)

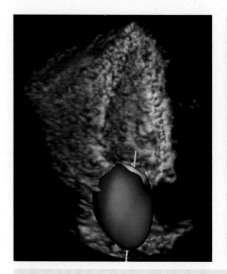
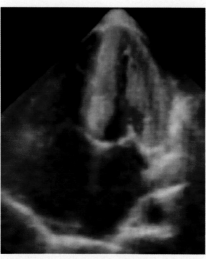
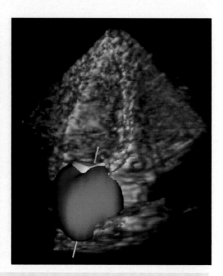

Figure 4-20. Visualization of the reconstructed LA cavity. Surface-rendered LA cavity reconstructed in three dimensions from a pyramidal 3DE dataset (middle, accompanying Video 4.20A) can be viewed from any desired angle (left and right panels, accompanying Video 4.20B). (Reprinted from Mor-Avi V, Yodwut C, Jenkins C, et al. Real-time 3D echocardiographic quantification of left atrial volume: Multicenter study for validation with magnetic resonance imaging. *J Am Coll Cardiol Img* 2012;5:769–777, with permission.)

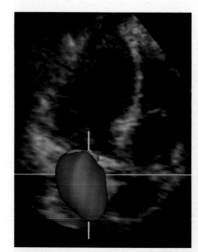
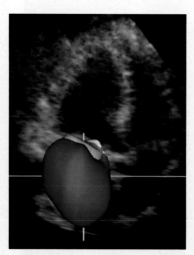
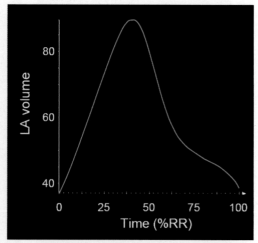

Figure 4-21. Three-dimensional evaluation of LA dynamics. Because 3D reconstruction of the LA surface is performed on each consecutive frame throughout the cardiac cycle, a dynamic display of the "beating" LA cast can be generated to facilitate the visualization of LA function (accompanying Video 4.22). Frames depicting minimal and maximal LAVs are shown along with the time curve of LAV over time (right). (Reprinted from Mor-Avi V, Yodwut C, Jenkins C, et al. Real-time 3D echo-cardiographic quantification of left atrial volume: Multicenter study for validation with magnetic resonance imaging. *J Am Coll Cardiol Img* 2012;5:769–777, with permission.)

Enlarged left atrium (LAVi>34 ml/m²):

		2DE		3DE	
		Normal	Abnormal	Normal	Abnormal
CMR	Normal	10	2	5	7
	Abnormal	28	60	7	81

accuracy=0.70   accuracy=0.86

Figure 4-22. Impact of imaging modality on the classification of LV diastolic function. Contingency tables for concordance between 2DE and 3DE classifications of LAV index as normal or abnormal against CMR classification, which was used as a reference. Threshold of 34 mL/m², recommended by the ASE guidelines, was used for all three modalities. Two-dimensional echocardiography classifications showed agreement with CMR in 70/100 patients, reflecting good intertechnique agreement. Three-dimensional echocardiography classifications agreed with CMR in 86/100 patients, indicating excellent agreement. Importantly, 2DE misclassified a larger number of atria as normal.

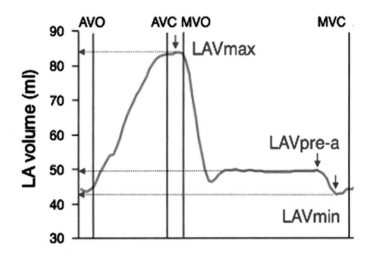

Reservoir function:
Expansion index = [(LAVmax - LAVmin) / LAV min] x 100%

Conduit function:
Passive emptying index = [(LAVmax - LAVpre-a) / LAVmax] x 100%

Booster function:
Active emptying index = [(LAVpre-a - LAVmin) / LAVmax] x 100%

Figure 4-23. Three-dimensional quantification of LA function. LAV over time curves can be used to measure indices of LA function: expansion index that describes LA reservoir function, passive emptying index that describes LA conduit function, and active emptying index that describes LA booster function. LAVmax, LAVmin, minimum and maximum volumes; LAVpre-a, volume just prior to atrial contraction; AVC, aortic valve closure; AVO, aortic valve opening; MVC, mitral valve closure; MVO, mitral valve opening. (Modified from Okamatsu K, Takeuchi M, Nakai H, et al. Effects of aging on left atrial function assessed by two-dimensional speckle tracking echocardiography. *J Am Soc Echocardiogr* 2009;22:70–75, with permission.)

References

1. Mertens LL, Friedberg MK. Imaging the right ventricle—current state of the art. *Nat Rev Cardiol* 2010;7:551–563.

2. Mangion JR. Right ventricular imaging by two-dimensional and three-dimensional echocardiography. *Curr Opin Cardiol* 2010;25:423–429.

3. Niemann PS, Pinho L, Balbach T, et al. Anatomically oriented right ventricular volume measurements with dynamic three-dimensional echocardiography validated by 3-Tesla magnetic resonance imaging. *J Am Coll Cardiol* 2007;50:1668–1676.

4. Tamborini G, Brusoni D, Torres Molina JE, et al. Feasibility of a new generation three-dimensional echocardiography for right ventricular volumetric and functional measurements. *Am J Cardiol* 2008;102:499–505.

5. Sugeng L, Mor-Avi V, Weinert L, et al. Multimodality comparison of quantitative volumetric analysis of the right ventricle. *JACC Cardiovasc Imaging* 2010;3:10–18.

6. Shiota T. 3D echocardiography: evaluation of the right ventricle. *Curr Opin Cardiol* 2009;24:410–414.

7. Gopal AS, Chukwu EO, Iwuchukwu CJ, et al. Normal values of right ventricular size and function by real-time 3-dimensional echocardiography: comparison with cardiac magnetic resonance imaging. *J Am Soc Echocardiogr* 2007;20:445–455.

8. Kjaergaard J, Petersen CL, Kjaer A, et al. Evaluation of right ventricular volume and function by 2D and 3D echocardiography compared to MRI. *Eur J Echocardiogr* 2006;7:430–438.

9. Kjaergaard J, Sogaard P, Hassager C. Quantitative echocardiographic analysis of the right ventricle in healthy individuals. *J Am Soc Echocardiogr* 2006;19:1365–1372.

10. Tamborini G, Marsan NA, Gripari P, et al. Reference values for right ventricular volumes and ejection fraction with real-time three-dimensional echocardiography: evaluation in a large series of normal subjects. *J Am Soc Echocardiogr* 2010;23:109–115.

11. Kjaergaard J, Hastrup SJ, Sogaard P, et al. Advanced quantitative echocardiography in arrhythmogenic right ventricular cardiomyopathy. *J Am Soc Echocardiogr* 2007;20:27–35.

12. Acar P, Abadir S, Roux D, et al. Ebstein's anomaly assessed by real-time 3-D echocardiography. *Ann Thorac Surg* 2006;82:731–733.

13. Grewal J, Majdalany D, Syed I, et al. Three-dimensional echocardiographic assessment of right ventricular volume and function in adult patients with congenital heart disease: comparison with magnetic resonance imaging. *J Am Soc Echocardiogr* 2010;23:127–133.

14. Scheurer M, Bandisode V, Ruff P, et al. Early experience with real-time three-dimensional echocardiographic guidance of right ventricular biopsy in children. *Echocardiography* 2006;23:45–49.

15. Tamborini G, Muratori M, Brusoni D, et al. Is right ventricular systolic function reduced after cardiac surgery? A two- and three-dimensional echocardiographic study. *Eur J Echocardiogr* 2009;10:630–634.

16. Nagueh SF, Appleton CP, Gillebert TC, et al. Recommendations for the evaluation of left ventricular diastolic function by echocardiography. *J Am Soc Echocardiogr* 2009;22:107–133.

17. Lang RM, Bierig M, Devereux RB, et al. Recommendations for chamber quantification: a report from the American Society of Echocardiography's Guidelines and Standards Committee and the Chamber Quantification Writing Group, developed in conjunction with the European Association of Echocardiography, a branch of the European Society of Cardiology. *J Am Soc Echocardiogr* 2005;18:1440–1463.

18. Avelar E, Durst R, Rosito GA, et al. Comparison of the accuracy of multidetector computed tomography versus two-dimensional echocardiography to measure left atrial volume. *Am J Cardiol* 2010;106:104–109.

19. Koka AR, Yau J, Van WC, et al. Underestimation of left atrial size measured with transthoracic echocardiography compared with 3D MDCT. *AJR Am J Roentgenol* 2010;194:W375–W381.

20. Kühl JT, Lønborg J, Fuchs A, et al. Assessment of left atrial volume and function: a comparative study between echocardiography, magnetic resonance imaging and multi slice computed tomography. *Int J Cardiovasc Imaging* 2012;28(5):1061–1071.

21. Jenkins C, Bricknell K, Marwick TH. Use of real-time three-dimensional echocardiography to measure left atrial volume: comparison with other echocardiographic techniques. *J Am Soc Echocardiogr* 2005;18:991–997.

22. Anwar AM, Soliman OI, Geleijnse ML, et al. Assessment of left atrial volume and function by real-time three-dimensional echocardiography. *Int J Cardiol* 2008;123:155–161.

23. Suh IW, Song JM, Lee EY, et al. Left atrial volume measured by real-time 3-dimensional echocardiography predicts clinical outcomes in patients with severe left ventricular dysfunction and in sinus rhythm. *J Am Soc Echocardiogr* 2008;21:439–445.

24. Artang R, Migrino RQ, Harmann L, et al. Left atrial volume measurement with automated border detection by 3-dimensional echocardiography: comparison with magnetic resonance imaging. *Cardiovasc Ultrasound* 2009;7:16.

25. Miyasaka Y, Tsujimoto S, Maeba H, et al. Left atrial volume by real-time three-dimensional echocardiography: validation by 64-slice multidetector computed tomography. *J Am Soc Echocardiogr* 2011;24:680–686.

26. Jiang L, Siu SC, Handschumacher MD, et al. Three-dimensional echocardiography. In vivo validation for right ventricular volume and function. *Circulation* 1994;89:2342–2350.

27. Okamatsu K, Takeuchi M, Nakai H, et al. Effects of aging on left atrial function assessed by two-dimensional speckle tracking echocardiography. *J Am Soc Echocardiogr* 2009;22:70–75.

28. Mor-Avi V, Yodwut C, Jenkins C, et al. Real-time 3D echocardiographic quantification of left atrial volume: Multicenter study for validation with magnetic resonance imaging. *J Am Coll Cardiol Img* 2012;5:769–777.

MITRAL VALVE: NORMAL ASPECTS

5

Benjamin H. Freed, Lynn Weinert, Roberto M. Lang

The natural history of mitral valve disease and its resultant mitral regurgitation (MR) depends on, to a large degree, the etiology as well as the severity at presentation. The causes are numerous and include myxomatous degeneration, rheumatic heart disease, mitral annular calcification, and connective tissue disorders. Ischemic MR, while common, has a different natural history related to both the effects of recurrent myocardial ischemia and the significant contribution of left ventricular (LV) remodeling to survival and function.[1]

In the 1960s, most cases of MR were caused by postinflammatory disease, whereas in the 1990s, inflammatory causes such as rheumatic disease (Fig. 5-27) accounted for only 3% of the cases.[2] Today, myxomatous degenerative disease (Fig. 5-12) is the most common etiology for MR in the United States.[3] The consequences of untreated MR are well known and include congestive heart failure, atrial fibrillation, and pulmonary hypertension. In one of the few studies describing the natural history of MR, Delahaye et al.[4] reported on 54 patients with severe, isolated MR due primarily to degenerative disease who were treated medically. The actuarial 5- and 8-year mortality rates were approximately 49% and 67%, respectively.

In 1808, Corvisart first described the treatment with diuretics and digitalis for MR.[5] This remained the only therapy for over 150 years. When surgical correction of this disorder came into vogue, it dramatically altered the natural history of MR and allowed patients to lead longer lives without symptoms. Even nowadays, it is still unclear how best to manage patients with MR. Currently, physicians rely heavily on management strategies that have evolved empirically and guidelines that have relied more on expert consensus opinion rather than on objective measures of efficacy and safety. The relative high morbidity and mortality rates associated with chronic MR make it imperative that evidence-based data drive how physicians manage these patients. To date, no large-scale randomized controlled clinical trial comparing different treatment strategies has ever been performed.

Recent improvements in surgical outcomes have modified the timing of surgery earlier in the natural history of appropriately selected patients with chronic nonischemic MR. This has forced clinicians to balance the upfront risks of surgery (death, stroke, bleeding, failure of repair) versus the delayed consequences of progressive LV volume overload (heart failure, atrial fibrillation, death), which, for some patients, may not develop for decades, if at all. Noninvasive imaging, especially echocardiography, plays a vital role in helping physicians make appropriate treatment recommendations. Many patients receive unnecessary valve replacements because the echocardiogram has not been considered in surgical referral and operative planning. Despite guideline recommendations for valve repair in degenerative valve disease when feasible, the current national repair rates generally approximate <60% of operated patients.[6]

In order to accurately assess the pathophysiology and severity of mitral valve disease, a systematic approach to identifying the disease process, localizing the lesion, and quantifying the degree of stenosis and/or regurgitation is essential (Figs. 5-2, 5-10, 5-11, 5-30 through 5-32). Real-time 3D (RT3D) using matrix 3D transesophageal echocardiogram (TEE) technology with its improved spatial resolution is particularly well suited for the study of the mitral valve apparatus given its complex morphology (Figs. 5-1 and 5-5).[7] It is quickly becoming an invaluable tool in both the diagnosis and treatment of mitral valve disease, providing critical information that helps guide therapeutic management decisions for both the clinician and surgeon.

The mitral valve annulus, leaflets, commissures, and subvalvular structures are best displayed when obtained in zoom mode to avoid stitch artifacts due to respiration and arrhythmias that may occur when using wide-angled acquisitions (Figs. 5-3 and 5-7).[8] This mode displays a small, magnified pyramidal volume of the mitral valve, which may vary from a 20 degrees × 20 degrees up to 90 degrees × 90 degrees depending on the density setting.[9] To simulate a surgeon's view of the valve (from left atrium to left ventricle while standing to the right of the patient), the 3D image is positioned with the aortic valve at the 12 o'clock position (Figs. 5-4, 5-8, and 5-9).[10]

While visualization of anatomy in its true 3D state is important, many physicians believe that the most significant value provided by RT3D TEE is the ability to provide accurate and reproducible quantification of annular diameters, annular nonplanarity, commissural lengths, leaflet surface areas, and aortic-to-mitral annular orientation (Figs. 5-33 through 5-36).[8] These measurements of the mitral valve apparatus may aid in better defining the pathophysiology of mitral valve disease and planning mitral valve surgery.

Diseases that affect the mitral valve are best described by defining the *etiology* of the disease, the specific *lesions* caused by the disease, and the *dysfunction* it creates of the mitral valve apparatus (Fig. 5-14). This "pathophysiologic triad" was first described by Carpentier et al.[11] in the early 1980s and is still extremely useful today in characterizing degenerative mitral valve regurgitation. For instance, Barlow's disease is a common type of degenerative disease of the mitral valve (Fig. 5-18). Typical lesions of this disease include multisegmental thickening of both leaflets, chordal elongation, and leaflet billowing. These lesions commonly result in mitral valve prolapse in which there is excess motion of the leaflet margin above the plane of the annulus. In the Carpentier classification scheme, prolapse is described as a type II dysfunction. A more detailed description of the Carpentier pathophysiologic triad is included below.

This chapter highlights the numerous advantages to using RT3D TEE in the management of mitral valve disease. Developing a methodical and systematic approach to diagnosing the mitral valve dysfunction will no doubt help in guiding therapeutic options for this challenging valvular disease.

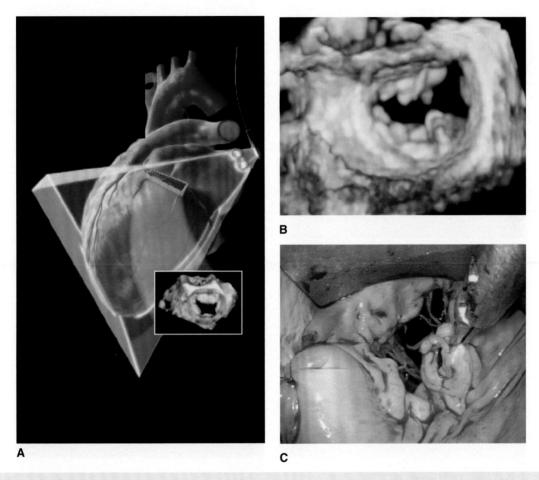

A

B

C

Figure 5-1. RT3D TEE imaging of the mitral valve. Matrix array technology using TEE allows acquisition of a 3D volume dataset that can be analyzed in real time.[12] The mitral valve annulus, leaflets, commissures, and subvalvular structures are best displayed in the zoom mode to avoid respiratory and stitch artifacts.[8] This mode displays a small, magnified pyramidal volume of the mitral valve (A). The mitral valve leaflets and their respective scallops are clearly visualized (B) in the anatomical orientation that is most similar to the surgeon's actual view of the valve (C) so that communication is facilitated between the imager and the surgeon regarding location and extent of various anatomic structures.

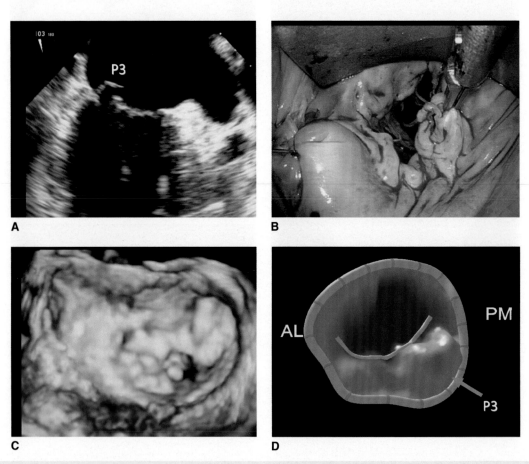

Figure 5-2. Localization and extent of flail component of mitral valve using RT3D TEE. In patients with MR, 2D TEE reveals a flail posterior leaflet as visualized here in the two-chamber view (A). Using RT3D TEE, the imager is able to further localize and determine the extent of the flail component of the mitral valve to the P3 scallop (B). These 3D images can be analyzed off-line for exact location and extent of the structural abnormality using software designed for quantitative analysis of the mitral apparatus (C). The images and 3D renderings allow the surgeon to accurately identify and repair the flail segment (D). P3, posteromedial mitral valve scallop; AL, anterolateral; PM, posteromedial.

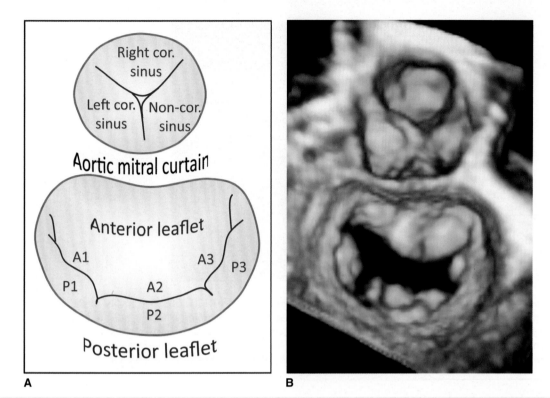

A   **B**

Figure 5-3. Anatomy of the mitral valve. In order to replicate the surgeon's intraoperative view of the mitral valve, the 3D image of the mitral valve is oriented so that the valve is visualized en face from the left atrium with the aortic valve directly above it at the 12 o'clock position.[9] A schematic diagram of the aortic and mitral valve in this orientation is shown in (A) with the corresponding 3D image shown in (B). The left and noncoronary cusps of the aortic valve are separated from the anterior leaflet of the mitral valve by a fibrous area known as the aortic–mitral curtain.[13] The anterior mitral leaflet has a semicircular shape and constitutes two-thirds of the valve area. The posterior mitral leaflet has a quadrangular shape and constitutes the remaining one-third of the valve area. The anterior and posterior leaflets are conjoined laterally and medially to form the anterolateral and posteromedial commissures, respectively. The commissures define a distinct area where the leaflets appose each other during systole. A1, anterolateral segment; A2, anterior–middle segment; A3, anteromedial segment; P1, posterolateral scallop; P2, posterior–middle scallop; P3, posteromedial scallop.

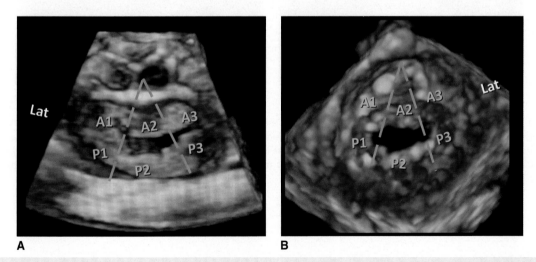

A   **B**

Figure 5-4. Scallops of the mitral valve leaflets. The anterior and posterior leaflets of the mitral valve can be divided into three separate segments or "scallops" in order to make it easier to identify specific mitral valve lesions. In (A), the mitral valve is viewed from the left atrium while (B) shows the mitral valve from the perspective of the left ventricle. The posterior mitral leaflet has two well-defined indentations that clearly demarcate the three scallops. The anterolateral scallop is defined as P1, the middle scallop is defined as P2, and the posteromedial scallop is defined as P3. The three opposing segments on the anterior leaflet are designated as A1 (anterior segment), A2 (middle segment), and A3 (posterior segment), respectively. P2 is the largest scallop with the greatest surface area making it the most vulnerable to prolapse.

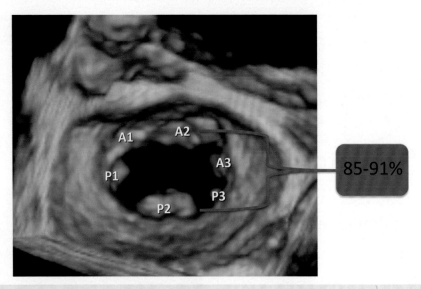

Figure 5-5. Acquisition and visualization of mitral valve scallops using RT3D TEE. The ability of RT3D TEE to visualize the mitral valve leaflets was studied in a population of 211 patients undergoing clinically indicated TEE exams.[14] Patients with atrial fibrillation were included while patients with prosthetic valves and/or post–mitral valve repair were excluded. Acquisition of 3D data was accomplished in approximately 10 minutes. In this figure, the mitral valve is viewed in diastole from the left atrial view. Excellent visualization of all scallops (85% to 91%) was obtained in this patient population.

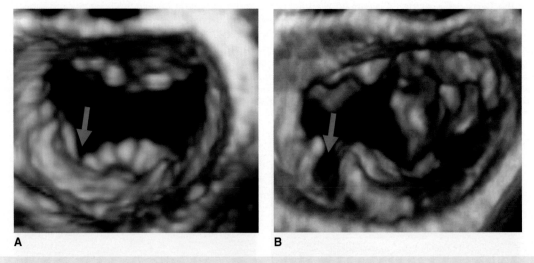

Figure 5-6. Scallop anatomy. RT3D TEE zoomed views of the mitral valve visualized from the left atrium are shown. The posterior leaflet scallops are defined by indentations as demonstrated by (A) in which the *arrow* represents a typical-looking indentation separating P1 from P2. Conversely, the mitral valve in (B) demonstrates the presence of a full cleft (*arrow*) between P1 and P2 with consequent MR and potential ramifications regarding surgical or percutaneous repair. P1, posterolateral scallop; P2, posterior middle scallop.

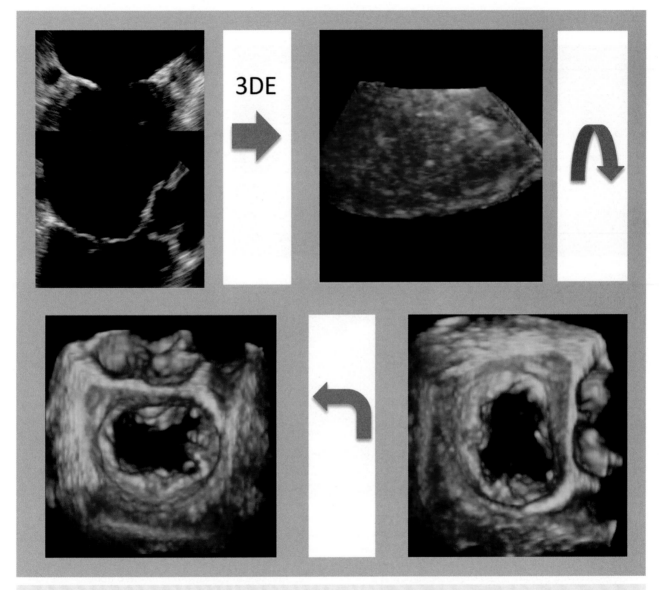

Figure 5-7. **RT3D TEE image acquisition of the mitral valve.** Starting with 2D TEE, the mitral valve is visualized in the three-chamber mid-esophageal view. With the entire mitral valve in the center of the image, a 3D image is obtained in zoom mode. The 3D image is then rotated 90 degrees to view the mitral and aortic valve en face from the left atrium. To replicate the surgeon's view, the 3D image is rotated 90 degrees counterclockwise so that the aortic valve is located in the 12 o'clock position.

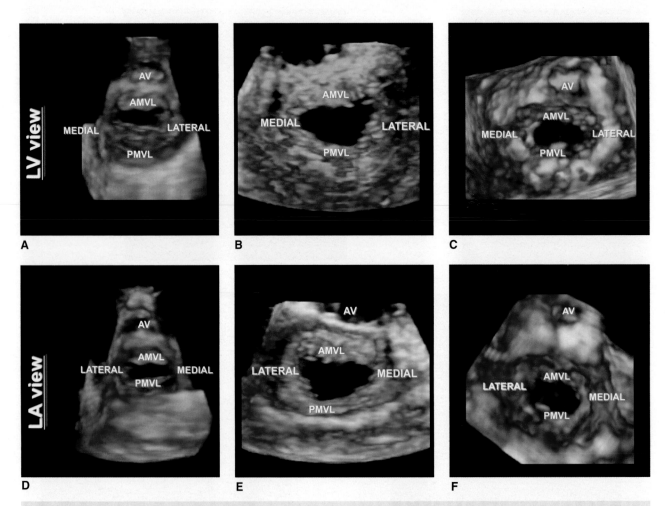

Figure 5-8. Various views of mitral valve. The morphology of the mitral valve can appear different depending on the size of the patient and structural abnormality, but the orientation of the valve should be consistent irrespective of perspective. Whether the mitral valve is viewed from the left ventricle (A–C) or left atrium (D–F), the aorta should always be positioned at 12 o'clock. Note that the anterolateral segment (P1) is located on the right side of the valve when viewed from the left ventricle and on the left side of the valve when viewed from the left atrium. AMVL, anterior mitral valve leaflet; PMVL, posterior mitral valve leaflet; AV, aortic valve; LV, left ventricle; LA, left atrium.

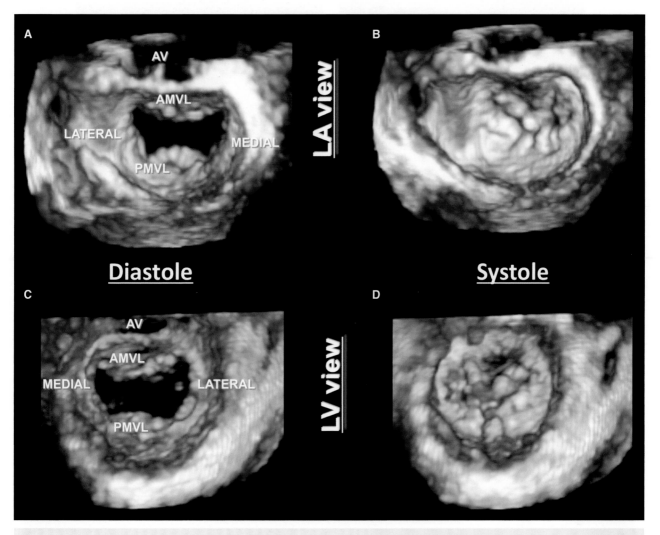

Figure 5-9. View of mitral valve in diastole and systole. The mitral valve is visualized in both diastole (A,C) and systole (B,D) from both the left atrial (A,B) and left ventricle (C,D) perspective. The scallops are best seen when the mitral valve is open in mid diastole. AMVL, anterior mitral valve leaflet; PMVL, posterior mitral valve leaflet; AV, aortic valve; LV, left ventricle; LA, left atrium.

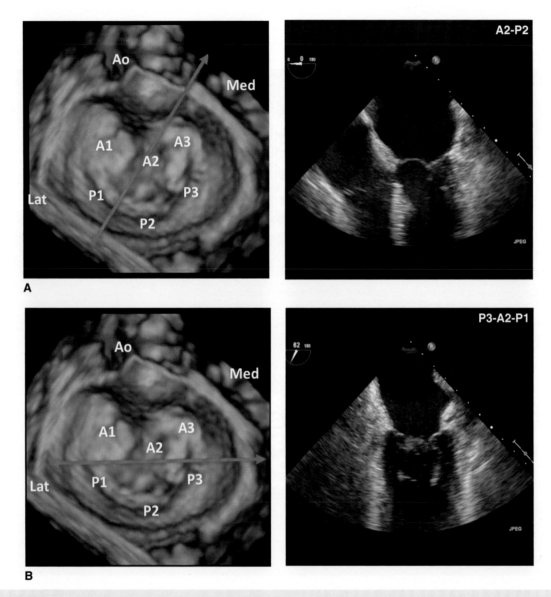

Figure 5-10. **Systematic interrogation of the mitral valve.** The first task for the imager is to determine whether the anterior leaflet, posterior leaflet, or both are abnormal. This is generally accomplished with the 2D TEE mid-esophageal four-chamber view. Once this is established, the imager is able to further refine the diagnosis by visualizing the mitral valve from multiple 2D TEE views. In the four-chamber view, the plane of the mitral valve (*red line*) is such that A2 is on the left and P2 is on the right (A). In the bicommissural view, P3 is on the left, A2 is in the middle, and P1 is on the right (B). All 3D mitral valve renderings are viewed from the left atrial perspective. A1, anterolateral segment; A2, anterior–middle segment; A3, anteromedial segment; P1, posterolateral scallop; P2, posterior–middle scallop; P3, posteromedial scallop; Lat, lateral; Med, medial; Ao, aorta.

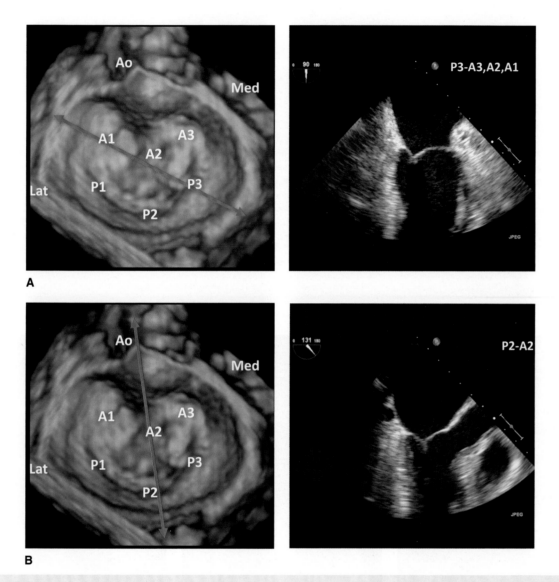

Figure 5-11. **Systematic interrogation of the mitral valve.** In the two-chamber view, the plane of the mitral valve (*red line*) is such that P3 is on the left and all three scallops of the anterior leaflet are on the right with A1 furthest to the right (A). By further rotating the transducer, the long-axis or three-chamber view shows P2 on the left and A2 on the right (B). All 3D mitral valve renderings are viewed from the left atrial perspective. A1, anterolateral segment; A2, anterior–middle segment; A3, anteromedial segment; P1, posterolateral scallop; P2, posterior–middle scallop; P3, posteromedial scallop; Lat, lateral; Med, medial; Ao, aorta.

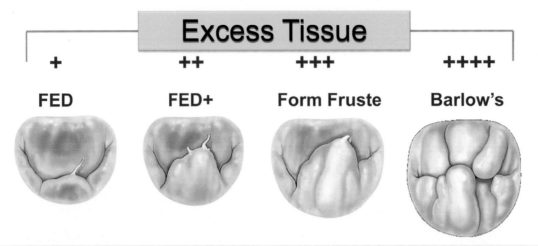

Figure 5-12. **Etiology of mitral valvular disease.** Mitral valve disease is due to either primary (direct) or secondary (indirect) causes. Examples of diseases that directly affect the mitral valve include congenital malformations, rheumatic disease, valvular tumors, and degenerative diseases. Examples of diseases that indirectly affect the mitral valve include ischemic and nonischemic dilated cardiomyopathy, hypertrophic obstructive cardiomyopathy, and infiltrative diseases. This slide illustrates the spectrum of diseases for mitral valve degenerative disease defined by the amount of excess pathologic tissue. On the left-hand side of the spectrum is fibroelastic deficiency (FED) with the least amount of excess tissue. On the right-hand side of the spectrum is Barlow's disease with the most excess tissue. FED+ and forme fruste are variations of FED and Barlow's disease and have an intermediate amount of excess pathologic tissue.[15]

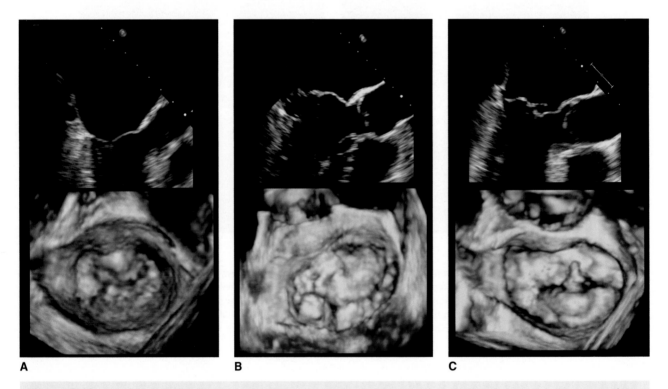

Figure 5-13. **2D and RT3D TEE examples of degenerative disease of the mitral valve.** 2D TEE three-chamber views of the mitral valve and their corresponding RT3D TEE image are shown. RT3D TEE is particularly useful at defining the type of lesion that develops as a result of the degenerative disease. A normal-appearing mitral valve is depicted in (A). Barlow's disease is demonstrated in (B). Note the large amount of excess myomatous tissue of both the anterior and posterior leaflet of the mitral valve. This lesion is a typical consequence of Barlow's disease. On the other end of the spectrum is FED, which results in very little excess tissue but is commonly associated with chordal elongation or rupture. An example of this is (C) in which FED has resulted in chordal rupture and P2 flail.

Type I (Nl Leaflet motion)

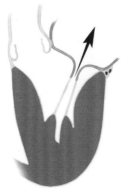

Annulus dilatation

Leaflet perforation

Type II (Increased leaflet motion)

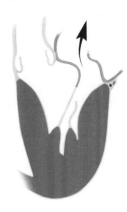

Ruptured chordae

Elongated chordae and/or papillary muscle

Rupture PM

Type IIIa (Systolic leaflet restriction)

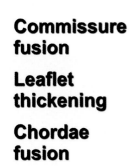

Commissure fusion

Leaflet thickening

Chordae fusion

Type IIIb (Diastolic leaflet restriction)

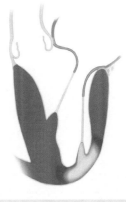

Ventricular dilatation

Ventricular dyskinesia

Figure 5-14. Classification of mitral valve dysfunction. No matter what the etiology of the mitral valve disease, each disease process results in one or more lesions. These lesions, in turn, lead to mitral valve dysfunction. Instead of classifying this dysfunction as simply mitral valve stenosis or regurgitation, Carpentier et al.[11] created a classification scheme for mitral valve dysfunction based on leaflet motion. Patients with normal leaflet motion are categorized as type I dysfunction. Type II dysfunction includes patients with increased leaflet motion such as prolapse or flail. Leaflet restriction during valve closure is defined as type IIIa dysfunction, and leaflet restriction during valve opening is defined as type IIIb dysfunction. The corresponding lesions for each type of dysfunction are listed and will be described in more detail in later figures. (Reused from Carpentier A. Cardiac valve surgery—the "French correction." *J Thorac Cardiovasc Surg.* 1983;86:323–337, with permission.)

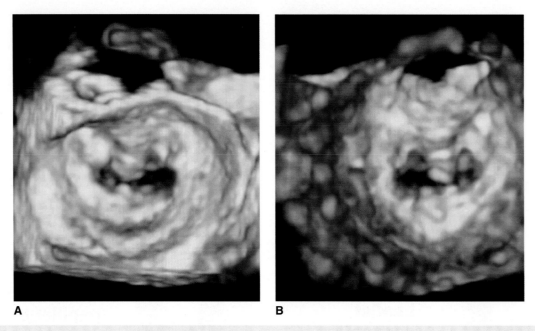

A   **B**

Figure 5-15. Type I dysfunction—annular dilatation. Dilated cardiomyopathy can result in mitral annular dilatation and what is commonly referred to as functional MR. RT3D TEE reveals that, while the leaflet motion is normal, the annulus is clearly stretched and dilated. This is shown from both the left atrial perspective (A) as well as the left ventricular perspective (B). Accompanying Video 5-1 corresponds to Figure 5-15.

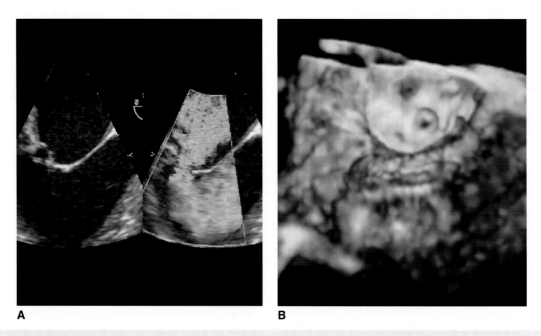

A   **B**

Figure 5-16. Type I dysfunction—leaflet perforation. 2D TEE shows that despite normal leaflet motion, there is severe MR due to a perforation of the posterior leaflet—a likely result of bacterial endocarditis (A). RT3D TEE clearly shows the perforation as a large crater-like structure in the posterior leaflet (B). Note that the rest of the valve appears normal underscoring the reason this type of dysfunction is categorized as type I. Accompanying Video 5-2 corresponds to Figure 5-16B.

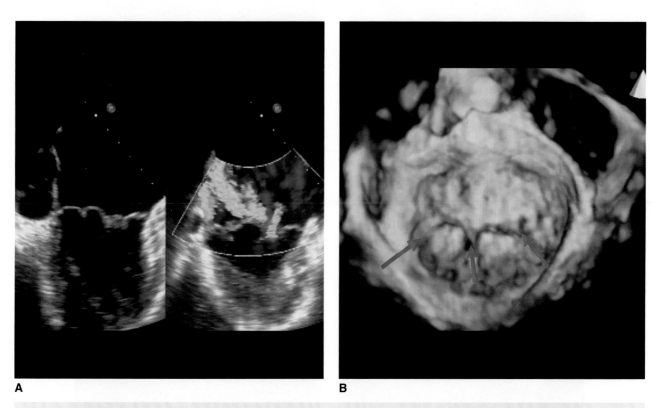

A

B

Figure 5-17. Type II dysfunction—bileaflet prolapse. 2D TEE of the mitral valve reveals thickened anterior and posterior leaflets due to excess tissue (A). Note the billowing nature of the leaflets. These lesions are consistent with Barlow's disease and commonly cause prolapse or excess leaflet motion. In this example, posterior leaflet prolapse is the cause of the severe MR. The RT3D TEE shows the classic bileaflet excess tissue of Barlow's disease (B). The *red arrows* outline the prolapse of the posterior leaflet.

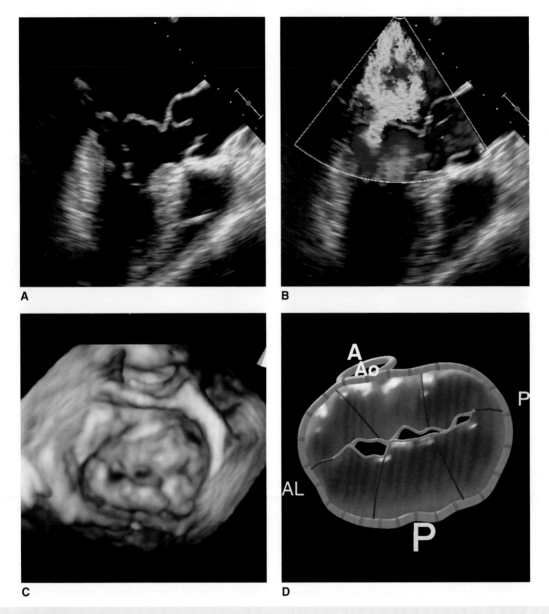

Figure 5-18. Barlow's Disease. In a three-chamber 2D TEE view, it is possible to visualize the bileaflet excess tissue and resultant multisegmental prolapse of the mitral valve (A). Clearly there is severe MR due to this type II dysfunction (B). The RT3D TEE view of the mitral valve better defines the anatomy, showing that, while both leaflets are affected, the entire posterior leaflet and the A3 segment are most involved (C). Accompanying Video 5-3 corresponds to Figure 5-18C. A 3D rendering of the mitral valve obtained from the corresponding RT3D TEE data set using software designed for quantitative analysis of the mitral apparatus delineates the scallops most affected (D). The *red area* of the parametric image represents prolapse. A, anterior; P, posterior; Ao, aorta; AL, anterolateral; PM, posteromedial.

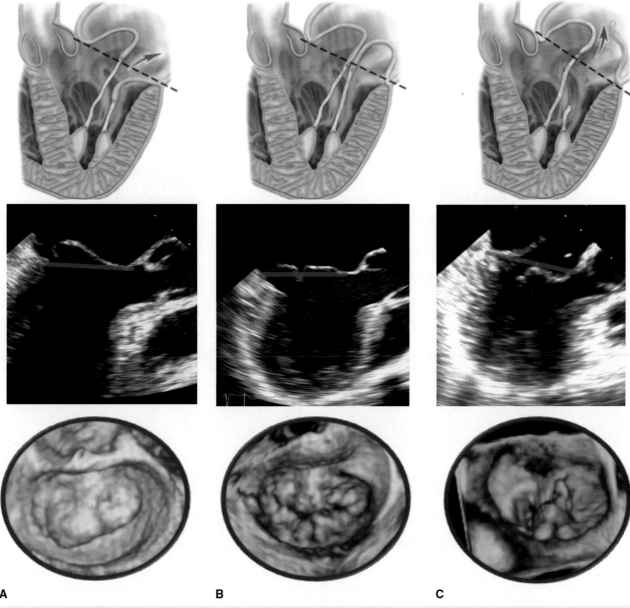

A   B   C

Figure 5-19. **Billowing versus prolapse.** When describing Barlow's disease, leaflet billowing and prolapse are often used interchangeably. However, these words do not have the same definition.[16] Leaflet billowing is a lesion of Barlow's disease and is diagnosed when there is systolic excursion of the leaflet body into the left atrium due to excess leaflet tissue, with the leaflet free edge remaining below the plane of the mitral annulus. Leaflet prolapse is the resulting dysfunction of Barlow's disease and should be diagnosed when the free edge of the leaflet overrides the plane of the mitral annulus during systole. This figure depicts the difference between prolapse, billowing, and flail. Leaflet prolapse is illustrated (A, **top**) with an example of anterior leaflet prolapse seen in this 2D TEE long-axis view (A, **middle**) and P2 prolapse as seen in this RT3D TEE view from the left atrium (A, **bottom**). Leaflet billowing is illustrated (B, **top**) with a 2D TEE long-axis view demonstrating bileaflet billowing of the mitral valve (B, **middle**) and a corresponding RT3D TEE example as seen from the left atrium (B, **bottom**). Finally, flail leaflet is illustrated (C, **top**) along with a 2D TEE long-axis view demonstrating flail valve due to chordae rupture (C, **middle**) and a RT3D TEE example of P2 flail as viewed from the left atrium (C, **bottom**).

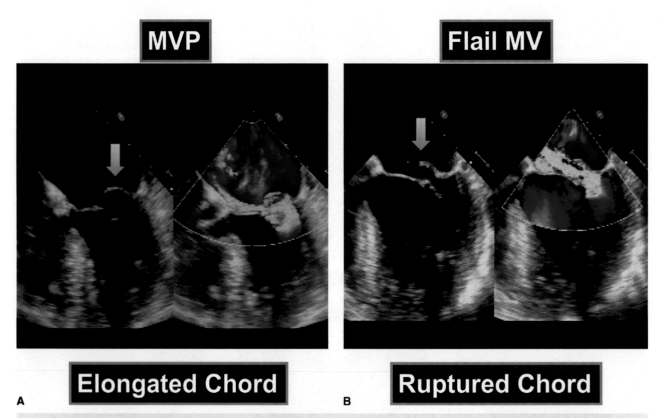

Figure 5-20. **Fibroelastic deficiency.** FED is, like Barlow's disease, a degenerative disease that affects the mitral valve. Unlike Barlow's disease, it is due to abnormal connective tissue structure/function, and is characterized by minimal excess tissue, and is typically unisegmental.[15] Whereas Barlow's disease is commonly diagnosed in younger patients, FED is usually a disease of older patients. A typical history is that of an older patient with a short history of MR due to chordal elongation resulting in leaflet prolapse (A) or chordal rupture resulting in flail leaflet (B). MVP, mitral valve prolapse; MV, mitral valve.

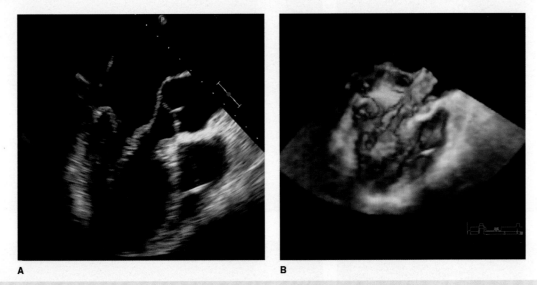

A   **B**

Figure 5-21. Type II dysfunction—posterior leaflet prolapse. The three-chamber 2D TEE view of the mitral valve reveals elongated chords of both the anterior and posterior leaflet (A). The corresponding RT3D TEE image shows the resultant posterior leaflet prolapse that is a common consequence of chordal elongation due to fibroelastic deficiency (B). Accompanying Video 5-4 corresponds to Figure 5-21B.

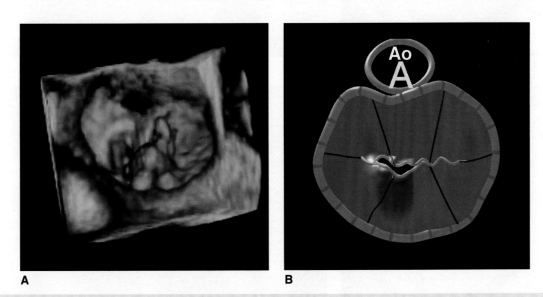

A   **B**

Figure 5-22. Type II dysfunction—posterior leaflet flail. The chordal tissue in FED is usually so thin, fragile, and overall unstable that chordal rupture is a common occurrence resulting in flail of the attached leaflet. The RT3D TEE view of the mitral valve demonstrates flail of a very discreet segment of the posterior leaflet (A). In this case, it is the P2 scallop. The focal nature of this lesion is very typical of FED. Software designed to display a parametric rendering of the mitral valve using the corresponding 3D data confirms that the P2 scallop is most affected (B). The *red area* of the parametric image represents flail. Ao, aorta; A, anterior.

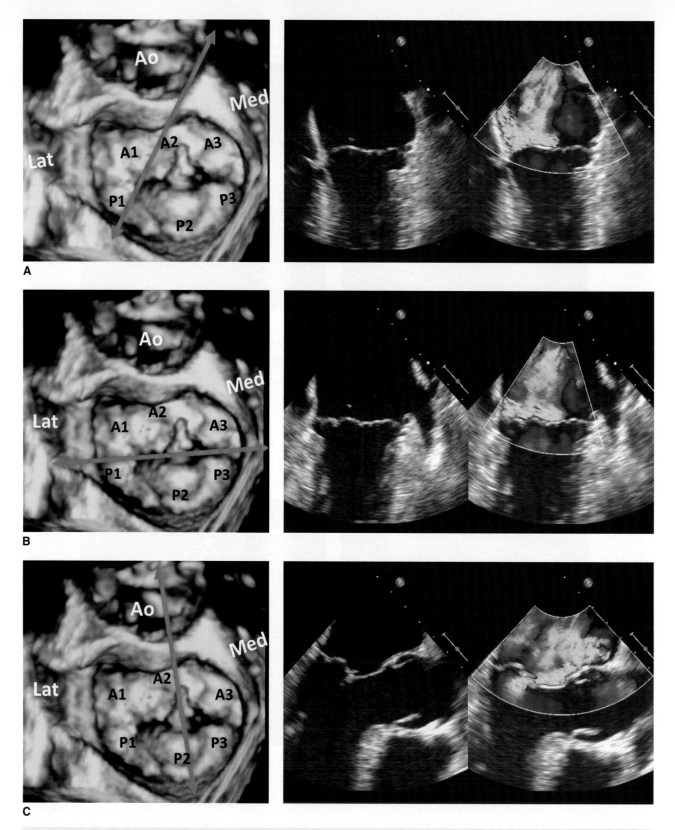

Figure 5-23. Systematic approach to diagnosing P2 flail of the mitral valve using RT3D TEE. In a five-chamber 2D TEE view depicting A2 on the left and P2 on the right, it is obvious that the posterior leaflet is most affected (A). The direction of the eccentric MR jet further demonstrates involvement of the posterior leaflet. Rotating the transducer approximately 90 degrees to the two-chamber view, P3 is on the left and the three scallops of the anterior leaflet are on the right (B). Although significant MR exists, it is difficult from this view to identify the exact lesion. Rotating the transducer an additional 30 degrees to the three-chamber view, P2 is now on the left and A2 is on the right (C). Here, the P2 flail is clearly evident with the resulting eccentric MR jet directed away from the lesion. The corresponding RT3D TTE image is represented for each view. The *red lines* represent the approximate cut planes from which the respective 2D TEE images were obtained. A1, anterolateral segment; A2, anterior–middle segment; A3, anteromedial segment; P1, posterolateral scallop; P2, posterior–middle scallop; P3, posteromedial scallop; Lat, lateral; Med, medial; Ao, aorta.

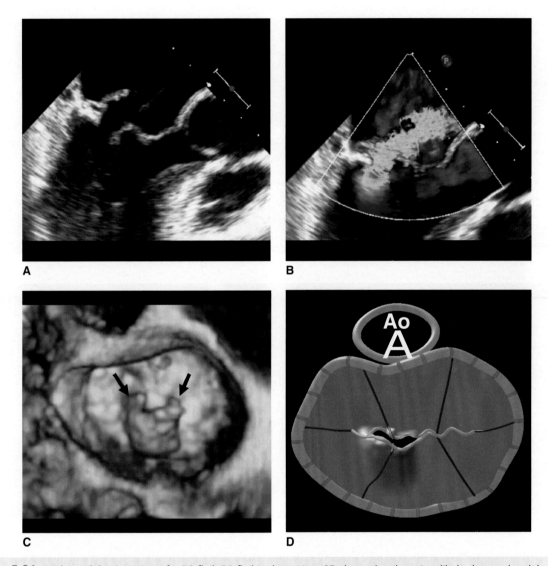

Figure 5-24. Multimodality imaging of a P2 flail. P2 flail is shown in a 2D three-chamber view likely due to chordal rupture (A). A significant amount of MR directed toward the anterior leaflet is visualized in (B). RT3D TEE better defines the anatomy of this mitral valve (C). Accompanying Video 5-5 corresponds to Figure 5-24C. Note that, while there is clear involvement of the P2 scallop (*black arrows*), the remainder of the valve appears normal. The 3D rendering of this valve shows that P2 is most affected (D). A, anterior; Ao, aorta.

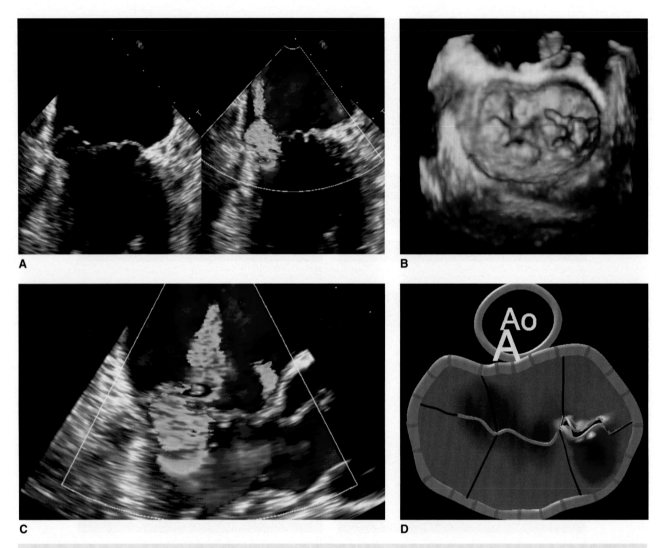

Figure 5-25. Multimodality imaging of a P3 flail. In this bicommissural 2D TEE view with the transducer rotated to approximately 60 degrees, P3 is depicted on left, A2 in the middle, and P1 on the right (A). The P3 scallop is clearly above the annular plane. The corresponding RT3D TEE image demonstrates the abnormal P3 segment and associated chordal rupture (B). Accompanying Video 5-6 corresponds to Figure 5-25B. A zoomed view of the mitral valve reveals significant MR due to the flail (C). A computerized representation of the valve shows how the lesion is isolated to the P3 scallop (D). Ao, aorta; A, anterior.

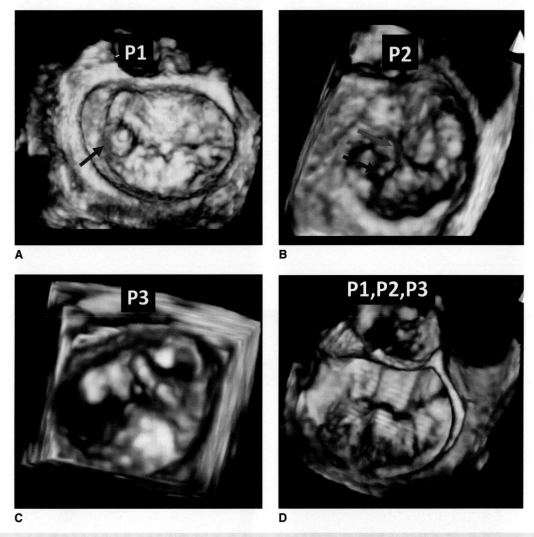

Figure 5-26. RT3D TEE examples of patients with prolapse and flail mitral valve. Degenerative diseases such as Barlow's disease and FED result in multiple types of lesions including excess myomatous tissue of the leaflets, chordal elongation, chordal thinning, and chordal rupture. These lesions typically lead to increased motion of the mitral valve leaflets causing prolapse and flail—a type II dysfunction of the mitral valve.[11] In (A), the posterior leaflet of the mitral valve appears thickened, and the P1 scallop appears to be prolapsed (*blue arrow*). Accompanying Video 5-7 corresponds to Figure 5-26A. In (B), the P2 scallop is flail (*blue arrow*) due to a ruptured chord (*red arrow*). Accompanying Video 5-8 corresponds to Figure 5-26B. This scenario is typical of a patient with FED. A flail scallop is also noted in (C) but, this time, RT3D TEE reveals that P3 is most affected. In (D), all three scallops of the posterior leaflet are prolapsed due to excessive myomatous tissue. This finding is consistent with Barlow's disease. P1, posterolateral scallop; P2, posterior–middle scallop; P3, posteromedial scallop.

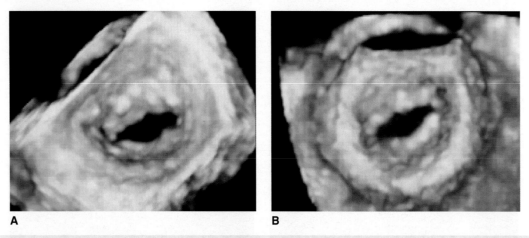

A   **B**

Figure 5-27. Type IIIA dysfunction—rheumatic mitral disease. Although the prevalence of rheumatic mitral valve disease has significantly diminished in the United States, it is still a major cause of mitral stenosis and regurgitation worldwide.[17] This disease results in lesions such as commissure fusion, leaflet thickening, and chordae fusion, which leads to mitral valve leaflet restriction primarily during systole. RT3D TEE helps the imager visualize the thickened leaflets and fused commissures both from the left atrial perspective (A) as well as the left ventricle perspective (B). Accompanying Video 5-9 corresponds to Figure 5-27.

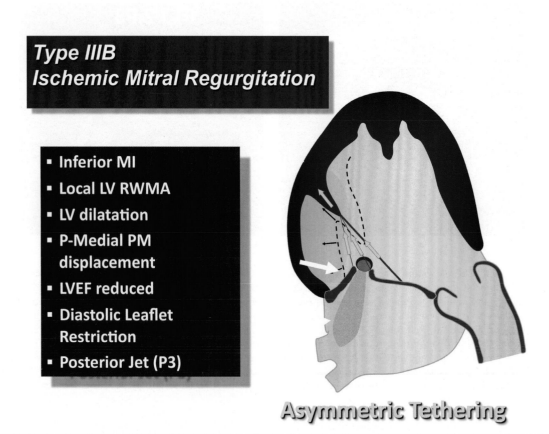

Figure 5-28. Type IIIB dysfunction—ischemic MR. In the Carpentier et al.[11] classification scheme, type IIIB dysfunction includes patients with leaflet restriction during diastole. A common cause of this type of dysfunction includes ischemic heart disease leading to lesions such as papillary muscle dysfunction or regional wall motion abnormalities in the left ventricle. A common scenario is a patient who suffers an inferior myocardial infarction with resultant posteromedial papillary muscle dysfunction and asymmetric tethering of the posterior leaflet. The anterolateral papillary muscle is less likely affected than the posteromedial papillary muscle in ischemic left ventricular dysfunction due to its dual coronary blood supply. The MR jet is typically directed posterior toward the dysfunctional papillary muscle. (Courtesy of Alain Berrebi, MD.)

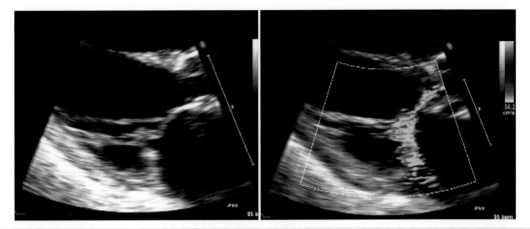

Figure 5-29. Asymmetric tethering of the posterior leaflet in type IIIB ischemic mitral regurgitation. In this 2D TTE image, there are several clues as to the etiology of this patient's MR. One clue is that the posteromedial papillary muscle is tethered and unable to coapt during systole likely due to ischemia of the right coronary artery. The right coronary artery is the only blood supply for this papillary muscle making it more vulnerable than the anterolateral papillary muscle. Another clue is that the resultant MR jet is eccentric and directed toward the restricted posterior mitral valve leaflet.

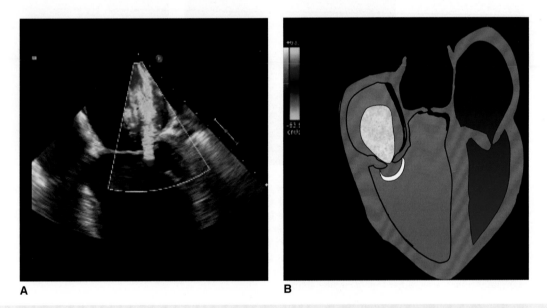

A   B

Figure 5-30. Quantification of MR. Determining the severity of MR by quantitative analysis is an important step in the management of mitral valve disease.[8] The flow convergence method is used most often, but 2D TEE typically requires many assumptions due to differences in orifice shape, size, and leaflet angle that lead to over- or underestimation of the degree of MR.[18] Volumetric imaging using RT3D TEE has been shown to overcome the limitations of 2D TTE providing better accuracy.[7] The 2D TEE image of the mitral valve demonstrates MR and the illustration (B) highlights one method of MR quantification—the proximal isovelocity surface area (PISA) technique.

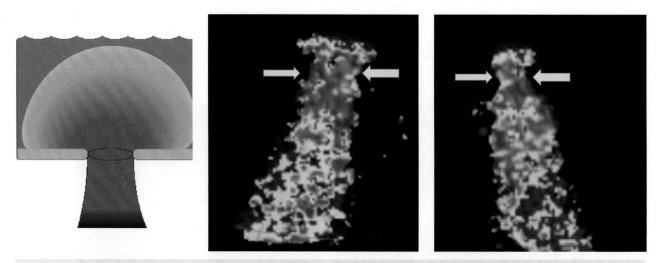

Figure 5-31. The use of RT3D TEE to better measure the degree of MR. With better visualization of the MR jet using RT3D TEE, a more suitable geometric model (hemielliptical rather than hemispheric) was applied for the measurement of MR using the PISA method.[19] In addition, the narrowest portion of the jet is easily visualized and measured in two orthogonal views demonstrating that the vena contracta area is more oval than circular. These corrections allow for more accurate measurements of the degree of MR and, therefore, better guide therapy. The illustration on the left depicts the classic way of using PISA by visualizing the proximal surface area as a hemisphere. The images in the middle and to the right reveal two orthogonal views of the vena contracta using RT3D TEE demonstrating the unequal radius. This results in a more accurate oval shape effective regurgitant orifice area rather than a circular shape.[8]

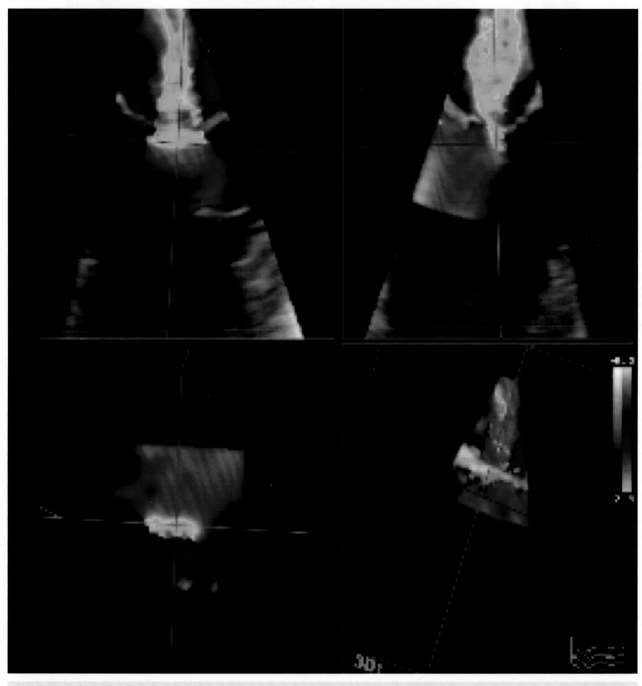

Figure 5-32. RT3D color flow imaging. Fully sampled matrix array probes are capable of performing 3D color flow imaging typically using ECG gating over seven cardiac cycles. This results in a volume dataset that accurately displays the necessary components for quantifying the MR jet.

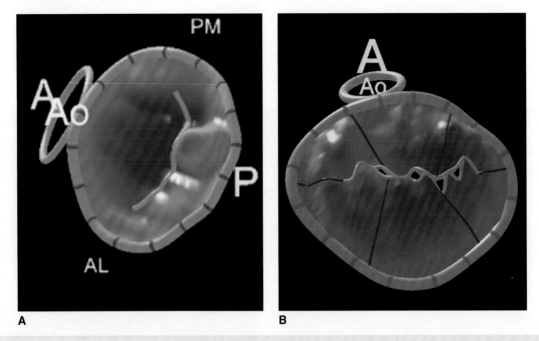

Figure 5-33. Volumetric quantification of the mitral valve: diagnosis from a single parametric image. Three-dimensional parametric maps transform the 3D images of the mitral valve into color-encoded topographic displays of mitral valve anatomy in which the color gradation indicates the distance of the leaflet from the mitral annular plane toward the left atrium.[20] In (A), note how the different color is isolated to P2 suggesting a unisegmental disease process such as fibroelastic deficiency. In (B), there are multiple areas of different colors suggesting a multisegmental disease process such as Barlow's disease. Ao, aorta; A, anterior; AL, anterolateral; PM, posteromedial; P, posterior.

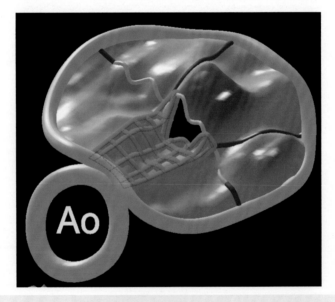

Figure 5-34. 3D rendering of mitral valve prolapse. In this figure, the *red area* indicates prolapse of the P2 scallop as well as some of the P1 scallop. The *green, hatched area* corresponds to the surface of P2. Note the disruption of the coaptation zone due to the prolapse. Ao, aorta. (Reused with permission from Lang RM, Tsang W, Weinert L, et al. Valvular heart disease: The value of 3-dimensional echocardiography. *J Am Coll Cardiol.* 2011;58(19):1933–1944.)

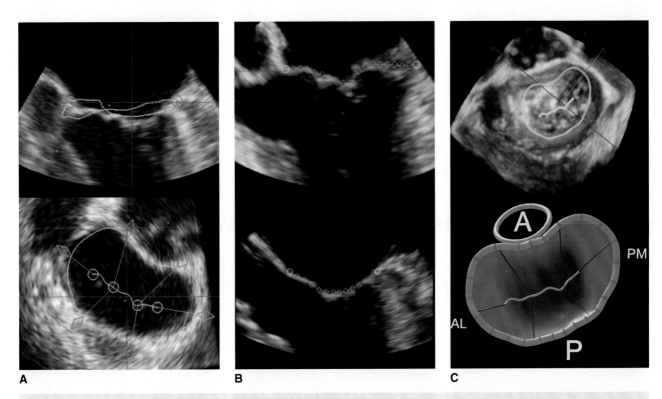

A   **B**   **C**

Figure 5-35. 3D morphologic analysis of a normal mitral valve. Volumetric analysis of the mitral valve using RT3D TEE allows for accurate measurements of the mitral valve apparatus and surrounding structures, which aid in surgical management.[10] The mitral annulus is manually drawn in one plane (A, top) and then repeated in multiple rotated planes and interpolated. The resultant 3D contour is superimposed on the en-face view of the valve to allow assessment of annular shape (A, bottom). The mitral valve leaflets are then manually traced from commissure to commissure in multiple parallel planes (B). The coaptation zone is then generated by these tracings and displayed on the original 3D image (C, top). The resultant surface area is displayed as a color-coded 3D rendered valve surface representing a topographical map of the mitral leaflets (C, bottom). Ao, aorta; A, anterior; AL, anterolateral; PM, posteromedial; P, posterior.

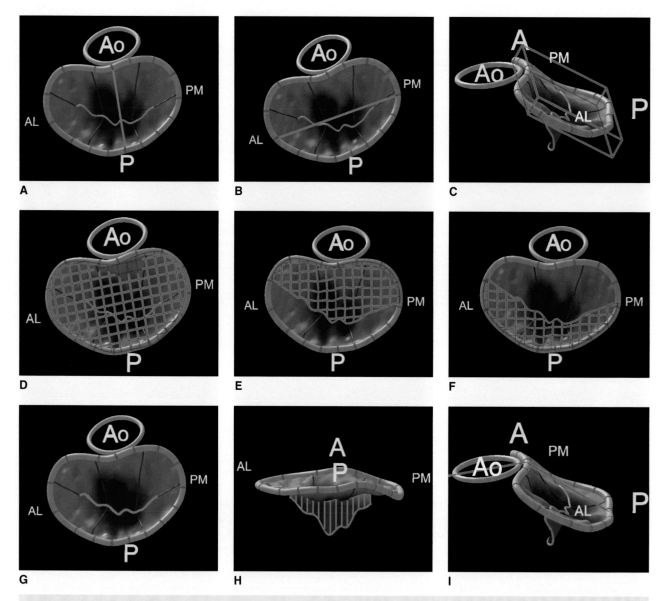

Figure 5-36. Quantitative analysis of the mitral valve apparatus using computer-generated 3D rendered surface area reconstruction. Quantifiable differences between degenerative diseases allow accurate classification of the etiology of mitral valve prolapse and determination of the anticipated complexity of repair. By using software designed to replicate the mitral valve surface area and its surrounding structures, the imager is able to calculate the anterior–posterior diameter (A), commissural diameter (B), and annular height (C). In addition, the aggregate surface area (D), the anterior leaflet surface area (E), the posterior leaflet surface area (F), the length of the coaptation line (G), the height of the coaptation line (H), and the angle between the mitral and aortic annular planes (I) can be quantified. Ao, aorta; AL, anterolateral; PM, posteromedial; P, posterior.

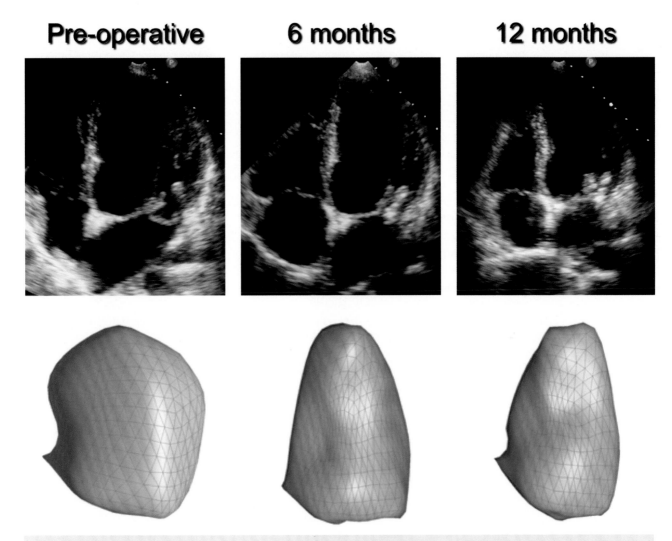

Pre-operative   6 months   12 months

Figure 5-37. Serial changes in left ventricular shape following mitral valve repair. RT3D TEE can also provide mechanistic insight into what happens anatomically to the left ventricle after mitral valve repair. In 50 patients with severe, asymptomatic mitral valve regurgitation who underwent mitral valve repair, RT3D TEE was performed the day before, as well as 6 and 12 months postsurgery.[21] The authors concluded that mitral valve repair significantly decreases left ventricular volume and alters the geometry from a spherical shape to a more conical, normal shape. This figure illustrates these changes showing the 2D TTE apical five-chamber views (top) and corresponding left ventricular endocardial surfaces (bottom) extracted from the RT3D TEE datasets in a patient who underwent mitral valve repair for severe, asymptomatic MR.

References

1. Yatteau RF, Peter RH, Behar VS, et al. Ischemic cardiomyopathy: the myopathy of coronary artery disease. Natural history and results of medical versus surgical treatment. *Am J Cardiol.* 1974;34:520–525.

2. Segal BL. Valvular heart disease, Part 2. Mitral valve disease in older adults. *Geriatrics.* 2003;58:26–31.

3. Adams DH, Anyanwu AC, Sugeng L, et al. Degenerative mitral valve regurgitation: surgical echocardiography. *Curr Cardiol Rep.* 2008;10:226–232.

4. Delahaye JP, Gare JP, Viguier E, et al. Natural history of severe mitral regurgitation. *Eur Heart J.* 1991; 12(suppl B):5–9.

5. Horton-Smith P. A clinical lecture on mitral regurgitation. *Clin J.* Creasy LE, ed. London: 1902:252–256.

6. Bonow RO, Carabello BA, Chatterjee K, et al. ACC/AHA 2006 Guidelines for the management of patients with valvular heart disease: a report of the American College of Cardiology/American Heart Association Task Force on Practice Guidelines. *Circulation.* 2006;114:e84–e231.

7. Lang RM, Tsang W, Weinert L, et al. Valvular heart disease. The value of 3-dimensional echocardiography. *J Am Coll Cardiol.* 2011;58:1933–1944.

8. O'Gara P, Sugeng L, Lang R, et al. The role of imaging in chronic degenerative mitral regurgitation. *JACC Cardiovasc Imaging.* 2008;1:221–237.

9. Freed BH, Sugeng L, Adams DH, et al. The role of echocardiography in the surgical management of degenerative mitral valve disease. In: Badano L, ed. *Textbook of real-time three dimensional echocardiography.* London, UK: Springer-Verlag; 2010:147–159.

10. Tsang W, Lang RM, Kronzon I. Role of real-time three dimensional echocardiography in cardiovascular interventions. *Heart.* 2011;97:850–857.

11. Carpentier A. Cardiac valve surgery—the "French correction." *J Thorac Cardiovasc Surg.* 1983;86:323–337.

12. Lang RM, Salgo IS, Anyanwu AC, et al. The road to mitral valve repair with live 3D transesophageal echocardiography. *Medicamundi.* 2008;52:37–42.

13. McCarthy KP, Ring L, Rana BS. Anatomy of the mitral valve: understanding the mitral valve complex in mitral regurgitation. *Eur J Echocardiogr.* 2010;11:i3–i9.

14. Sugeng L, Shernan SK, Salgo IS, et al. Live 3-dimensional transesophageal echocardiography: initial experience using the fully-sampled matrix array probe. *J Am Coll Cardiol.* 2008;52:446–449.

15. Anyanwu AC, Adams DH. Etiologic classification of degenerative mitral valve disease: Barlow's disease and fibroelastic deficiency. *Semin Thorac Cardiovasc Surg.* 2007;19:90–96.

16. Carpentier A, Adams DH, Filsoufi F. Pathophysiology, preoperative valve analysis, and surgical indications. In: Carpentier A, Adams DH, Filsoufi F, eds. *Reconstructive valve surgery: from valve analysis to valve reconstruction.* Maryland Heights, MO: Saunders-Elsevier; 2010:43–53.

17. Steer AC, Carapetis JR. Prevention and treatment of rheumatic heart disease in the developing world. *Nat Rev Cardiol.* 2009;6:689–698.

18. Bhave NM, Lang RM. Quantitative echocardiographic assessment of native mitral regurgitation: two- and three-dimensional techniques. *J Heart Valve Dis.* 2011;20:483–492.

19. Chandra S, Salgo IS, Sugeng L, et al. A three-dimensional insight into the complexity of flow convergence in mitral regurgitation: adjunctive benefit of anatomic regurgitant orifice area. *Am J Physiol Heart Circ Physiol.* 2011;301:H1015–H1024.

20. Tsang W, Weinert L, Sugeng L, et al. The value of three-dimensional echocardiography derived mitral valve parametric maps and the role of experience in the diagnosis of pathology. *J Am Soc Echocardiogr.* 2011;24:860–867.

21. Maffessanti F, Caiani EG, Tamborini G, et al. Serial changes in left ventricular shape following early mitral valve repair. *Am J Cardiol.* 2010;106:836–842.

THREE-DIMENSIONAL ECHOCARDIOGRAPHY FOR DEGENERATIVE MITRAL VALVE DISEASE

6

Stanton K. Shernan

Although the concept of three-dimensional (3D) echocardiography was first introduced in the early 1970s, its utility for defining mitral valve (MV) pathology has only recently acquired appropriate recognition.[1–6] Primary areas of interest have included the utility of 3D echocardiography in preoperative surgical planning, intraoperative assessment of the surgical procedure, and postoperative early and long-term follow-up to determine the need for further intervention.[7–8]

The Carpentier classification scheme describes mechanisms of mitral apparatus disease associated with mitral regurgitation (MR) according to three types of leaflet motion: Type I disorders refer primarily to normal mitral leaflet motion with MR due most commonly to a dilated annulus but also include perforations and clefts. Type III disorders are reserved for leaflets that exhibit restrictive motion either in both systole and diastole (type IIIA: rheumatic heart disease) or only during systole (type IIIB: acute/chronic ischemia, dilated cardiomyopathy; functional MR). Type II disease describes patients with excessive motion, which occurs occasionally with either endocarditis or ruptured papillary muscles, but more commonly in patients with degenerative mitral valve disease (DMVD). DMVD is the most frequent cause of MR in the United States, occurring in 4% to 5% of the population.[9,10] While only 10% to 15% of patients with MV prolapse develop progressive MR, an even smaller percentage actually requires surgery.[9–12]

Several etiologies of classic DMVD have been described including Marfan's disease, myxomatous degeneration (Barlow's), and fibroelastic deficiency (FED). The echocardiographic hallmark of all of these disorders is the presence of excessive leaflet motion due to prolapse or a flail leaflet(s), hence the reference to the "floppy mitral valve." The diagnosis of a flail leaflet is usually not difficult, due to the predictable appearance of ruptured chords and a regurgitant jet that is directed away from the involved leaflet segment (Figs. 6-1 through 6-4). However, the definition of prolapse has received more attention. Ideally, prolapse refers to systolic billowing or atrialization of at least part of a mitral leaflet above the annulus and is often associated with leaflet thickening[13,14] (Fig. 6-5). A more specific criterion for diagnosis of prolapse may be to include free-edge or marginal prolapse of any leaflet segment seen in any cross section, because clinically relevant prolapse generally involves elongation and/or rupture of primary chords. Some of the controversy regarding the diagnosis of mitral prolapse has focused on differences in appearance of the mitral apparatus due to the saddle shape of the normal annulus, with its higher points in the anteroposterior plane. Thus, the leaflets may appear to "prolapse" in the midcommissural view (lateral–medial diameter) or even four-chamber view compared to the midesophageal five-chamber or long-axis view (anteroposterior diameter)[13–17] (Fig. 6-6). Consequently, a more specific definition of abnormal prolapse refers to billowing at base of the leaflet when it exceeds 2 mm above the annular plane in a long-axis view (≈130 degrees in midesophageal plane by transesophageal echocardiographic [TEE]) and 5 mm in four-chamber view (0 degree midesophageal plane). In addition, tethering of one leaflet may produce the appearance of prolapse ("pseudoprolapse") in the other leaflet even when there is no actual elevation above the annulus[18] (Figs. 6-7 and 6-8). Similar to an isolated flail leaflet, single leaflet prolapse may also be associated with an eccentric jet directed away from the affected leaflet segment (Fig. 6-9). Alternatively, bileaflet prolapse may be associated with more of a single central jet if there is equal insufficiency and prolapse from both leaflets or two jets having opposite trajectories when the location of prolapse occurs at different positions along the line of coaptation[19] (Fig. 6-10).

The two main etiologies of DMVD are Barlow's disease and FED.[20] While echocardiography cannot be used to determine histology, there are additional ultrasonographic characteristics that tend to distinguish different etiologies of DMVD. In addition, while the echocardiographic hallmark of these disorders is excessive leaflet motion (i.e., type II), there may be multiple concurrent mechanisms for the observed MR including annular dilatation[21,22] (Fig. 6-11).

Barlow's disease results in myxoid degeneration of the MV, which is associated with infiltration of acid mucopolysaccharide material and architectural disorganization of elastin and collagen, creating excess tissue in multiple valve segments, chordal thickening and elongation, annular dilation, and a vulnerability to annular calcification (Fig. 6-12). Leaflet malcoaptation at the commissures and functional indentations or even clefts commonly occur concurrently in MVs affected by myxomatous degeneration and may be difficult to diagnose with conventional two-dimensional (2D) echocardiography yet are often easily visualized with standard 3D echocardiographic views (Fig. 6-13). Chordal rupture is less common than in FED.

In contrast, FED results from loss of mechanical integrity due to abnormalities of connective tissue structure and/or function, leading to chordal thinning, elongation, and/or rupture, with classic findings of prolapse and MR of varying severity. The prolapsing segment, often the middle segment of the posterior leaflet, may be thickened and distended, while the remaining segments of the valve may be normal or translucent and even abnormally thin (Figs. 6-14 through 6-17). Thus, while DMVD can often be distinguished from the normal leaflet by significant differences in leaflet billowing height, Barlow's valve generally has greater billowing volume than the FED valve due to more extensive involvement[23] (Figs. 6-18 and 6-19).

The noninvasive assessment of DMVD may have important implications for triaging patients and perioperative planning. While the FED valve may require a more straightforward repair with either resection of the involved leaflet or a chordal procedure, the Barlow's valve usually requires a more extensive procedure to restore the optimal functional geometry of the mitral apparatus. Increasing degrees of complexity are easily defined by 3D echocardiography and should prompt preferential referral of a patient, in whom a MV repair is warranted, to a specialized MV surgery center of excellence.[24] (Figs. 6-20 through 6-25). Thus, a comprehensive appreciation for normal MV shape and motion, as well the changes associated with pathology of the MV apparatus, has important implications for patients with DMVD undergoing MV repair. The details of the surgical procedure including selection of partial ring versus rigid or flexible band (Fig. 6-26) and a "resect versus respect" must be appreciated in order to anticipate rare yet still prevalent acute iatrogenic complications including persistent insufficiency, stenosis, or systolic anterior motion (SAM) of the subvalvular apparatus (Fig. 6-27 and 6-28). In addition, the efforts made toward reestablishing normal annular geometry and the consequential redistribution of stress to components of the MV apparatus may have important implications on longer-term durability of the repair especially considering that progression of the initial etiologies that may continue postoperatively[25–29] (Figs. 6-29 and 6-30).

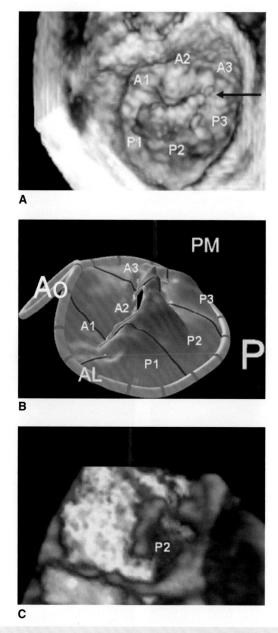

Figure 6-1. Flail posterior leaflet of the mitral valve (MV). A. Three-dimensional transesophageal echocardiographic (3D TEE) en-face image from the left atrial (LA) perspective, demonstrating a flail middle segment (P2) of the posterior leaflet of the MV with ruptured chords (*blue arrow*). B. Parametric image (Q-labs; Philips Healthcare, Inc.) of the MV demonstrating a flail middle segment (P2) of the posterior leaflet with ruptured chords (*blue arrow*). C. Three-dimensional TEE image showing eccentric color flow Doppler jet of mitral regurgitation associated with a flail middle segment (P2) of the posterior leaflet of the MV (*blue arrow*). A1, anterolateral segment; A2, middle segment of the anterior leaflet; A3, anteromedial segment; P1, posterolateral segment; P3, posteromedial segment; AL, anterolateral commissure; PM, posteromedial commissure; Ao, aortic valve; P, posterior. See Videos 6.1A and 6.1B.

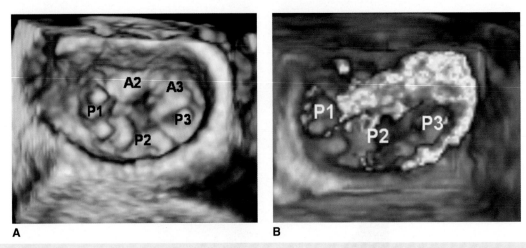

A   B

Figure 6-2. Flail posterior leaflet of the mitral valve (MV). A: Three-dimensional TEE image of flail posterior leaflet lateral scallop (P1) associated with ruptured chordae. B. Accompanying color flow Doppler image demonstrating a regurgitant jet directed along the anterior leaflet and annulus before swirling back around the posteromedial commissure. A2, middle segment of the anterior leaflet; A3, anteromedial segment; P2, middle segment of the posterior leaflet; P3, posteromedial segment. See Videos 6.2A and 6.2B.

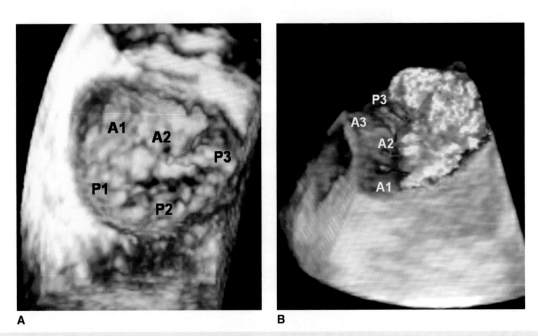

A   B

Figure 6-3. Flail posterior leaflet of the mitral valve (MV). A. Three-dimensional TEE image of a posteromedial (P3) flail of the MV associated with ruptured chordae. B. Accompanying color flow Doppler image demonstrating an eccentric regurgitant jet. A1, anterolateral segment; A2, middle segment of the anterior leaflet; A3, anteromedial segment; P1, posterolateral segment; P2, middle segment of the posterior leaflet. See Videos 6.3A and 6.3B.

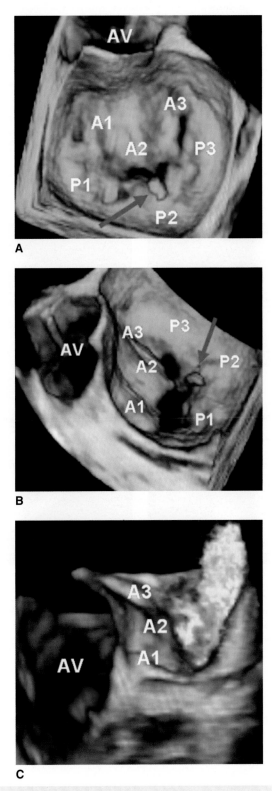

Figure 6-4. Flail anterior leaflet of the mitral valve (MV). A,B. Three-dimensional TEE images of a flail middle segment of the anterior leaflet (A2) with associated ruptured chords (*red arrows*). C. Accompanying color flow Doppler showing an eccentric regurgitant jet cascading over the posterior leaflet. The patient received a MV replacement. A1, anterolateral segment; A3, anteromedial segment; P1, posterolateral segment; P2, middle segment of the posterior leaflet; P3, posteromedial segment; AV, aortic valve. See Videos 6.4A and 6.4B.

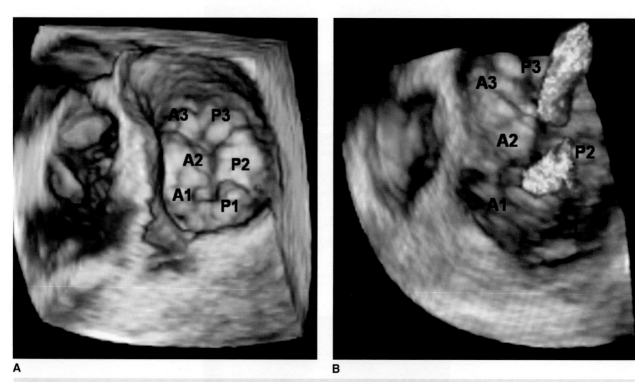

A   **B**

Figure 6-5. **Myxomatous degeneration of the mitral valve (MV). A.** Three-dimensional TEE image demonstrating prolapsing of multiple segments of the posterior and anterior leaflets. **B.** Color flow Doppler demonstrating significant two jets of mitral regurgitation. A1, anterolateral segment; A2, middle segment of the anterior leaflet; A3, anteromedial segment; P1, posterolateral segment; P2, middle segment of the posterior leaflet; P3, posteromedial segment. See Videos 6.5A and 6.5B.

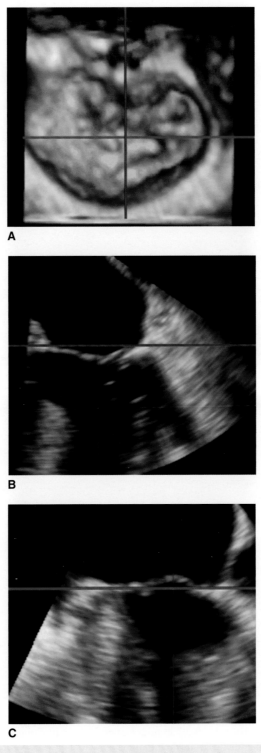

Figure 6-6. Mitral valve prolapse. Prolapse refers to systolic billowing or atrialization of at least part of a mitral valve (MV) leaflet above the annulus and is often associated with leaflet thickening. Some controversy regarding the diagnosis of mitral prolapse has focused on differences in appearance of the mitral apparatus due to the saddle shape of the normal annulus, with its higher points in the anteroposterior plane. A. Three-dimensional TEE en-face view of a normal MV from the LA perspective. B. The leaflets do not appear to prolapse in the midesophageal five-chamber 2D view (anteroposterior diameter). C. However, the leaflets may appear to "prolapse" in the midcommissural 2D TEE view (lateral–medial diameter). See Videos 6.6A through 6.6C.

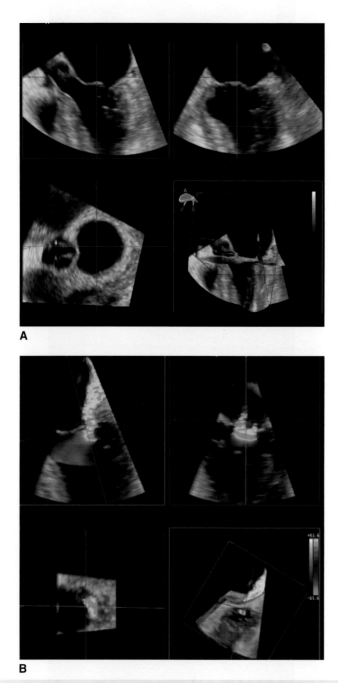

A

B

Figure 6-7. Pseudoprolapse of the mitral valve (MV) anterior leaflet. Tethering of one leaflet may produce the appearance of prolapse (pseudoprolapse) in the other leaflet even when there is no actual elevation above the annulus. A. Two-dimensional TEE image showing pseudoprolapse of the anterior leaflet relative to a restricted posterior leaflet. B. Accompanying 2D TEE color flow Doppler image showing that similar to an isolated flail leaflet, single leaflet pseudoprolapse of the overriding anterior leaflet may also be associated with an eccentric jet directed away from the affected leaflet segment. See Videos 6-7A and 6-7B.

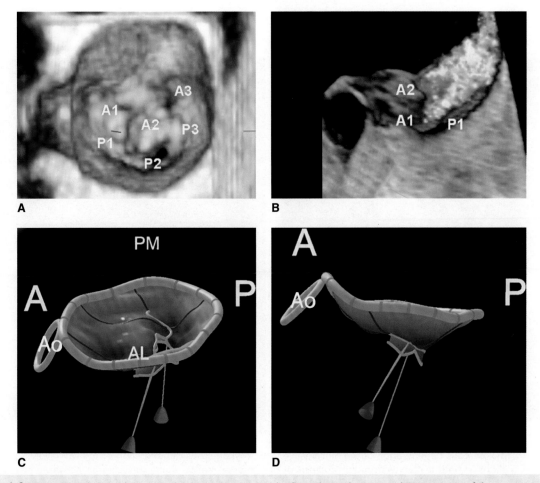

Figure 6-8. **Pseudoprolapse of the mitral valve (MV) anterior leaflet.** Three-dimensional TEE images of the same MV shown in Figure 6-7 with pseudoprolapse of the anterior leaflet. A. Three-dimensional TEE en-face view of the MV demonstrating an overriding, pseudoprolapsing anterior leaflet relative to a restricted posterior leaflet. B. Three-dimensional TEE color flow Doppler view showing the eccentric jet of MR. C,D. Parametric images (Q-labs, Philips Healthcare, Inc.) of the same valve. A1, anterolateral segment; A2, middle segment of the anterior leaflet; A3, anteromedial segment; P1, posterolateral segment; P2, middle segment of the posterior leaflet; P3, posteromedial segment; Ao, aortic valve; AL, anterolateral commissure; PM, posteromedial commissure; A, anterior; P, posterior. See Videos 6-8A and 6-8B.

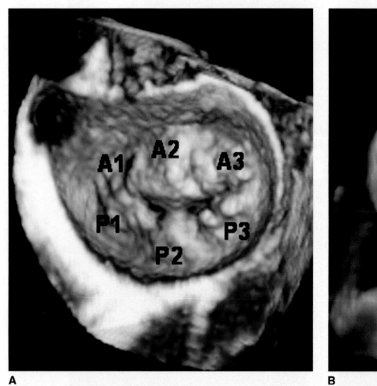

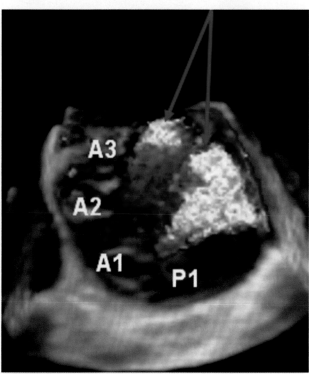

A

B

Figure 6-9. Myxomatous degeneration of the mitral valve (MV). Myxomatous degeneration of the MV involving prolapse of multiple scallops in both leaflets with more prolapse of the anterior leaflet, thus producing an eccentric jets of mitral regurgitation. A. An en-face 3D TEE image of the MV demonstrates relatively more prolapse of the anterior leaflet compared to the posterior leaflet. B. Accompanying color flow Doppler image demonstrating eccentric regurgitant jets (*arrows*). A1, anterolateral segment; A2, middle segment of the anterior leaflet; A3, anteromedial segment; P1, posterolateral segment; P2, middle segment of the posterior leaflet; P3, posteromedial segment. See Videos 6-9A and 6-9B.

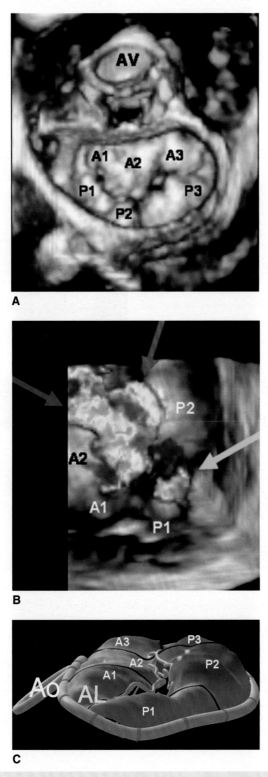

Figure 6-10. **Myxomatous degeneration of the MV. A.** Three-dimensional TEE image of a MV with myxomatous degeneration showing prolapse primarily of the middle (A2) and medial (A3) anterior leaflet segments, as well as the middle (P2) segment of the posterior leaflet. **B.** Color flow Doppler images show separate regurgitant jets associated with each prolapsing leaflet ("cross swords" pattern of anterior leaflet prolapse—*blue arrow* and posterior leaflet prolapse—*red arrow*) as well as a jet associated with a functional, deep indentation or cleft between P2 and the lateral scallop (P1) of the posterior leaflet (*yellow arrow*). **C.** Parametric image (Q-labs; Philips Healthcare, Inc.) of the same valve. A1, anterolateral segment; P3, posteromedial segment; Ao, aortic valve; AL, anterolateral commissure. See Videos 6-10A and 6-10B.

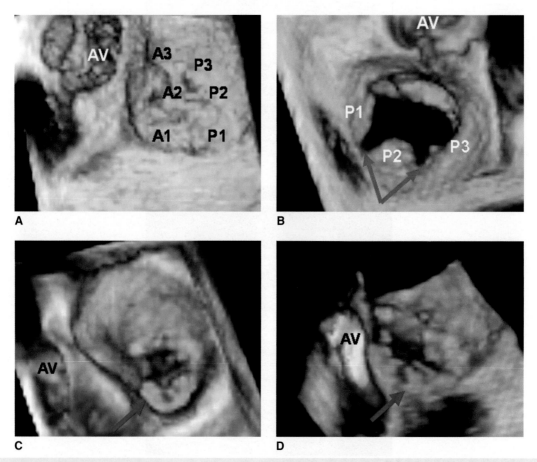

Figure 6-11. **Myxomatous degeneration of the mitral valve (MV).** Myxomatous degeneration of the MV in addition to posterior leaflet indentations and annular dilatation. A. Three-dimensional TEE image demonstrating diffuse yet mild prolapse of multiple MV scallops in both leaflet along with annular dilatation. B. Indentations or clefts (*red arrows*) are also shown in both the lateral and medial side of the middle scallop of the posterior leaflet (P2). C. Postrepair 3D TEE images showing a ring annuloplasty (*blue arrows*) and (D) the absence of significant MR. A1, anterolateral segment; A2, middle segment of the anterior leaflet; A3, anteromedial segment; P1, posterolateral segment; P2, middle segment of the posterior leaflet; P3, posteromedial segment; AV, aortic valve. See Videos 6-11A and 6-11B. C. Postrepair 3D TEE images showing a ring annuloplasty (*blue arrows*) and (D) the absence of significant MR. A1, anterolateral segment; A2, middle segment of the anterior leaflet; A3, anteromedial segment; P1, posterolateral segment; P2, middle segment of the posterior leaflet; P3, posteromedial segment; AV, aortic valve. See Videos 6-11A and 6-11B.

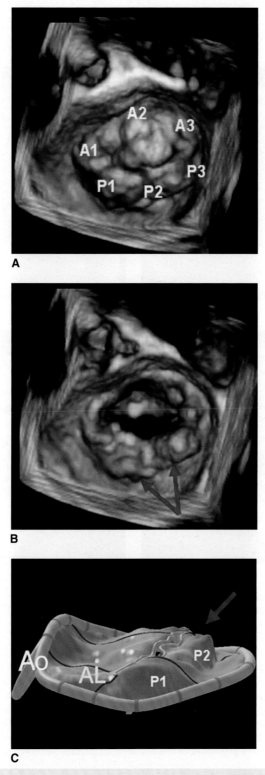

Figure 6-12. Myxomatous degeneration of the mitral valve (MV). A. Three-dimensional TEE en-face view of a MV showing diffuse prolapse of multiple leaflet segments during systole. B. In the same valve, the posterior leaflet remains in a fixed "prolapsed" state (*blue arrows*) even during diastole consistent with mitral annular calcification extending into the body of the leaflet. C. Parametric image (Q-labs; Philips Healthcare, Inc.) of the same valve. A1, anterolateral segment; A2, middle segment of the anterior leaflet; A3, anteromedial segment; P1, posterolateral segment; P2, middle segment of the posterior leaflet; P3, posteromedial segment; AL, anterolateral commissure. See Videos 6-12A and 6-12B.

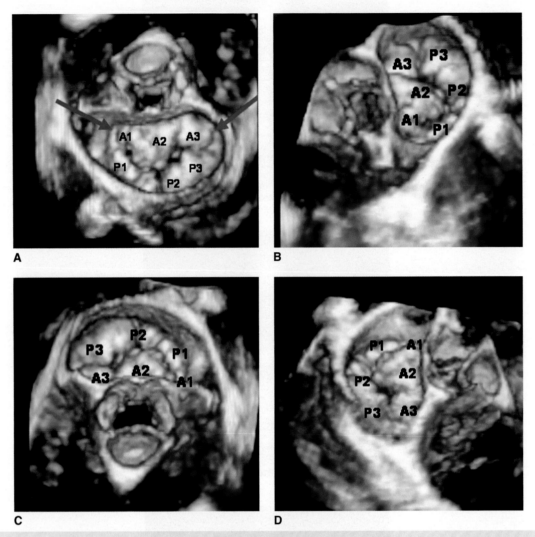

Figure 6-13. Orientation of 3DE images of the mitral valve (MV). The orientation of 3D echocardiographic image of the MV can facilitate the visualization and identification of prolapsing scallops. A. This 3D TEE en-face view of the MV from the left atrial (LA) perspective displays the anterior leaflet on the top of the image below the aortic valve (AV) and the posterior leaflet beneath, with the anterolateral commissure (ALC) on the left side of the image (*blue arrow*) and the posteromedial commissure (PMC) on the right side of the image (*red arrow*). The lateral segments (A1,P1), middle segments (A2,P2), and medial segments (A3,P3) are oriented from the left side to the right side of the image. In this image orientation, the direction of prolapsing is toward the viewer. This view is also known as the "cardiac surgeon's view" as it displays the MV leaflets in the same orientation as seen intraoperatively by the cardiac surgeon upon its exposure through a LA incision. Beginning with the LA en-face view, consecutive counterclockwise rotations, and alignment of the MV annulus parallel to the viewing plane, may facilitate visualization of prolapsing scallops since the direction of prolapsing toward the LA is now toward the top of the image, while diastolic movement is downward toward the left ventricle (LV). B. A 90-degree counterclockwise rotation of the image from the LA en-face view and alignment of the MV annulus parallel to the viewing plane displays the ALC, A1, and P1 in the near field. C. Further counterclockwise rotation by 90 degree displays the anterior leaflet in the near field below the posterior leaflet. D. A final counterclockwise rotation by 90 degrees displays the PMC, A3, and P3 in the near field. See Videos 6-10A and 6-10B.

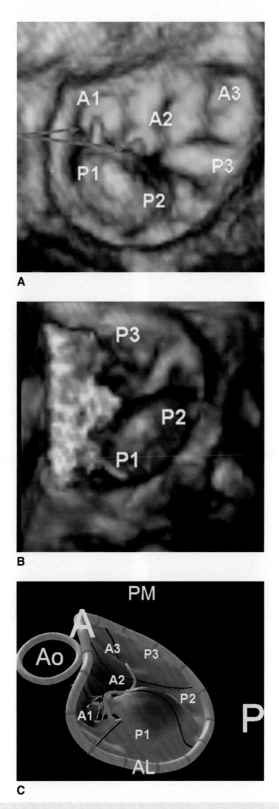

Figure 6-14. Fibroelastic deficiency (FED) of the mitral valve. FED results from loss of mechanical integrity due to abnormalities of connective tissue structure and/or function, leading to chordal thinning, elongation, and/or rupture, with classic findings of prolapse and MR of varying severity. The prolapsing segment, often the middle segment of the posterior leaflet (P2), may be thickened and distended, while the remaining segments of the valve may be normal or translucent and even abnormally thin. A. Three-dimensional TEE image of a P2 flail of the MV with ruptured chords (*red arrows*). B. Color flow Doppler image demonstrating an eccentric regurgitant jet cascading over the anterior leaflet. C. Parametric image (Q-labs; Philips Healthcare, Inc.). A1, anterolateral segment; A2, middle segment of the anterior leaflet; A3, anteromedial segment; P1, posterolateral segment; P2, middle segment of the posterior leaflet; P3, posteromedial segment; AL, anterolateral commissure. PM, posteromedial commissure; Ao, aortic valve; A, anterior; P, posterior. See Videos 6-14A and 6-14B.

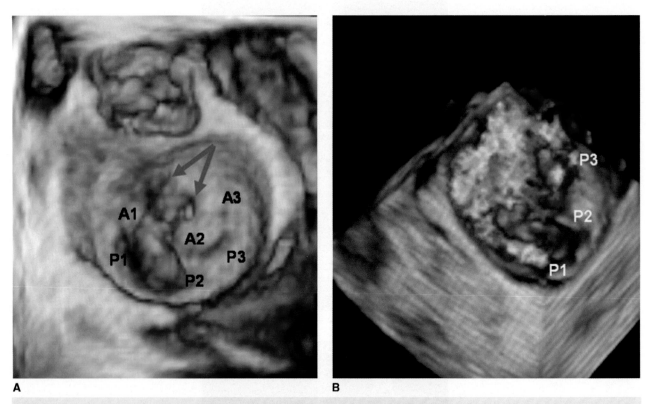

A

B

Figure 6-15. Fibroelastic deficiency of the mitral valve. A. Three-dimensional TEE image demonstrating flail posterior leaflet middle (P2) segment associated with ruptured chordae (*blue arrows*). B. Accompanying color flow Doppler image demonstrating a regurgitant jet cascading over the anterior leaflet. A1, anterolateral segment; A2, middle segment of the anterior leaflet; A3, anteromedial segment; P1, posterolateral segment; P3, posteromedial segment. See Videos 6-15A and 6-15B.

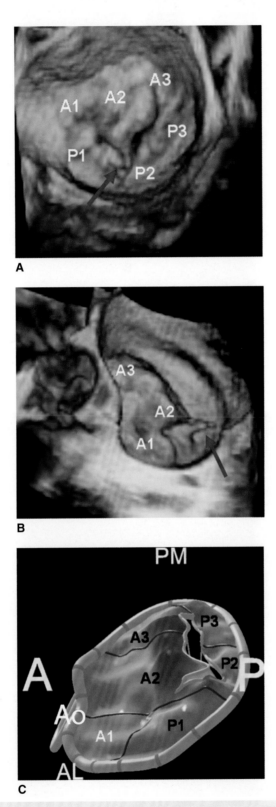

Figure 6-16. Flail anterior leaflet of the mitral valve. A,B. Three-dimensional TEE images of a flail middle scallop of the anterior leaflet (A2) with associated ruptured chords (*arrows*). C. Parametric image of the same valve showing the A2 flail. A1, antero-lateral segment; A3, anteromedial segment; P1, posterolateral segment; P2, middle segment of the posterior leaflet; P3, pos-teromedial segment. A, anterior; P, posterior; AL, anterolateral commissure; PM, posteromedial commissure. See Video 6-16.

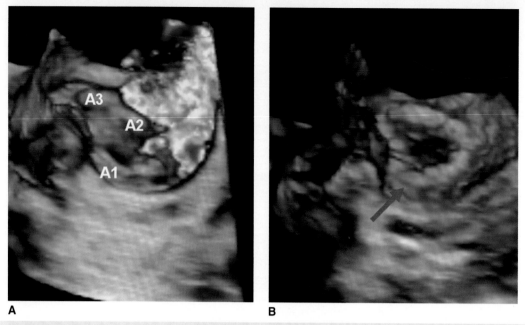

A   B

Figure 6-17. Flail anterior leaflet of the mitral valve (MV). A. Color flow Doppler of the same MV shown in Figure 6-16, showing an eccentric regurgitant jet cascading over the posterior leaflet. B. Post repair color flow Doppler image demonstrating a resection of the flail segment along with an annuloplasty band (*arrows*) and an edge-to-edge repair. A1, anterolateral segment; A2, middle segment of the anterior leaflet; A3, anteromedial segment. See Videos 6-17A and 6-17B.

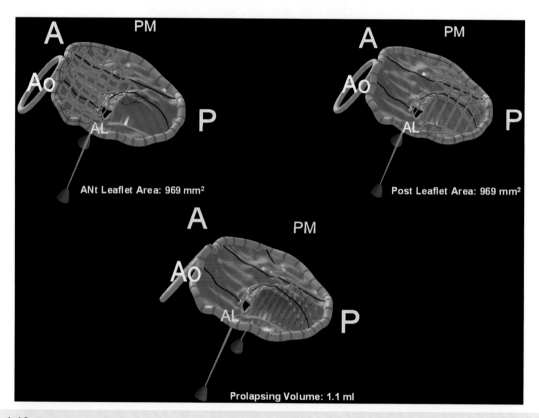

Figure 6-18. Parametric images of the mitral valve. Parametric images of a MV showing the leaflet area and prolapsing volume in a patient with fibroelastic deficiency and an isolated flail of the posterolateral and medial flail segments. Anterior and posterior leaflet areas as well as prolapsing volume are considerable smaller than similar values in patients with myxomatous degeneration as shown in Figure 6-19. AL, anterolateral commissure; PM, posteromedial commissure; A, anterior; P, posterior; Ao, aortic valve. See Videos 6-15A and 6-15B.

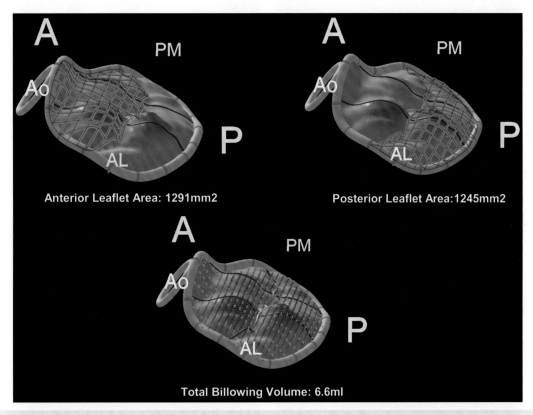

Figure 6-19. Parametric images of the mitral valve. Parametric images of a MV showing the leaflet area and prolapsing volume in a patient with myxomatous degeneration and prolapse of multiple leaflet segments. Anterior and posterior leaflet areas as well as prolapsing volume are considerable larger than similar values in patients with fibroelastic deficiency as shown in Figure 6-18. AL, anterolateral commissure; PM, posteromedial commissure; A, anterior; P, posterior; Ao, aortic valve. See Videos 6-20A through 6-20C.

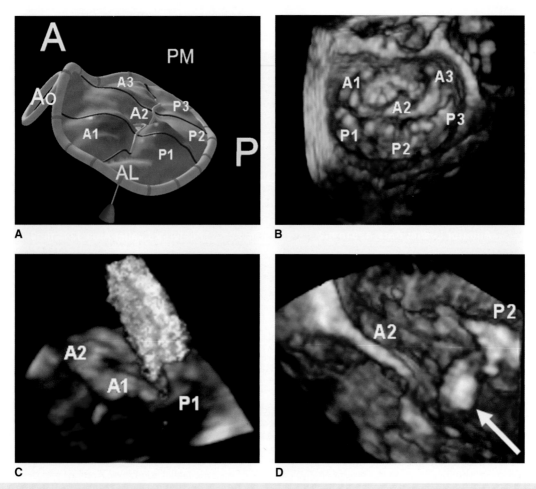

Figure 6-20. Myxomatous degeneration of the mitral valve (MV). A,B. Parametric image and 3D TEE en-face image of a MV demonstrating prolapsing of the posterolateral (P1) and middle (P2) scallops along with anterolateral (A1) prolapse. C. Color flow Doppler demonstrating significant MR. D. A MV repair involving a P1 and P2 foldoplasty (*arrow*) was performed along with a ring annuloplasty. A2, middle segment of the anterior leaflet; A3: anteromedial segment; P3, posteromedial segment; AL, antero-lateral commissure; PM, posteromedial commissure; A, anterior; P, posterior; Ao, aortic valve. See Videos 6-20A through 6-20C.

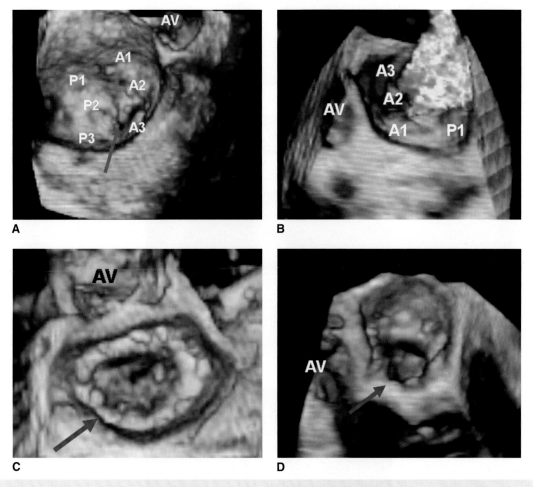

Figure 6-21. Flail anterior leaflet of the mitral valve. A. Three-dimensional TEE image of a flail middle scallop of the anterior leaflet (A2) with associated ruptured chords (*red arrow*) and annular dilatation. B. Accompanying color flow Doppler showing an eccentric regurgitant jet cascading over the posterior leaflet. C. The MV was repaired with neochords to the anterior leaflet and a full annuloplasty ring (*blue arrows*). D. Postrepair color flow Doppler image showing no residual mitral regurgitation. A1, anterolateral segment; A3, anteromedial segment; P1, posterolateral segment; P2, middle segment of the posterior leaflet; P3, posteromedial segment; AV, aortic valve. See Videos 6-21A through 6-21D.

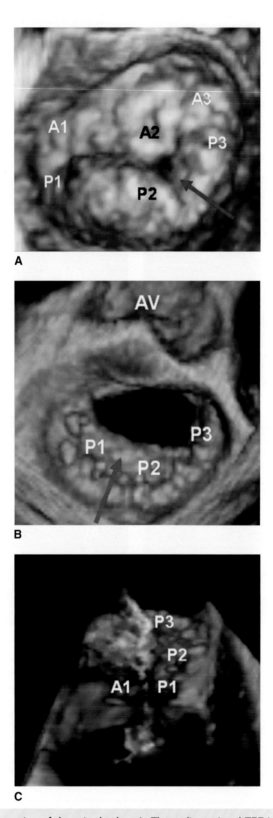

Figure 6-22. Myxomatous degeneration of the mitral valve. A. Three-dimensional TEE image demonstrating prolapsing of the middle (P2) scallop with a deep indentation (*blue arrow*) as well as prolapsing of the posterolateral scallop (P1). B. MV repair involving a P1 and P2 foldoplasty (*red arrow*) and P2 cleft repair along with a ring annuloplasty was performed. C. Following the repair, color flow Doppler demonstrated only trace residual mitral regurgitation. A1. anterolateral segment; A2, middle segment of the anterior leaflet; A3, anteromedial segment; P3, posteromedial segment. See Videos 6-22A through 6-22C.

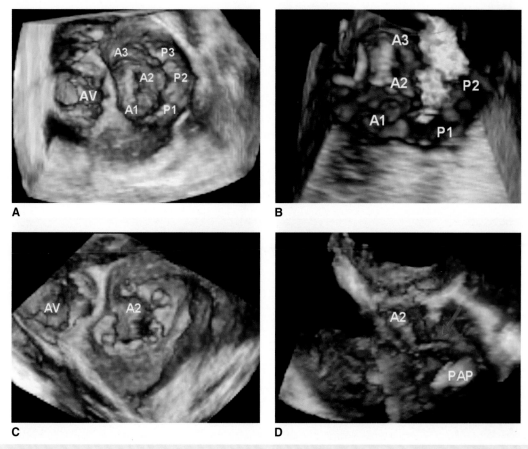

Figure 6-23. Myxomatous degeneration of the mitral valve. A. Three-dimensional TEE image demonstrating prolapsing of a very elongated and redundant middle scallop of the anterior leaflet (A2) and prolapse of the lateral scallop (P1) of the MV posterior leaflet. B. Color flow Doppler demonstrating significant mitral regurgitation. C,D. A MV repair involving placement of multiple neochords to A1 and A2 (*red arrow*) and a P1 foldoplasty, and an annuloplasty band was performed. A1, antero-lateral segment; A3, anteromedial segment; P2, middle segment of the posterior leaflet; P3, posteromedial segment; PAP, papillary muscle. See Videos 6-23A through 6-23D.

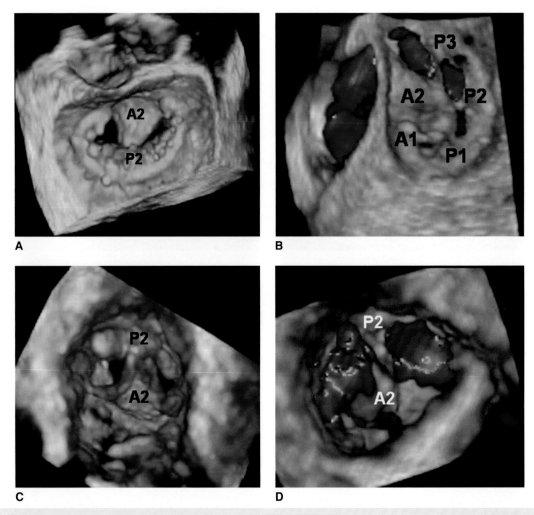

Figure 6-24. Mitral valve repair in a patient with myxomatous degeneration of the mitral valve (MV). A. Three-dimensional TEE en-face view of the MV following a repair involving a posterolateral (P1) and middle segment of the posterior leaflet (P2) resection, along with a ring annuloplasty and an edge-to-edge repair between the lateral side of the middle scallops, A2 and P2. B. Following the repair, color flow Doppler demonstrated only trace residual mitral regurgitation. C. Three-dimensional TEE view of the postrepair MV from the left ventricular perspective showing the edge-to-edge repair between the lateral side of the middle scallops, A2 and P2. D. Color flow Doppler 3D TEE view of the postrepair MV from the left ventricular perspective showing the edge-to-edge repair between the lateral side of the middle scallops, A2 and P2. A1, anterolateral segment; A3, anteromedial segment; P1, posterolateral segment; P3, posteromedial segment. See Videos 6-5A, 6-5B, 6-24A through 6-24D.

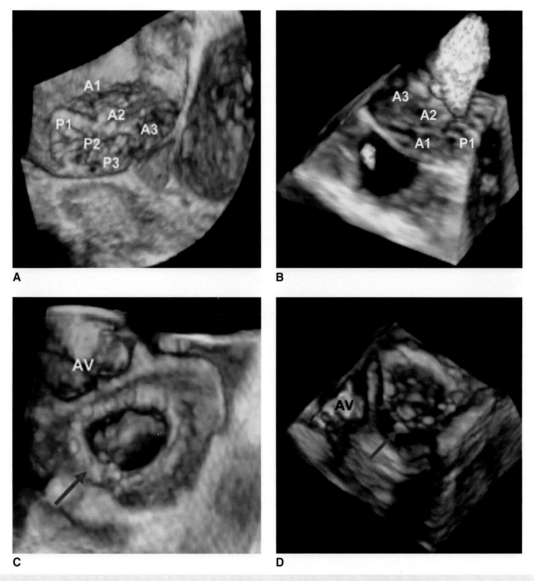

Figure 6-25. Myxomatous degeneration of the mitral valve. A. Three-dimensional TEE image demonstrating prolapsing of the middle scallop of the anterior leaflet (A2) and a dilated annulus of the MV. B. Color flow Doppler demonstrating significant mitral regurgitation. C. A MV repair involving an annuloplasty band (*blue arrows*) was performed. D. Following the repair, color flow Doppler demonstrated only trace residual mitral regurgitation. A1, anterolateral segment; A3, anteromedial segment; P1, posterolateral segment; P2, middle segment of the posterior leaflet; P3, posteromedial segment; AV, aortic valve. See Videos 6-25A through 6-25D.

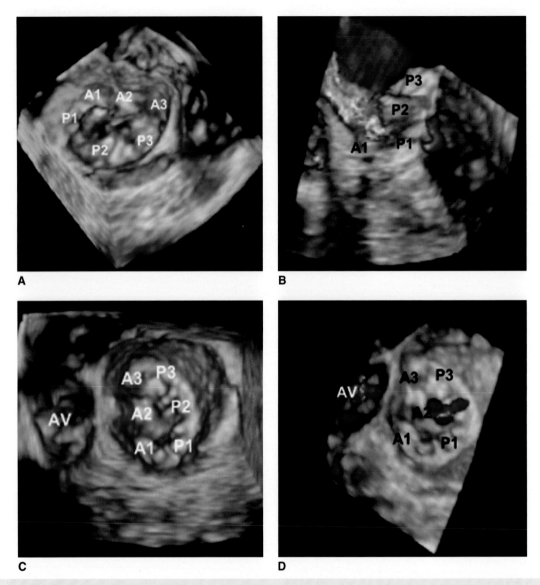

Figure 6-26. Myxomatous degeneration of the mitral valve (MV). A. Flail middle scallop (P2) with ruptured chords and pro-lapsed lateral scallop (P1) of the posterior leaflet of the MV. B. Color flow Doppler demonstrating regurgitant jet. C. MV repair included a resection of P2 and a P1 foldoplasty. D. Color flow Doppler demonstrated only trace mitral regurgitation. AV, aortic valve; A1, anterolateral segment; A2, middle segment of the anterior leaflet; A3, anteromedial segment; P3, posteromedial segment; AV, aortic valve. See Videos 6-26A through 6-26D.

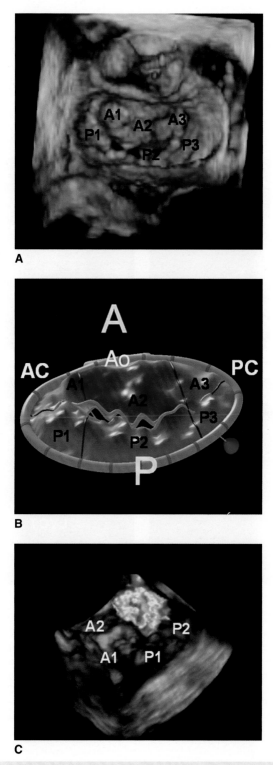

Figure 6-27. Myxomatous degeneration of the mitral valve. A,B. Three-dimensional TEE image and accompanying parametric image showing myxomatous degeneration of the lateral side of the MV, with greater prolapse in the lateral segments (A1 and P1) compared to the middle segments (A2 and P2), and relatively little involvement of the medial segments (A3 and P3). Elongation and excessive redundancy of the lateral scallops of the anterior and posterior leaflets (A1 and P1) may be a risk factor for systolic anterior motion (SAM) and left ventricular outflow tract obstruction (LVOTO) following MV repair. C. Accompanying color flow Doppler image demonstrating an eccentric regurgitant jets. AC, anterolateral commissure; PC,posteromedial commissure; A, anterior; P, posterior. See Videos 6-27A and 6-27B.

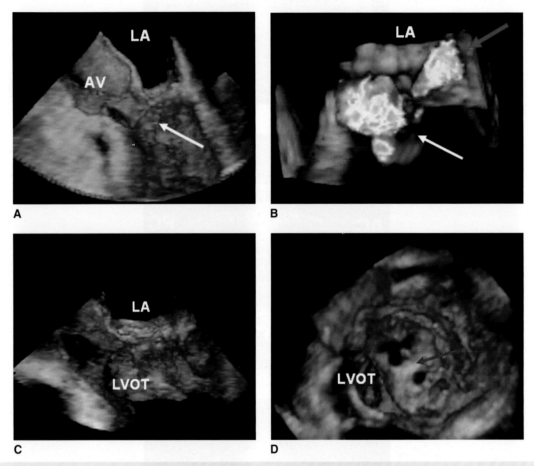

Figure 6-28. Mitral valve repair of myxomatous degeneration of the mitral valve (MV). Mitral valve repair in the same patient shown in Figure 6-27, with asymmetric myxomatous degeneration of the MV. A. In this case, despite a P2 resection and annuloplasty ring, refractory systolic anterior motion (SAM) of the MV subvalvular apparatus (*white arrows*) along with left ventricular outflow tract obstruction (LVOTO) developed after weaning from cardiopulmonary bypass. B. Color flow Doppler demonstrating the mitral regurgitant jet (*red arrow*) during SAM and LVOTO. C. Cardiopulmonary bypass was reestablished, and edge-to-edge repair (i.e., "Alfieri stitch") was performed on the lateral side of A2 and P2, thus eliminating the SAM and LVOTO. D. Three-dimensional TEE view from the left ventricular perspective showing edge-to-edge suture (*blue arrow*) between the anterior and posterior leaflet. LA, left atrium. See Videos 6-28A through 6-28C.

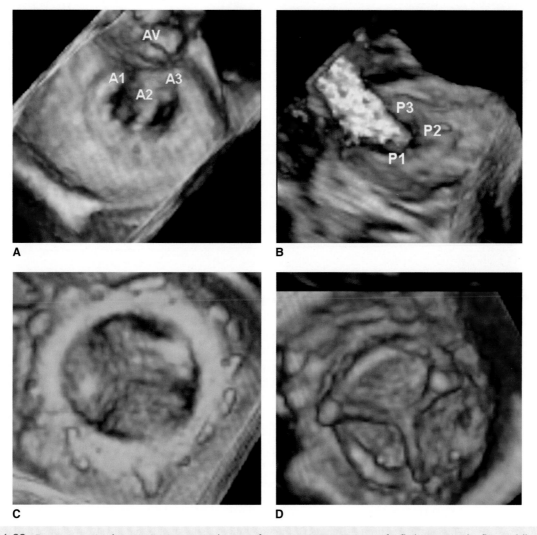

Figure 6-29. Recurrent mitral regurgitation several years after a previous resection of a flail posterior leaflet middle scallop (P2) and annuloplasty band mitral valve (MV) repair. A. Three-dimensional TEE en-face image from the left atrial perspective showing significant retraction of the posterior leaflet and limited coaptation with the anterior leaflet. B. Accompanying color flow Doppler image showing significant mitral regurgitation. C. Postoperative TEE 3D image showing en-face views of the bioprosthetic valve from both the left atrium and left ventricular (D) perspectives. A1, anterolateral segment; A2, middle segment of the anterior leaflet; A3, anteromedial segment; P1, posterolateral segment; P2, middle segment of the anterior leaflet; P3, posteromedial segment; AV, aortic valve. See Videos 6-29A through 6-29C.

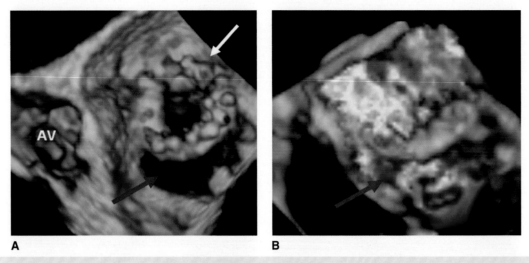

A   **B**

Figure 6-30. Mitral valve (MV) annuloplasty band dehiscence several years after MV repair. A. Three-dimensional TEE image demonstrating an annuloplasty band (*white arrow*) that has dehisced (*blue arrow*) along the lateral aspect. B. Color flow Doppler demonstrating significant mitral regurgitation (*blue arrow*) at the site of dehiscence. AV, aortic valve. See Videos 6-30A and 6-30B.

References

1. Lang R, Badano L, Tsang W, et al. EAE/ASE Recommendations for image acquisition and display using three-dimensional echocardiography. *J Am Soc Echocardiogr*. 2012;25:3–46.

2. Sugeng L, Shernan S, Salgo I, et al. Real-time three-dimensional transesophageal echocardiography using fully-sampled matrix array probe. *J Am Coll Cardiol*. 2008;52;446–449.

3. Sugeng L, Shernan S, Weinert L, et al. Real-time three-dimensional transesophageal echocardiography in valve disease: comparison with surgical findings and evaluation of prosthetic valves. *J Am Soc Echocardiogr*. 2008;12:1347–1354.

4. Mor-Avi V, Sugeng L, Lang R. Real-time 3-dimensional echocardiography: an integral component of the routine echocardiographic examination in adult patients? *Circulation*. 2009;119:314–329.

5. Salcedo E, Quaife R, Seres T, et al. A framework for systematic characterization of the mitral valve by real-time three-dimensional transesophageal echocardiography. *J Am Soc Echocardiogr*. 2009;22:1087–1099.

6. Vegas A, Meineri, M. Three-dimensional transesophageal echocardiography is a major advance for intra-operative clinical management of patients undergoing cardiac surgery: a core review. *Anesth Analg*. 2010;110:1548–1573.

7. Fischer G, Anyanwu A, Adams D. Intra-operative classification of mitral valve dysfunction: the role of the anesthesiologist in mitral valve reconstruction. *J Cardiothorac Vasc Anesth*. 2009;23:531–543.

8. Grewal J, Suri R, Mankad S, et al. Real-time 3-dimensional echocardiography mitral annular dynamics in myxomatous valve disease: new insights with real-time 3-dimensional echocardiography. *Circulation*. 2010;121;1423–1431.

9. Mills WR, Barber JE, Skiles JA, et al. Clinical, echocardiographic, and biomechanical differences in mitral valve prolapse affecting one or both leaflets. *Am J Cardiol*. 2002;89(12):1394–1399.

10. Michelena H, Topilsky Y, Suri R, et al. Degenerative mitral valve regurgitation: understanding basic concepts and new developments. *Postgrad Med*. 2011;123:56–69.

11. Foster E. Mitral regurgitation due to degenerative mitral-valve disease. *N Engl J Med*. 2010;363:156–165.

12. Freed L, Levy D, Levine R, et al. Prevalence and clinical outcome of mitral-valve prolapse. *N Engl J Med*. 1999;341:1–7.

13. Shah P. Current concepts in mitral valve prolapse. Diagnosis and management. *J Cardiol*. 2010;56:125–133.

14. Shah P. Echocardiographic diagnosis of mitral valve prolapse. *J Am Soc Echocardiogr*. 1994;7:286–293

15. Salgo I, Gorman J, Gorman R, et al. Effect of annular shape on leaflet curvature in reducing mitral leaflet stress. *Circulation*. 2002;106:711–717.

16. Levine R, Handschumacher M, Sanfilippo A, et al. Three-dimensional echocardiographic reconstruction of the mitral valve, with implications for the diagnosis of mitral valve prolapse. *Circulation*. 1989;80:589–598.

17. Levine R, Triulzi M, Harrigan P, et al. The relationship of mitral annular shape to the diagnosis of mitral valve prolapse. *Circulation*. 1987;75:756–767.

18. Shah P, Raney AA. Echocardiography in mitral regurgitation with relevance to valve surgery. *J Am Soc Echocardiogr*. 2011;24:1086–1091.

19. Beeri R, Streckenbach S, Isselbacher E, et al. The crossed swords sign: insights into the dilemma of repair in bileaflet mitral valve prolapse. *J Am Soc Echocardiogr*. 2007;20:698–702.

20. O'Gara P, Sugeng L, Lang R, et al. The role of imaging in chronic degenerative mitral regurgitation. *JACC Cardiovasc Imaging*. 2008;2:221–237.

21. Fornes P, Heudes D, Fuzellier J, et al. Correlation between clinical and histologic patterns of degenerative mitral valve insufficiency: a histomorphometric study of 130 excised segments. *Cardiovasc Pathol*. 1999;8(2):81–92.

22. Biaggi P, Gruner C, Jedrzkiewicz S, et al. Assessment of mitral valve prolapse by 3D TEE angled views are key. *JACC Cardiovasc Imaging*. 2011;4:94–97.

23. Chandra S, Salgo I, Sugeng L, et al. Characterization of degenerative mitral valve disease using morphologic analysis of real-time three-dimensional echocardiographic images objective insight into complexity and planning of mitral valve repair. *Circ Cardiovasc Imaging*. 2011;4:24–32.

24. Anyanwu A, Adams D. Etiologic classification of degenerative mitral valve disease: Barlow's disease and fibroelastic deficiency. *Semin Thorac Cardiovasc Surg*. 2007;19:90–96.

25. Maffessanti F, Marsan N, Tamborini G, et al. Quantitative analysis of mitral valve apparatus in mitral valve prolapse before and after annuloplasty: a three-dimensional intra-operative transesophageal study. *J Am Soc Echocardiogr*. 2011;24:405–413.

26. Lawrie G. Structure, function, and dynamics of the mitral annulus: importance in mitral valve repair for myxomatous mitral valve disease. *Methodist Debakey Cardiovasc J*. 2010;6:8–14.

27. Zekry S, Nagueh S, Little S, et al. Comparative accuracy of two- and three-dimensional transthoracic and transesophageal echocardiography in identifying mitral valve pathology in patients undergoing mitral valve repair: initial observations. *J Am Soc Echocardiogr*. 2011;24:1079–1085.

28. Vergnat M, Jackson BM, Cheung AT, et al. Saddle-shape annuloplasty increases mitral leaflet coaptation after repair for flail posterior leaflet. *Ann Thorac Surg*. 2011;92:797–804.

29. Mahmood F, Subramaniam B, Gorman J, et al. Three-dimensional echocardiographic assessment of changes in mitral valve geometry after valve repair. *Ann Thorac Surg*. 2009;88:1838–1844.

ISCHEMIC MITRAL REGURGITATION

7

Sonal Chandra, Masaaki Takeuchi, Roberto M. Lang

Ischemic mitral regurgitation (IMR) is a pathophysiologic outcome of ventricular remodeling or structural imbalance arising from ischemia. It falls in the broad category of "functional MR" whereby MR from abnormal valve closure occurs in the context of impaired ventricular function.[1] A normally functioning mitral valve (MV) is physiologically dependent on its anatomic relationships with the left ventricle. Etiologically, chordal or papillary muscle rupture (a surgical emergency) is often mechanistically responsible for acute IMR, while the more commonly occurring chronic IMR ensues from ischemic cardiomyopathy–left ventricular (LV) remodeling and dysfunction. The focus of this chapter is primarily chronic IMR, which as defined by Borger et al.[2] requires myocardial infarction as the inciting factor resulting in segmental wall motion abnormalities due to presence of coronary artery disease in the underlying territory; however, the valve and the subvalvular apparatus are originally structurally intact. IMR occurs in roughly 20% to 25% of patients with myocardial infarction.[3,4]

The mortality and morbidity of IMR have been well established in the epidemiologic studies. There is a direct relationship between presence of IMR and heart failure and/or death with IMR severity irrespective of the degree of LV systolic function.[4–7] MR is found in over 50% of patients undergoing coronary artery bypass grafting, and while the scope of this clinical entity is significant, it is expected to worsen in the future as the population ages.[2,8] A sequela of myocardial infarction, presence of even mild IMR can initiate or worsen the LV remodeling process. The adverse remodeling occurs in part from MR's impact on the LV loading conditions, which increases the diastolic wall stress resulting in eccentric hypertrophy with LV dilatation and failure.[9,10] A logical corollary would be to reverse or stop the remodeling process. Hence, several surgical and/or percutaneous approaches have been proposed and tried based on the geometric changes in the MV and LV. This chapter focuses on three-dimensional echocardiography's (3DE) role in assessing MV structure, function, and insights conferred on the ongoing surgical quest addressing IMR.

MECHANISMS

In IMR, it has been demonstrated that abnormal MV kinematics results from displaced papillary muscle(s), apical tethering of chords, and/or annular dilation (Fig. 7-1). There is a wide spectrum of geometric distortions that result in a regurgitant MV. The question is whether the ventricular contribution to deranged kinematics is a consequence of abnormal ventricular function or shape. Three-dimensional echocardiography with its higher spatial resolution has demonstrated that the anatomic shifts in annular–papillary muscle relationships lead to abnormal leaflet tension, which arises from changes in LV size and shape rather than function. Three-dimensional echocardiography–derived measurements confirmed an increase in MV annular area and tethering distance in setting of LV dilation (Fig. 7-2), but not when LV systolic function was reduced without accompanying dilation.[11]

When compared with 2D, 3D reconstruction of the MV allows accurate quantification of mitral anatomy. The 3D approach is especially accurate and useful in direct calculation of annular

135

geometry, leaflets angles, interpapillary muscle distance, tenting volume, surface of the leaflets, and dynamic assessment of MV (Fig. 7-3).

ANNULUS

While most IMR patients manifest some degree of annular and subvalvular remodeling, annular size and shape vary widely. This regional heterogeneity in annular geometry was demonstrated by 3DE.[12,13] In 3D studies, the IMR group compared to their normal counterparts demonstrated larger annular area and circumference, but subgroup comparison of anterior versus inferior infarct demonstrated larger annular indices in the former, including the length of the posterior annulus. Some patients maintained a nearly normal saddle-shaped annulus, while in others, especially in the anterior infarct group, severe annular flattening was demonstrated.

Undersized annuloplasty rings have become the preferred treatment with the idea that they increase leaflet coaptation and therefore decreasing regurgitation. Annuloplasty strategies aiming to restore the saddle shape of the mitral annulus by use of flexible or semirigid rings have not been necessarily effective at addressing MR successfully. While ring annuloplasty is effective in treating annular dilatation, it does not always improve coaptation and indeed may potentiate leaflet tethering (Video 7-2).[14] Video 7-2 demonstrates posterior displacement of coaptation zone and restriction of the posterior leaflet status post annuloplasty. Unfortunately, this therapeutic approach is associated with a 30% recurrence rate of significant IMR at 6 months after surgery with even higher rates of recurrence in the long term.[15–17] For patients with IMR, this lack of durability is likely to contribute to the difficulty in demonstrating a survival advantage of MV repair compared with either medical management or revascularization alone.[18,19]

Undersized annuloplasty exacerbates leaflet tethering. Posterior leaflet augmentation with less severe annular reduction increases leaflet curvature and decreases tethering.[20] Developments in 3DE have made it possible to glean 3D MV annular changes dynamically throughout the cardiac cycle (Figs. 7-4 and 7-5). Normal MV configurative changes from hyperbolic paraboloid in systole to a flatter configuration during diastole can increase leaflet curvature and therefore minimize leaflet stress (Fig. 7-6).[21] Commonly employed annuloplasty strategies at their best aim to statically hold the annulus in a certain 3D configuration or immobilize the posterior leaflet. We know that saddle-shaped annuloplasty rings provide better leaflet coaptation geometry than flat rings.[22] Three-dimensional echocardiography's assessment of MV dynamics may facilitate a better understanding of valvular stress distribution and thereby lead to better durability of MV repair.

LEAFLETS AND CHORDS

The common mechanistic outcome in IMR is an incomplete coaptation resulting from a combination of apically restricted leaflet in patients with LV dysfunction and altered leaflet geometry (Figs. 7-7 and 7-8). Although leaflet motion is typically restricted, it can be excessive or a combination of both. Tethering (Fig. 7-9) between the affected papillary muscle and the opposite mitral annulus decreases leaflet curvature and results in increased leaflet and chordal stress. This exacerbation of abnormal leaflet geometry may contribute to the suboptimal repair results for IMR.

Quantitative echocardiographic parameters measuring leaflet deformation, as a result of tethering, can offer mechanistic clues along with prognostic information on the durability of certain MV approaches. These parameters include tenting height, which is the vertical distance between the annulus and the leaflet coaptation point.[23,24] Tenting area is the region bordered by the annulus and the leaflets (Fig. 7-10). Tenting volume, a parameter measured by 3DE, encompasses many of the 2D measurements, including tenting and annular area (Figs. 7-11 and 7-12). It is less susceptible to foreshortening and therefore may serve as a marker of severity in IMR.[25]

In chronically tethered mitral leaflets in ischemic ventricles, MV leaflet surface area as measured by 3DE reconstruction increased on average by 35%.[26] Patients with greater valve adaptation to the tethered valve geometry had less MR but did not entirely overcome the demands of the tethered geometry. Interestingly, leaflet expansion has been demonstrated to be more a function of an increase in annular circumference rather than elongation from insertion to tip; two-dimensional echocardiography (2DE) is unable to discern these changes in length. Three-dimensional echocardiography can serve as the means of quantifying these MV adaptive changes, that is, increase in leaflet area to mechanical stress when suitable pharmacologic or surgical strategies enhancing this process are applied.[27] Three-dimensional echocardiography has demonstrated that leaflet enlargement was not elicited when papillary muscles were realigned, implicating the use for particular surgical approaches modifying ventricular wall or papillary geometry.

ASSESSING SEVERITY OF MITRAL REGURGITATION

With IMR, there is an increased mortality even in it is mild form; however, there exists a direct relationship between severity and decreased survival.[7,8] Consequently, accurate quantification of MR severity denotes clinical course. Planimetry of the regurgitant orifice area (ROA) in patients with MR is not feasible because of the complex, nonplanar 3D geometry of the orifice. Accordingly, indirect measurements are used to determine ROA using Doppler measurements of the proximal flow convergence (FC). Three-dimensional vena contracta area (VCA) provides a single, directly visualized, and reliable measurement of ROA, which classifies MR severity comparable to current clinical practice utilizing the American Society of Echocardiography–recommended 2D integrative method. Direct assessment of VCA using RT3DE revealed significant asymmetry of VCA in ischemic MR demonstrating the reason behind poor estimation of EROA by single VC width measurements.[28] The 3D VCA method accurately grades MR severity in comparison to 2D proximal isovelocity surface area (PISA) method by avoiding the geometric and flow assumptions and therefore independent of etiology and orifice shape (Figs. 7-13 and 7-14).[29] Two-dimensional FC, specifically PISA assessment, is predicated on the hypothetical hemispherical shape, which is not always strictly hemispherical and therefore leads to underestimation or overestimation of the flow rate. Three-dimensional computational fluid dynamics model has demonstrated that as the regurgitant orifice gets larger but remains circular, the convergence zones become oblate spheroidal (flattened) near the orifice and prolate ellipsoidal (elongated) far from the orifice. It is known from 3D studies that the orifice is often not circular but frequently hemiellipsoidal or even irregularly shaped (Fig. 7-15). Such altered morphology of the orifice is likely to lead to either under- or overestimation of effective ROA. Since planimetry of the ROA in patients with MR is not feasible because of the complex, nonplanar 3D geometry of the orifice, 3D-anatomic regurgitant orifice area (AROA) may provide a reasonable alternative to determine the severity of MR. Three-dimensional measurement of AROA is feasible even in patients with complex MV pathology, including those with flail, overlapping leaflets and eccentric jets (Fig. 7-16).[30]

Three-dimensional echocardiography's adjunct and at times primary role in understanding the specific mechanisms of IMR is demonstrated below. Particularly, insights into mitral geometry and dynamics and its impact on MV repair are explored.

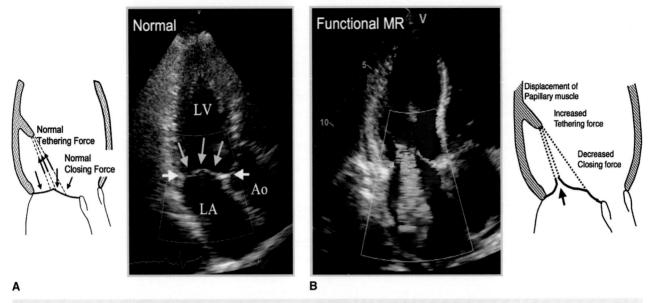

A   B

Figure 7-1. Ischemic MR: Mechanism. A. Normal mitral valve anatomy as depicted by illustration and 2DE results in normal kinematics. The *yellow arrows* point to normal coaptation of leaflets. B. Abnormal mitral valve kinematics results from displaced papillary muscle(s), apical tethering of chords, and/or resultant annular dilation.

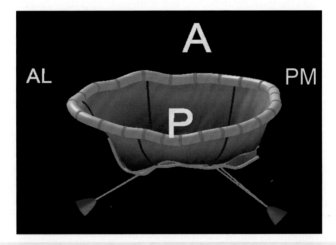

Figure 7-2. Analysis of the mitral valve apparatus using computer-generated 3D-rendered surface map. This color-coded, 3D-rendered surface map of an ischemic mitral valve is demonstrating funnel-shaped deformity (loss of saddle shape), displacement of the coaptation zone, and increase in annulus-to-papillary muscle tethering length and annular dilation. Accompanying Video 7-1 demonstrates the abnormal leaflet function as a result of these geometric derangements. A, anterior; P, posterior; PM, posteromedial.

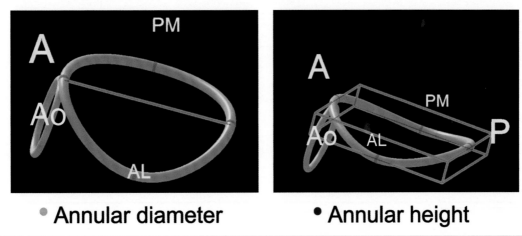

Figure 7-3. Quantitative analysis of the mitral valve apparatus using 3D-rendered surface area map. When compared with 2D, 3D reconstruction of the MV allows an accurate quantification of mitral anatomy. The 3D approach is especially accurate and useful in direct calculation of the annular geometry, leaflets angles, interpapillary muscle distance, tenting volume, and surface of the MV leaflets. A, anterior; AL, anterolateral; Ao, aorta; P, posterior; PM, posteromedial.

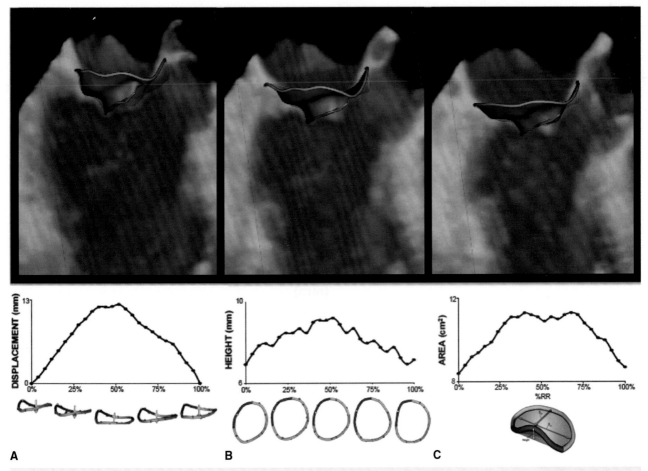

Figure 7-4. Annular dynamics. Developments in 3DE have made it possible to glean 3D MV annular changes dynamically throughout the cardiac cycle. Three-dimensional echocardiography facilitates dynamic measurements of annular displacement (A), changes in annular height (B) and annular area (C) throughout the cardiac cycle.

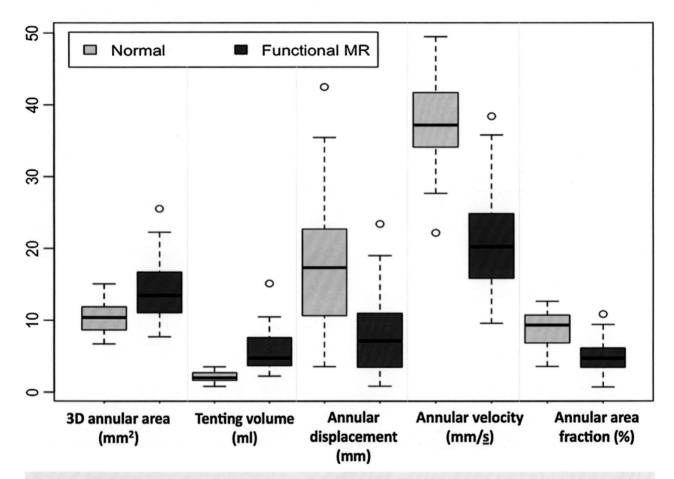

Figure 7-5. Quantification of annular geometry and dynamics in ischemic MR. Graphical representation of differences in mitral annular geometry and dynamics between normal (*yellow*) and functional MR (ischemic MR, *green*) in a cohort of 20 patients (10 normal, 10 with ischemic MR) quantified using 3DE (unpublished data). Annular parameters measured using 3D software include 3D area, tenting volume, displacement, velocity, and area fraction. There is an increase in annular area and tenting volume but a significant decline in displacement, velocity, and area fraction.

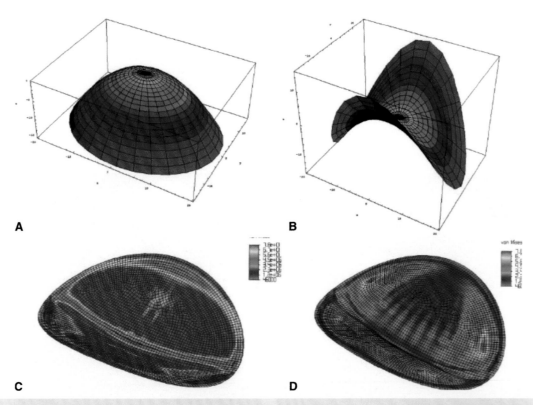

A   B

C   D

Figure 7-6. Annular dynamics in ischemic MR. Normal MV configurative changes from hyperbolic paraboloid in systole to a flatter configuration during diastole can increase leaflet curvature and therefore minimize leaflet stress. **Top panels:** Plot of an elliptic billowing leaflet model and hyperbolic paraboloid (A) or nonplanar annulus model (B) as fundamental shapes, not leaflets. The hue of the shapes varies by curvature using differential geometry. The configuration in **top right panel** represents minimal surface area. **Bottom left panel (C)** represents a plot of mitral phantom leaflets without billowing, demonstrating stresses by von Mises distortion energy theory. **Bottom right panel (D)** is a plot of mitral phantom leaflet with billowing demonstrating stresses by von Mises distortion energy theory. Note the decrease in stress for the curved leaflets in **bottom right panel.** (Reproduced from Salgo IS, Gorman JH III, Gorman RC, et al. Effect of annular shape on leaflet curvature in reducing mitral leaflet stress. *Circulation* 2002;106:711–717, with permission.)

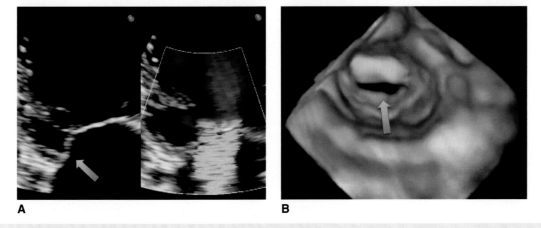

A   B

Figure 7-7. **Restricted leaflet in ischemic MR.** The common mechanistic outcome in IMR is an incomplete coaptation resulting from a combination of apically restricted leaflet in patients with LV dysfunction and altered leaflet geometry. A. Two-dimensional echocardiography demonstrating restricted posterior leaflet (*arrow,* **left panel**) resulting in severe mitral regurgitation (**right panel**). B. Restricted leaflet motion during systole (*arrow*) resulting in a regurgitant orifice is evident on an en-face 3D view of the valve from the left atrial perspective. The accompanying Video 7-3 demonstrates valve motion demonstrating restricted posterior leaflet on the **right panel** and ensuing MR from improper coaptation on the **left panel.**

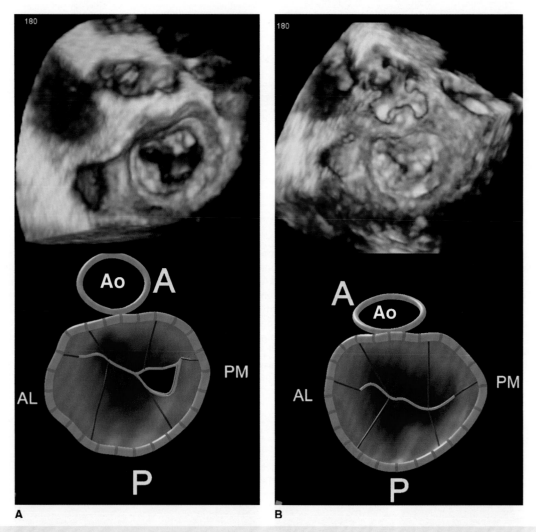

Figure 7-8. Three-dimensional configurations of an ischemic MV and its representative parametric maps. A. Restricted posterior leaflet on en-face 3D view of the valve from the left atrial perspective (top panel). The regurgitant orifice size, location, and shape resulting from distortion in leaflet geometry is visualized as an interrupted coaptation line on a color-coded 3D-rendered surface representing a topographical map of the mitral apparatus (bottom). B. Normal mitral valve in an en-face 3D view of the valve from the left atrial perspective (top) and the 3D-rendered surface map without a regurgitant orifice (bottom).

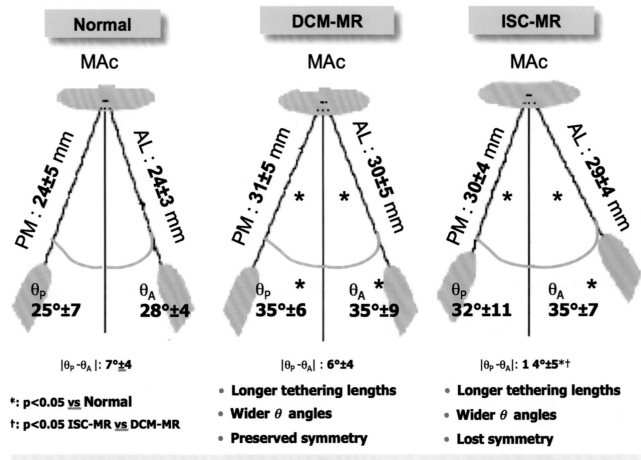

Figure 7-9. Graphic representation of the 3D papillary muscles geometry measured in the three groups of patients (DCM—dilated cardiomyopathy with MR and ISC—ischemic MR and normal MV). This figure demonstrates examples of mitral annulus motion, velocity, and papillary three-dimensional position obtained in representative control subjects and in patients with ischemic and dilated cardiomyopathy with mitral regurgitation. The dilated and ischemic MR groups had significantly longer tethering length, compared to normal subjects, both in posteromedial and anterolateral papillary muscles. In patients with DCM, the symmetry of the papillary muscle position was preserved, whereas in ischemic patients significant asymmetry of the papillary muscles was noted. Accompanying Video 7-4 demonstrates this excessive MV motion in an IMR patient with a ruptured chord. Accompanying Video 7-5 demonstrates this tethering resulting in significant MR in the long-axis view. This tethering, between the affected papillary muscle and the opposite mitral annulus, decreases leaflet curvature and results in increased leaflet and chordal stress. MA, mitral annulus; PM and AL, posteromedial and anterolateral papillary muscle tethering length; MAC, mitral annulus center. (Courtesy of Dr. F. Veronesi.)

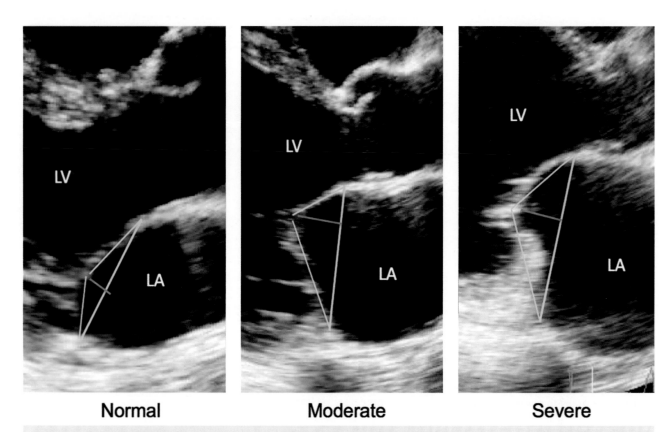

Normal **Moderate** **Severe**

Figure 7-10. **MV tenting parameters—tenting height in 2D.** In this figure, the tenting area is the region bordered by the annulus and the leaflets and is outlined in *yellow*. The tenting height (*red line*) extends from the annulus to the coaptation point. The apex of the triangle represents leaflet coaptation. LA, left atrium; LV, left ventricle.

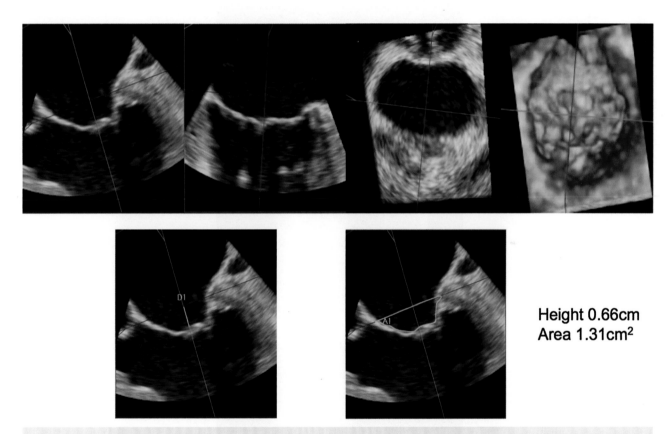

Height 0.66cm
Area 1.31cm²

Figure 7-11. MV tenting parameters—tenting height in 3D. Three-dimensional echocardiography-derived multiplanar reformations of the annulus and mitral valve leaflets permit accurate measurements of annular height and area.

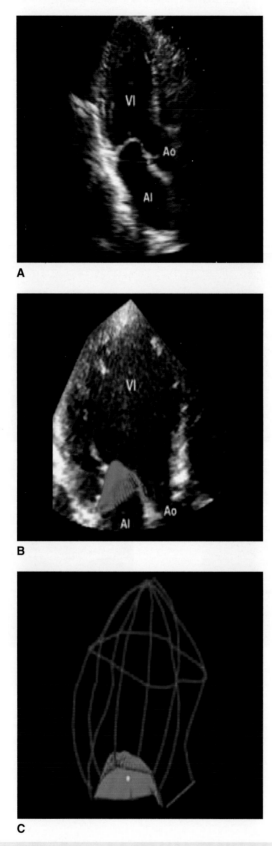

Figure 7-12. MV tenting parameters—tenting volume. A. Two-dimensional echocardiography measurement of tenting area is limited by asymmetry especially in ischemic MR, making single plane studies less than optimal. Three-dimensional echocardiography enables the measurement of tenting volume. B. Two-dimensional view of a plane demonstrating 3D reconstruction of MV (in *green*). C. Three-dimensional reconstruction of tenting volume (*green*) along with left ventricle (*red*) and mitral annulus (*blue*). (Reproduced from Solis J, Sitges M, Levine RA, et al. Three-dimensional echocardiography. New possibilities in mitral valve assessment. *Rev Esp Cardiol* 2009;62:188–198, with permission.)

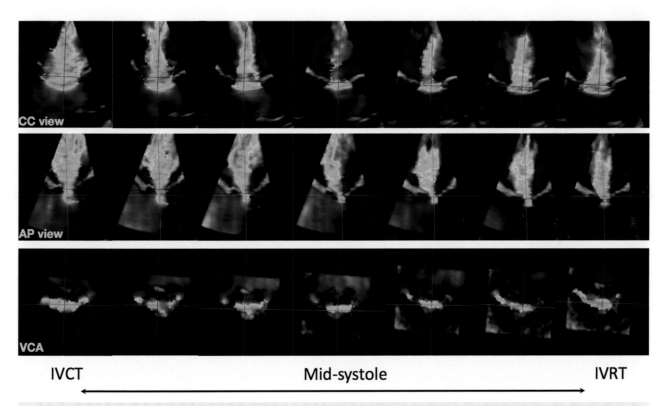

CC view

AP view

VCA

IVCT　　　　　　　　　　Mid-systole　　　　　　　　　　IVRT

Figure 7-13. **Quantifying 3D vena contracta.** Reproducible measurements of phasic changes in VCA are feasible with 3DE. CC, intercommissural; AP, anterior–posterior; VCA, vena contracta area; IVCT, isovolumetric contraction time; IVRT, isovolumetric relaxation time.

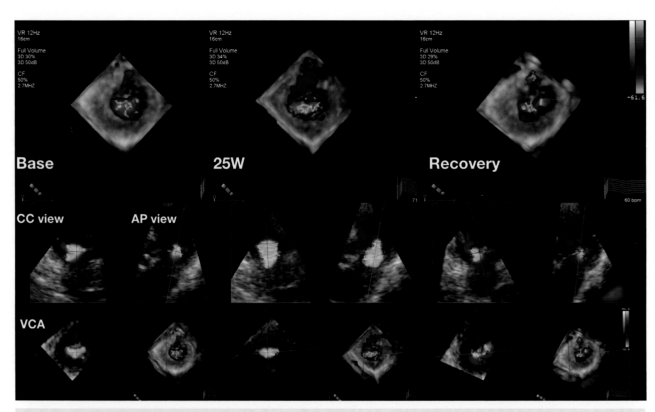

Figure 7-14. Dynamic changes in 3D vena contracta with exercise. Three-dimensional assessment of vena contracta (VC) revealed dynamic changes in ischemic mitral regurgitation at rest (left), exercise (middle), and recovery (right). Orthogonal views (middle panels) demonstrate variable VC diameters; corresponding cross-sectional views (bottom panel with *yellow arrows*) demonstrate VCA allowing accurate assessment of MR severity at maximal exertion. CC, intercommissural; AP, anteroposterior; W, watts.

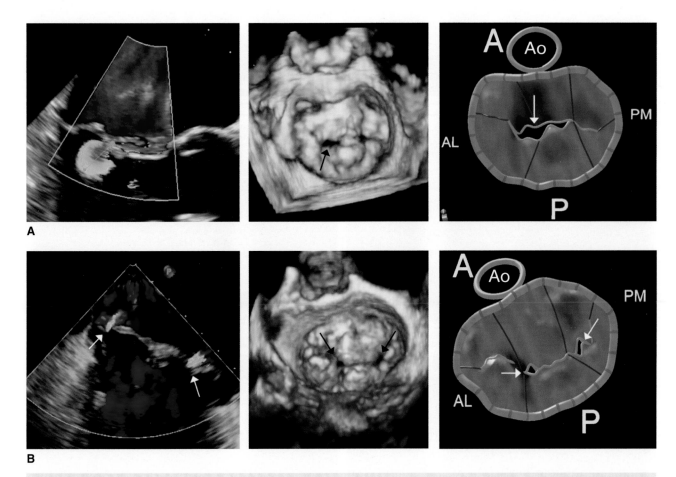

Figure 7-15. **Complexity of effective regurgitant orifices in mitral regurgitation and challenges posed by conventional 2D techniques. A.** This figure depicts difficulty with quantification of flow convergence with distorted valvular geometry as noted in the 3D en-face view of the MV (**top middle panel**). There is a complex 3D shape to the regurgitant orifice as noted in the color-coded 3D-rendered surface (**top right panel**) and distorted flow convergence geometry where proximal isovelocity surface area geometric assumptions could be potentially inapplicable. **B.** This panel represents the difficulty in quantification posed by presence of two separate regurgitant jets, which can occur in either myxomatous and/or ischemic MR (**left bottom,** *arrows*). Individual orifices are evident in 3D (**middle bottom panel**) and the color-coded 3D-rendered surface (**right bottom panel**). Video 7-6 demonstrates the complex shape and presence of multiple MR orifices at the coaptation zone of the A1-A2 and P1-P2 segments and a commissural orifice at A3 and P3 coaptation zone. (Reproduced from Chandra S, Salgo IS, Sugeng L, et al. A three-dimensional insight into the complexity of flow convergence in mitral regurgitation: adjunctive benefit of anatomic regurgitant orifice area. *Am J Physiol Heart Circ Physiol* 2011;301:H1015–H1024, with permission.)

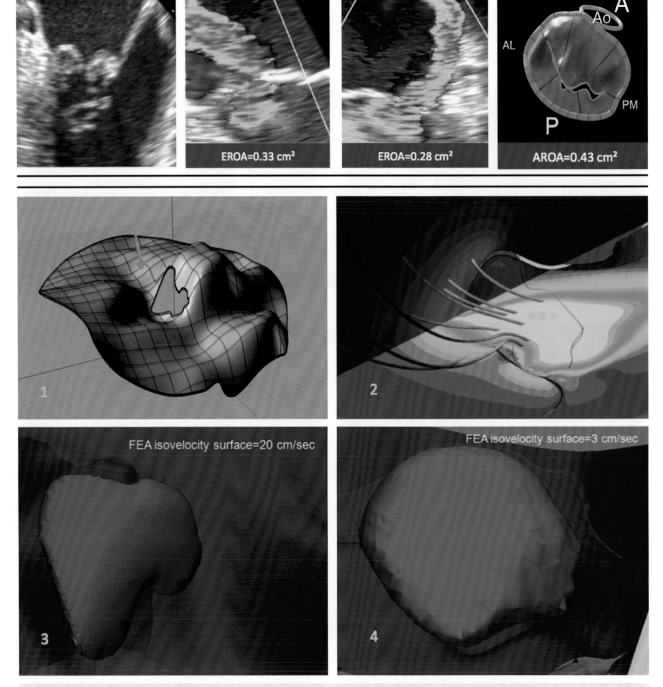

Figure 7-16. Difficulty with quantification of flow convergence (FC) in the presence of severely distorted valvular geometry. A. The overlapping leaflets result in a complex 3D shape of the regurgitant orifice as noted in the color-coded 3D-rendered surface and distorted FC geometry, causing considerable discrepancy between FC and 3D volumetric measurements of anatomic ROA due to invalid PISA geometric assumptions. B. Three-dimensional model of a mitral valve reconstructed from 3DTEE using MVQ software (*1*). Note the noncircular, nonplanar regurgitant orifice (*arrow*). The geometry was modeled to simulate regurgitant blood flow in 3D space (*2*). At the FC zone closer to the asymmetric orifice, the isovelocity contour is flattened and nonhemispherical (*3*). Farther away from the orifice, the isovelocity contour becomes more spherically symmetric (*4*). This 3D simulation demonstrates the nature of the transition in general and the lack of hemisphericity near the irregular orifice. (Reproduced from Chandra S, Salgo IS, Sugeng L, et al. A three-dimensional insight into the complexity of flow convergence in mitral regurgitation: adjunctive benefit of anatomic regurgitant orifice area. *Am J Physiol Heart Circ Physiol* 2011;301:H1015–H1024, with permission).

References

1. Levine RA, Schwammenthal E. Ischemic mitral regurgitation on the threshold of a solution: from paradoxes to unifying concepts. *Circulation* 2005;112(5):745–758.

2. Borger MA, Alam A, Murphy PM, et al. Chronic ischemic mitral regurgitation: repair, replace or rethink? *Ann Thorac Surg* 2006;81(3):1153–1161.

3. Birnbaum Y, Chamoun AJ, Conti VR, et al. Mitral regurgitation following acute myocardial infarction. *Coron Artery Dis* 2002;13(6):337–344.

4. Lamas GA, Mitchell GF, Flaker GC, et al.; Survival and Ventricular Enlargement Investigators. Clinical significance of mitral regurgitation after acute myocardial infarction. *Circulation* 1997;96(3):827–833.

5. Bursi F, Enriquez-Sarano M, Nkomo VT, et al. Heart failure and death after myocardial infarction in the community: the emerging role of mitral regurgitation. *Circulation* 2005;111(3):295–301.

6. Grigioni F, Detaint D, Avierinos JF, et al. Contribution of ischemic mitral regurgitation to congestive heart failure after myocardial infarction. *J Am Coll Cardiol* 2005;45(2):260–267.

7. Grigioni F, Enriquez-Sarano M, Zehr KJ, et al. Ischemic mitral regurgitation: long-term outcome and prognostic implications with quantitative Doppler assessment. *Circulation* 2001;103(13):1759–1764.

8. Trichon BH, Felker GM, Shaw LK, et al. Relation of frequency and severity of mitral regurgitation to survival among patients with left ventricular systolic dysfunction and heart failure. *Am J Cardiol* 2003;91(5):538–543.

9. Carabello BA. Mitral valve regurgitation. *Curr Probl Cardiol* 1998;23(4):202–241.

10. Spinale FG, Ishihra K, Zile M, et al. Structural basis for changes in left ventricular function and geometry because of chronic mitral regurgitation and after correction of volume overload. *J Thorac Cardiovasc Surg* 1993;106(6):1147–1157.

11. Otsuji Y, Handschumacher MD, Schwammenthal E, et al. Insights from three-dimensional echocardiography into the mechanism of functional mitral regurgitation: direct in vivo demonstration of altered leaflet tethering geometry. *Circulation* 1997;96(6):1999–2008.

12. Vergnat M, Jassar AS, Jackson BM, et al. Ischemic mitral regurgitation: a quantitative three-dimensional echocardiographic analysis. *Ann Thorac Surg* 2011;91(1):157–164.

13. Watanabe N, Ogasawara Y, Yamaura Y, et al. Mitral annulus flattens in ischemic mitral regurgitation: geometric differences between inferior and anterior myocardial infarction: a real-time 3-dimensional echocardiographic study. *Circulation* 2005;112(9 suppl):I458–I462.

14. Kuwahara E, Otsuji Y, Iguro Y, et al. Mechanism of recurrent/persistent ischemic/functional mitral regurgitation in the chronic phase after surgical annuloplasty: importance of augmented posterior leaflet tethering. *Circulation* 2006;114(1 suppl):I529–I534.

15. McGee EC, Gillinov AM, Blackstone EH, et al. Recurrent mitral regurgitation after annuloplasty for functional ischemic mitral regurgitation. *J Thorac Cardiovasc Surg* 2004;128(6):916–924.

16. Hung J, Papakostas L, Tahta SA, et al. Mechanism of recurrent ischemic mitral regurgitation after annuloplasty: continued LV remodeling as a moving target. *Circulation* 2004;110(11 suppl 1):II85–II90.

17. Crabtree TD, Bailey MS, Moon MR, et al. Recurrent mitral regurgitation and risk factors for early and late mortality after mitral valve repair for functional ischemic mitral regurgitation. *Ann Thorac Surg* 2008;85(5): 1537–1542; discussion 1542–1543.

18. Mihaljevic T, Lam BK, Rajeswaran J, et al. Impact of mitral valve annuloplasty combined with revascularization in patients with functional ischemic mitral regurgitation. *J Am Coll Cardiol* 2007;49(22):2191–2201.

19. Diodato MD, Moon MR, Pasque MK, et al. Repair of ischemic mitral regurgitation does not increase mortality or improve long-term survival in patients undergoing coronary artery revascularization: a propensity analysis. *Ann Thorac Surg* 2004;78(3):794–799; discussion 794–799.

20. Robb JD, Minakawa M, Koomalsingh KJ, et al. Posterior leaflet augmentation improves leaflet tethering in repair of ischemic mitral regurgitation. *Eur J Cardiothorac Surg* 2011;40:1501–1507.

21. Salgo IS, Gorman JH III, Gorman RC, et al. Effect of annular shape on leaflet curvature in reducing mitral leaflet stress. *Circulation* 2002;106(6):711–717.

22. Jensen MO, Jensen H, Levine RA, et al. Saddle-shaped mitral valve annuloplasty rings improve leaflet coaptation geometry. *J Thorac Cardiovasc Surg* 2011;142(3):697–703.

23. Messas E, Guerrero JL, Handschumacher MD, et al. Paradoxic decrease in ischemic mitral regurgitation with papillary muscle dysfunction: insights from three-dimensional and contrast echocardiography with strain rate measurement. *Circulation* 2001;104(16):1952–1957.

24. Silbiger JJ. Mechanistic insights into ischemic mitral regurgitation: echocardiographic and surgical implications. *J Am Soc Echocardiogr* 2011;24(7):707–719.

25. Song JM, Fukuda S, Kihara T, et al. Value of mitral valve tenting volume determined by real-time three-dimensional echocardiography in patients with functional mitral regurgitation. *Am J Cardiol* 2006;98(8): 1088–1093.

26. Chaput M, Handschumacher MD, Tournoux F, et al. Mitral leaflet adaptation to ventricular remodeling: occurrence and adequacy in patients with functional mitral regurgitation. *Circulation* 2008;118(8):845–852.

27. Dal-Bianco JP, Aikawa E, Bischoff J, et al. Active adaptation of the tethered mitral valve: insights into a compensatory mechanism for functional mitral regurgitation. *Circulation* 2009;120(4):334–342.

28. Kahlert P, Plicht B, Schenk IM, et al. Direct assessment of size and shape of noncircular vena contracta area in functional versus organic mitral regurgitation using real-time three-dimensional echocardiography. *J Am Soc Echocardiogr* 2008;21(8):912–921.

29. Zeng X, Levine RA, Hua L, et al. Diagnostic value of vena contracta area in the quantification of mitral regurgitation severity by color Doppler 3D echocardiography. *Circ Cardiovasc Imaging* 2011;4(5):506–513.

30. Chandra S, Salgo IS, Sugeng L, et al. A three-dimensional insight into the complexity of flow convergence in mitral regurgitation: adjunctive benefit of anatomic regurgitant orifice area. *Am J Physiol Heart Circ Physiol* 2011;301(3):H1015–H1024.

Wendy Tsang, David A. Roberson, Roberto M. Lang

Over the past few decades, improvements in transesophageal three-dimensional (3D) echocardiography have created a highly effective tool for the visualization and evaluation of prosthetic valves and prosthetic annuloplasty rings.[1] This improvement has mainly been achieved through the ability to obtain nontraditional en-face views when using 3D echocardiography.[2] The en-face view from 3D imaging allows visualization of the entire prosthetic valve from a "superior" and/or "inferior" perspective. To date, this has had the greatest impact on the assessment of prosthetic valves in the mitral and aortic positions and, to a lesser degree, the tricuspid valve.

PROSTHETIC VALVE ASSESSMENT

With the use of 3D transesophageal echocardiography (TEE), it has been shown that in most patients with normal mitral mechanical (Figs. 8-1, 8-4, 8-5, 8-8, 8-26) or bioprosthetic valves (Figs. 8-9, 8-24, 8-25, 8-27), visualization of the prosthetic ring, leaflets, and struts from either the left atrium or ventricular perspective can be achieved.[3] The ability to use en-face views from 3D TEE imaging to assess both the "superior" and "inferior" aspects of an implanted valve presents an important advantage of 3D over 2D TEE.[4] This is because with 2D TEE, visualization of the ventricular aspect of a prosthetic mitral valve is always limited by acoustic shadowing, thus precluding complete examination of the prosthetic valve.[3] Three-dimensional TEE also improves the assessment of patients with repaired mitral valves (Figs. 8-16, 8-18, 8-19, 8-23). Three-dimensional TEE en-face views allow easy visualization of the implanted ring and the native anterior leaflet. However, it must be noted that there continues to be limitations with the complete visualization of the native posterior leaflet with 3D TEE.

The leaflets of aortic mechanical or bioprosthetic valves are frequently poorly visualized with 3D TEE irrespective of perspective.[3] This is because the aortic valve leaflets lie far from the transducer, and the thin aortic valve leaflets lie oblique to the angle of incidence of the ultrasound beam.[4] This same reason also explains why tricuspid valve leaflets are poorly visualized on 3D echocardiography (Figs. 8-23, 8-24, 8-25).[5] In comparison, both the aortic and tricuspid prosthetic valve rings are easily visualized on 3D TEE regardless of the en-face perspective.

COMPLICATIONS OF PROSTHETIC VALVES

The use of en-face 3D echocardiographic views provides incremental information in the assessment of prosthetic valves for infective endocarditis and paravalvular regurgitation.[6] In prosthetic valve endocarditis, 3D TEE imaging has been shown to identify vegetations not seen on 2D TEE.[7,8] However, it must be still stated that due to the frame rate limitations of 3D TEE, small mobile vegetations and intermittent prosthesis leaflet immobilization by thrombus (Figs. 8-6) or infection are still better appreciated on 2D TEE. However, the strength of 3D TEE lies in its ability to characterize a mass beyond noting its presence or absence. For example, 3D TEE can help differentiate loose suture material from vegetation (Figs. 8-13 and 8-14). As well, the rocking motion of a partially dehisced valve is well appreciated with 3D imaging.

With respect to paravalvular regurgitation, 3D imaging not only assists with determining the site, size, and number of paravalvular defects but also helps determine whether the defect is better suited for surgical or percutaneous approach to closure.[9,10] The location, shape, and area of the dehiscence site can be identified, and accurate quantification of the dehisced area and regurgitant jets can be performed using multiplanar imaging or 3D color modes (Figs. 8-7, 8-15, 8-17, 8-20, 8-21).[11,12] The relationship between the site of dehiscence and other anatomic structures is also better appreciated on 3D imaging.

Three-dimensional imaging has helped determine that the location of prosthetic mitral valve dehiscence is usually located in the posterior portion of the annulus due to four possible mechanisms.[13] These mechanisms include (1) poor suturing of the posterior mitral valve annulus because of its location in the far surgical field, thus providing a limited window for the surgeon to maneuver; (2) superficial suturing in that region since the surgeon is attempting to avoid harming the circumflex artery; (3) difficulties attaining proper suturing due to the higher prevalence of calcifications and fibrosis in that region; and (4) pulling of the posterior portion of the annulus by the anterior portion, which is restricted in motion after being sewn into the inflexible mitral fibrosa.

If a percutaneous approach is chosen, 3D TEE helps guide both the route of approach and the choice of closure device.[14,15] As well, with a single field of view, 3D TEE permits monitoring of all intracardiac catheters and their relationship to important cardiac structures during the procedure. Once the procedure is complete, 3D TEE can assess both the location and the function of the newly introduced occluder device as well as the function of the prosthetic valve.

LIMITATIONS IN 3D IMAGING OF PROSTHETIC VALVES

Three-dimensional zoom mode is one of the major imaging modes used to assess prosthetic valves. However, while traditional 3D zoom provides images with high spatial resolution, it is at the expense of temporal resolution. Frame rates are typically <10 Hz, which limits 3D of fast moving structures such as vegetations. Newly introduced software allowing frame rate acquisition of up to 30 Hz combined with single-beat full-volume acquisitions currently results in images that require short acquisition times while simultaneously minimizing stitch artifact and improving image resolution. In TTE, this type of acquisition has been shown to provide similar accuracy to RT3D imaging data acquired using conventional four-beat acquisition.

The introduction of single-beat full-volume acquisition techniques also circumvents issues relating to suboptimal images with stitching artifacts due to poor ECG triggering in patients with arrhythmias. However, it must be recognized that at this time, single-beat imaging does not have the same temporal resolution available with multibeat acquisitions. Overall, wide-angle multibeat acquisition is still required to increase temporal resolution to obtain frame rates >30 Hz. However, the risk of stitch artifacts may be increased due to the requirement for multiple cardiac samplings over four to seven beats. This frequently results in this type of artifacts in more than 70% of the cases. However, these generally do not compromise the diagnostic yield of the test. Users must be particularly aware of this limitation in the acquisition of color Doppler datasets as the acquisition spans seven cardiac cycles. In the operating room, stitch artifact can be eliminated by briefly interrupting the respirator during image acquisition.

SUMMARY

Overall, 3D TEE imaging allows clinically useful visualization of prosthetic valve components such as leaflets, rings, and struts of all prosthetic valves irrespective of position. Three-dimensional TEE imaging is particularly useful for the assessment of mechanical mitral and aortic valves where 2D images of the ventricular side of these prostheses are often of poor quality due to acoustic shadowing. Finally, one additional important point in using 3D TEE for the assessment of prosthetic valves is that it does not substantially lengthen the TEE procedural time. Acquisition times for 3D TEE imaging routinely require approximately 10 additional minutes.

In this chapter, we demonstrate the use of 3D TEE for the assessment of prosthetic valves, annuloplasty rings, and their associated complications such as prosthetic valve endocarditis and paravalvular regurgitation.

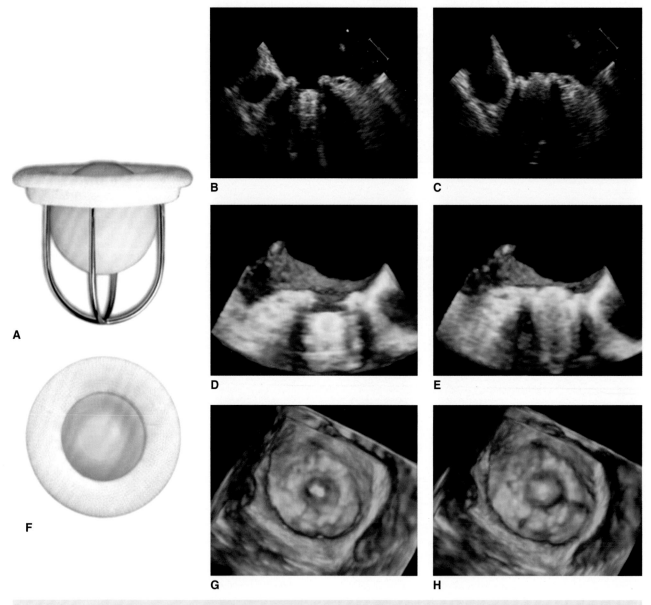

A

B

C

D

E

F

G

H

Figure 8-1. **Normal Starr-Edwards ball-and-cage mitral valve.** Side (A) and en-face cage base (F) profile of a Starr-Edwards ball-and-cage mitral valve. The valve consists of a circular sewing ring, a cage made of two metal arches, and a silastic ball. When the left ventricle contracts during systole, the ball moves against the base of the cage forming a seal and thus preventing blood flow through the valve into the left atrium. During diastole, the ball falls back into the cage, allowing blood to flow through the valve. On 2D TEE, the ball can be seen moving into the cage during diastole (B) and against the cage base during systole (C). With 3D TEE, not only can the ball's motion be appreciated during diastole (D) and systole (E) but also the entire ring apparatus can be visualized en face (G,H). Accompanying Video 8-1A corresponds to Panels D and E. Accompanying Video 8-1B corresponds to Panels G and H.

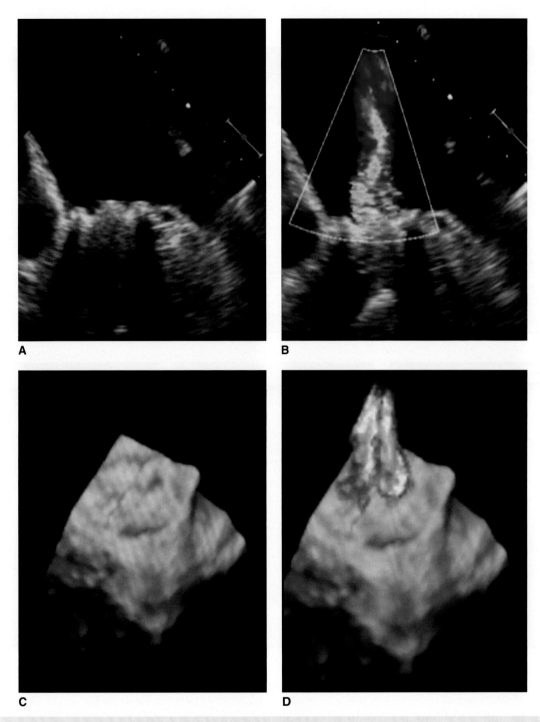

Figure 8-2. Image of a degenerative Starr-Edwards ball-and-cage mitral valve. While ball-and-cage valves have good durability, over time the silastic ball may shrink due to wear and tear. This is known as ball variance and results in a poor seal of the ball against the base of the cage with resultant regurgitation through the valve. While this may be visualized on 2D transesophageal echocardiographic imaging of the valve during systole without and with color (A,B), on 3D TEE, the circumferential nature of the color jet can easily be appreciated with en-face imaging of the base of the prosthetic valve without and with color (C,D). Accompanying Video 8-2 corresponds to Panels A and B.

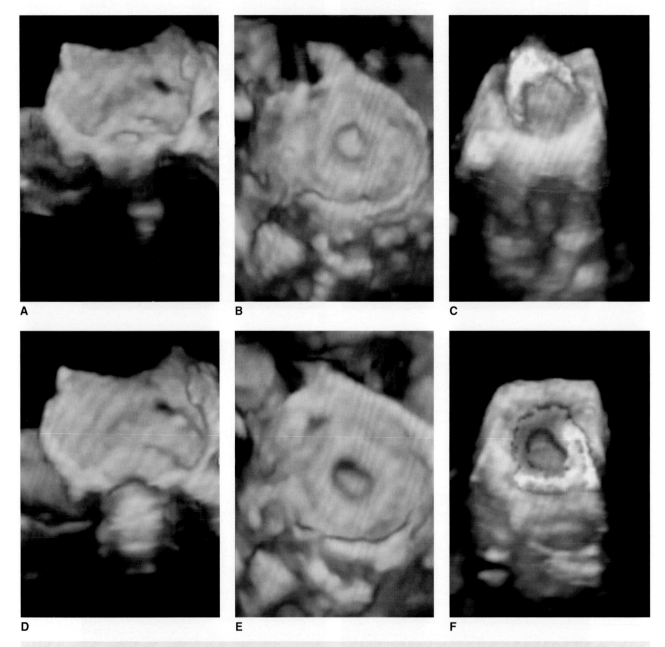

Figure 8-3. Three-dimensional echocardiographic images of a degenerative Starr-Edwards ball-and-cage mitral valve. In this series of 3D transesophageal echocardiographic images of a Starr-Edwards mitral valve, the ball is seen moving during systole (A,B) and diastole (D,E) in the cage. Note the eccentric jet of mitral regurgitation during systole (C). As well, blood flow through the valve in diastole is asymmetrical around the edges of the ball (F). Thus, Doppler gradients measured across this valve should be done around the periphery of the ball where the flow velocities are the highest. Finally, the area behind the ball during blood flow is relatively stagnant, which may lead to thrombus formation. Accompanying Video 8-3 corresponds to Panels C and F.

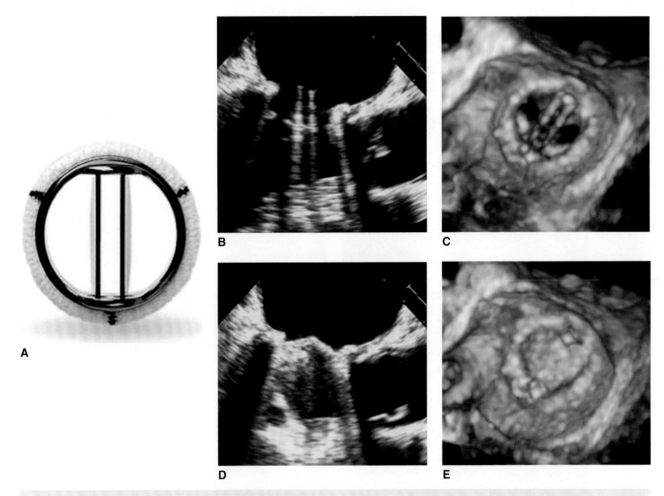

Figure 8-4. Normal St. Jude bileaflet mechanical mitral valve. Image of a St. Jude bileaflet mechanical mitral valve (A). The valve is composed of two semilunar discs attached to a rigid circular ring by hinges. During diastole, three orifices are created as the leaflets swing open to form a 75-degree to 90-degree angle to the prosthetic valve ring. The parallel orientation of the two leaflets can be visualized with 2D TEE (B). With 3D TEE, the en-face view of the prosthetic valve (C) allows the entire valve to be seen in a single image. In systole, the leaflets swing away from each other and coapt against the circular ring, preventing blood flow through the valve. The leaflets in their "closed" position can be seen in a single plane on 2D echocardiography (D) or in their entirety using an en-face view on 3D echocardiography (E). Accompanying Video 8-4 corresponds to Panel 8-4 C and E.

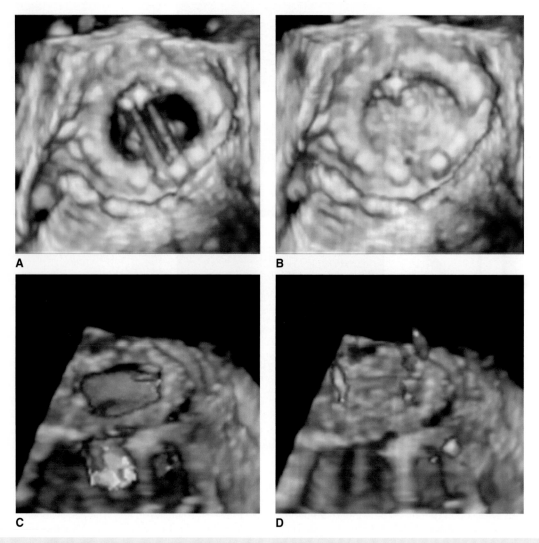

Figure 8-5. Normal motion of a St. Jude bileaflet mechanical mitral valve. Zoomed 3D transesophageal echocardiographic en-face image of a bileaflet mechanical mitral valve during diastole (A) and systole (B). With 3D transesophageal echocardiographic color imaging, normal flow through the valve in diastole can be seen (C). During systole, the flushing jets at the hinge regions of the valve can be seen (D).

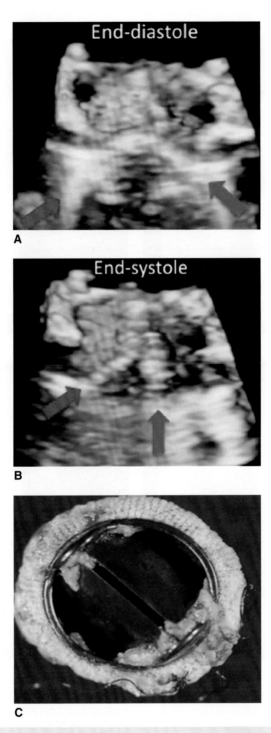

Figure 8-6. Restriction of normal mechanical mitral valve leaflet motion by thrombus. In this 3D transesophageal echo-cardiographic image of a bileaflet mechanical mitral valve, one leaflet demonstrates preserved motion (*blue arrow*) during diastole (A) and systole (B), while the other leaflet has reduced motion (*red arrow*) resulting in valvular stenosis. After the valve was excised, thrombus at the hinge regions of the valve is found to have restricted motion of the leaflet (C).

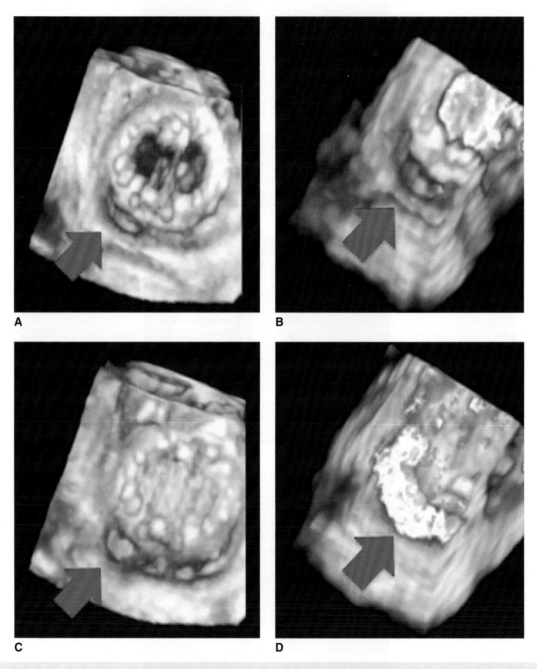

A

B

C

D

Figure 8-7. Paravalvular dehiscence of a mechanical mitral valve. In this series of 3D transesophageal echocardiographic images, a bileaflet mechanical mitral valve is presented as visualized en face from the left atrium. A paravalvular dehiscence with regurgitation (*red arrows*) is demonstrated. The area and size of the dehiscence can be assessed during diastole (A) and systole (C). When color is added to the 3D image, blood flow is seen passing mostly through the valve during diastole (B). However, while there is no blood flow through the valve during systole, there is a significant jet of regurgitation through the dehiscence site (D).

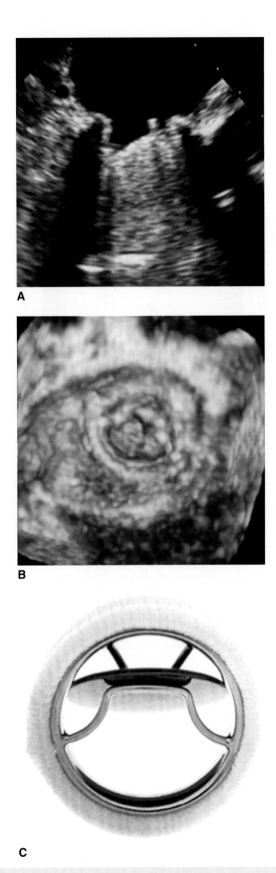

Figure 8-8. Normal single-tilting disc mechanical valve. Two-dimensional transesophageal echocardiographic image of a single-tilting disc valve in the mitral valve position during diastole (A). When viewed en face from the left atrial perspective using 3D transesophageal echocardiographic data, the hinge of the valve is easily visualized (B) and is comparable to the actual appearance of the valve (C).

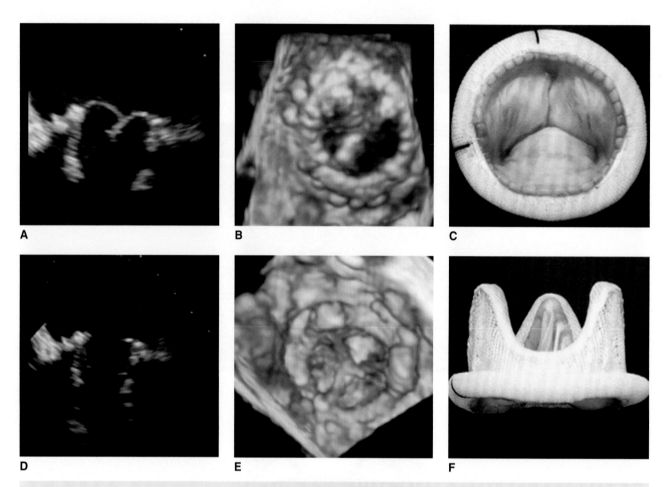

Figure 8-9. Normal bioprosthetic mitral valve. Two-dimensional transesophageal echocardiographic images of a bioprosthetic mitral valve during systole (A) and diastole (D). On 3D transesophageal echocardiographic imaging, from the en-face left atrial perspective, the prosthetic ring and leaflets can be seen (B). When viewed en face from the left ventricular perspective, the three valve struts, valve ring, and leaflet commissures can be visualized (E). These 3D echocardiographic images provide an accurate portrayal of the bioprosthetic valve when compared to its actual appearance (C,F).

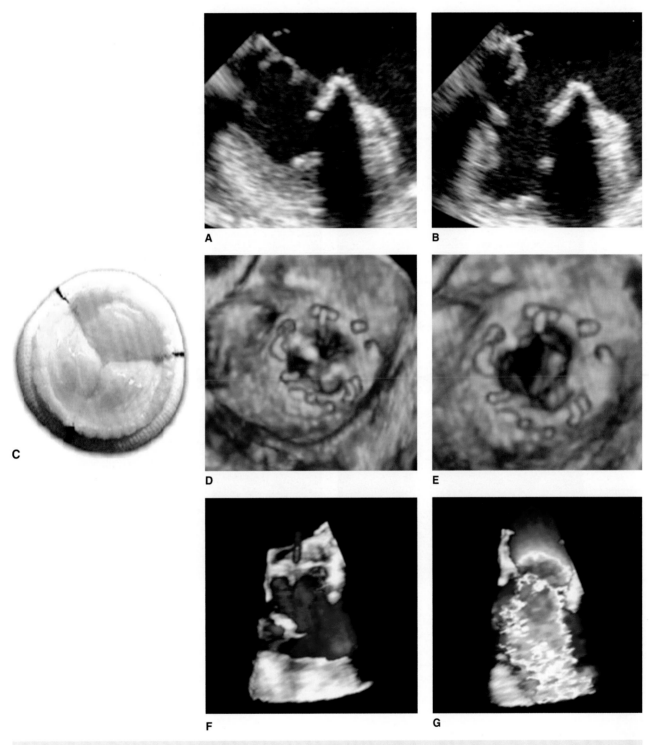

Figure 8-10. Imaging of an undersized bioprosthetic mitral valve. Two-dimensional transesophageal echocardiographic images of an undersized bioprosthetic mitral valve during systole (A) and diastole (B). When compared to the actual appearance of the bioprosthetic valve (C), the 3D transesophageal echocardiographic images in systole (D) and diastole (E) are realistic. In most patients, the prosthetic valve ring can easily be seen on 3D echocardiography, while the leaflets are more difficult to visualize. The 3D transesophageal echocardiographic color images demonstrate no valvular regurgitation during systole (F); however, there is flow convergence during diastole indicating stenosis (G).

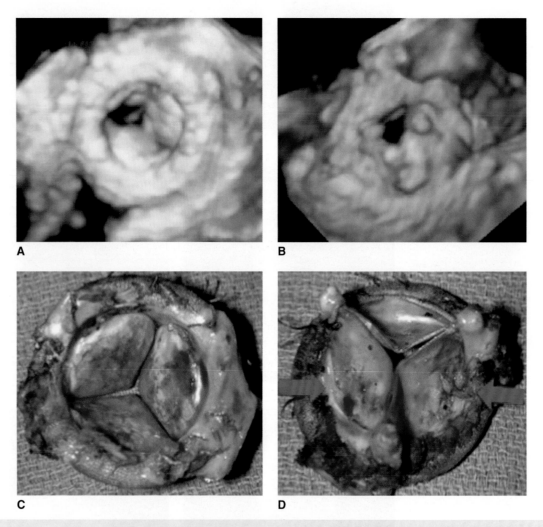

A

B

C

D

Figure 8-11. Calcification with restriction of bioprosthetic mitral valve leaflet motion. A bioprosthetic mitral valve is presented as seen en face from the left atrial (A) and left ventricular (B) perspectives during diastole. These 3D transesophageal echocardiographic images demonstrate that two of the three leaflets are relatively immobile, which resulted in stenosis. Accompanying Video 8-11 corresponds to Panels A and B. Surgical images of the excised valve from the left atrial (C) and left ventricular (D) side, shows extensive calcification of the two leaflets (*arrows*, D) on the left ventricular side of the valve causing their immobility.

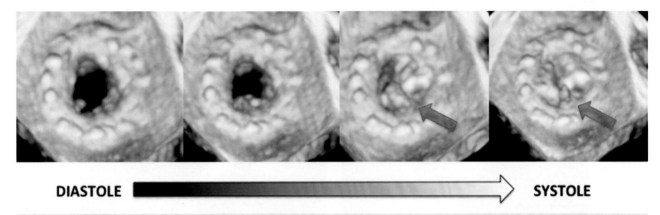

DIASTOLE ⟶ **SYSTOLE**

Figure 8-12. **Flail bioprosthetic mitral valve leaflet.** This series of 3D transesophageal echocardiographic images of a bioprosthetic mitral valve as viewed from the left atrium demonstrates identification of the flail leaflet (*arrows*) as the valve cycles from diastole to systole.

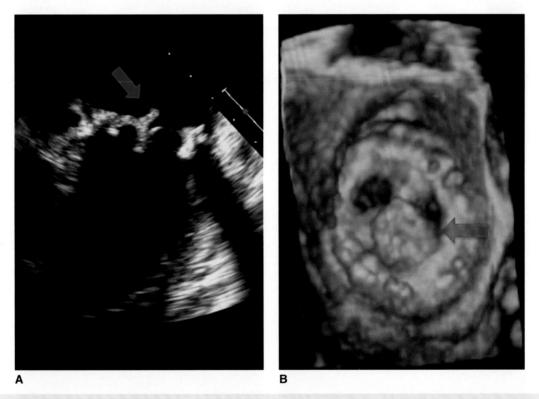

A   B

Figure 8-13. **Bioprosthetic mitral valve vegetation.** This 2D transesophageal echocardiographic image demonstrates the presence of a vegetation on the bioprosthetic mitral valve (A). Accompanying Video 8-13A corresponds to Panel A. With 3D TEE, the size of the vegetation can be appreciated when view en face from the left atrial perspective (B). Accompanying Video 8-13B corresponds to Panel B. It must be noted that 2D echocardiography is still superior in identifying the presence or absence of a small vegetation, whereas 3D echocardiography offers more information on assessing vegetation size and structural involvement.

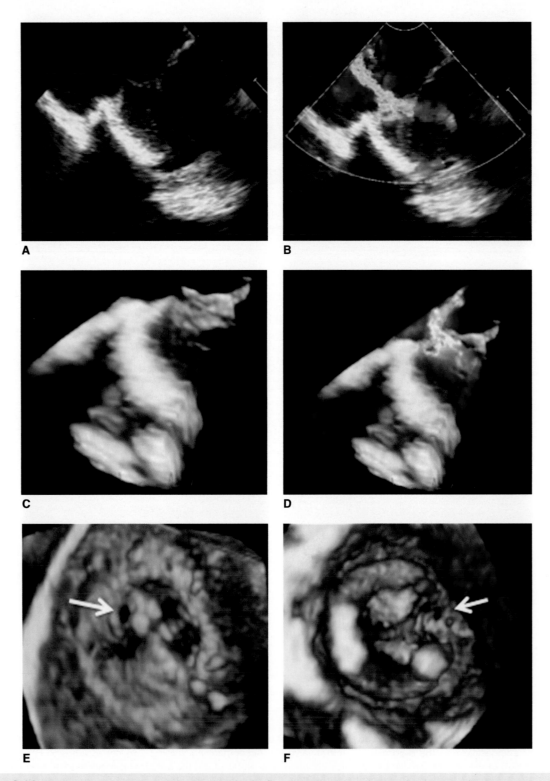

Figure 8-14. **Perforation of a bioprosthetic mitral valve leaflet.** Two-dimensional (A) and color Doppler (B) transesophageal echocardiographic image demonstrating perforation of a bioprosthetic mitral valve leaflet. The same view is presented for a 3D (C) and 3D color Doppler (D) transesophageal echocardiographic dataset. En-face views of the bioprosthetic mitral valve, from the left atrial (E) and the left ventricular (F) perspectives, allow the entire area of the perforation to be visualized (*white arrow*). Accompanying Video 8-14 corresponds to Panels E and F.

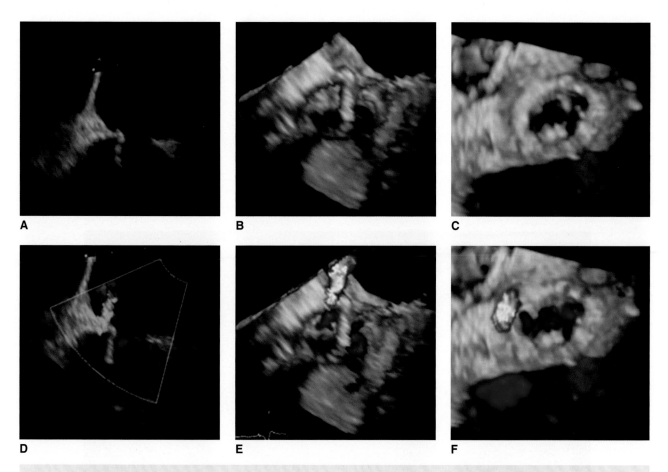

Figure 8-15. Paravalvular dehiscence of a bioprosthetic mitral valve. In this series of images, paravalvular regurgitation of a bioprosthetic mitral valve can be seen. The top row of images demonstrates the anatomy, and the lower row uses color to demonstrate the regurgitation. On 2D TEE, in the midesophageal two-chamber view, a paravalvular leak is identified (A,D). With 3D TEE, the leak can be seen (B,E); however, with the en-face view from the left atrial perspective, the entire site of the leakage can be appreciated (C,F). Accompanying Video 8-15 corresponds to Panels C and F.

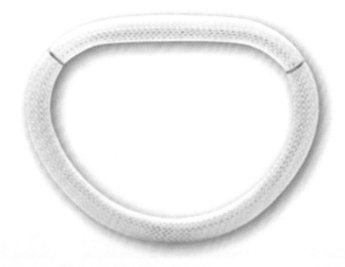

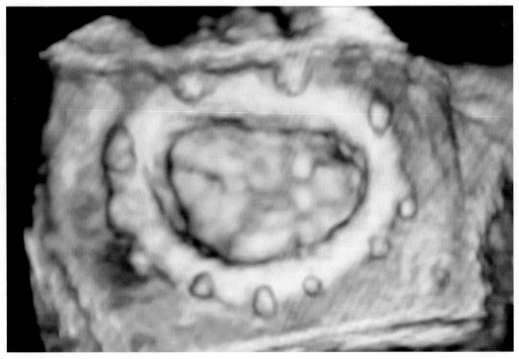

Figure 8-16. **Normal Carpentier-Edwards Physio mitral annuloplasty ring.** The top image demonstrates the actual appearance of a Carpentier-Edwards Physio mitral annuloplasty ring. The bottom image demonstrates how 3D TEE allows the entire ring to be visualized, and its appearance reflects its true structure.

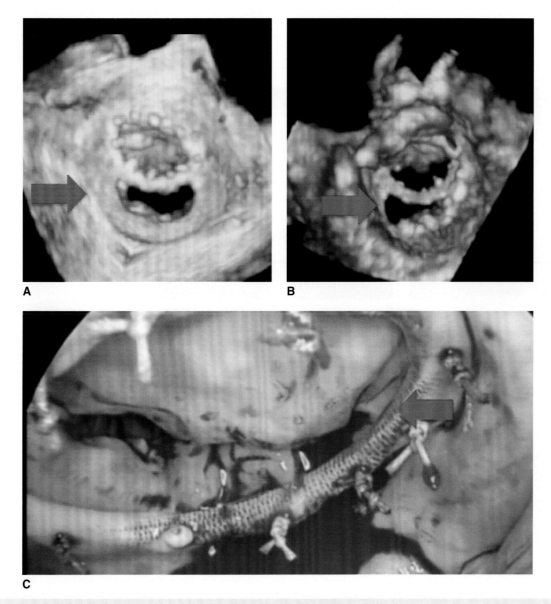

A

B

C

Figure 8-17. **Dehiscence of a Carpentier-Edwards Physio ring.** Dehiscence (*arrows*) of a Carpentier-Edwards Physio ring in the posterior region the mitral annulus as visualized en face from the left atrial (A) and left ventricular (B) perspectives. Accompanying Videos 8-17A and B corresponds to Panels A and B. The intraoperative image demonstrates how the 3D echocardiographic images reflect the true pathology (C).

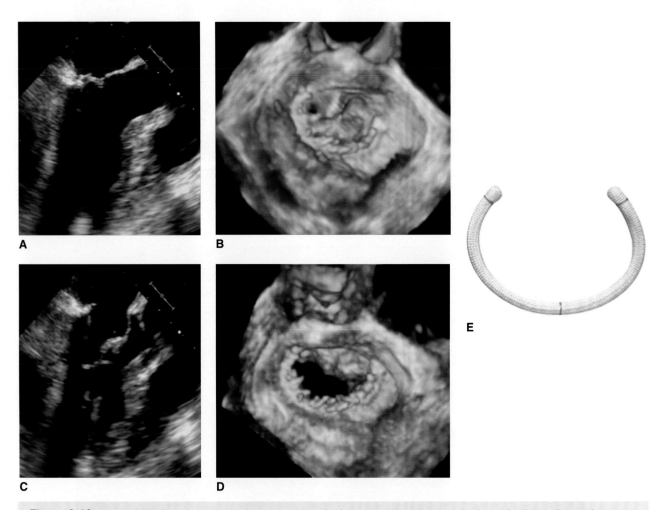

Figure 8-18. Normal Medtronic Duran AnCore mitral annuloplasty ring. On 2D transesophageal echocardiographic imaging, the semicircular nature of the Medtronic Duran AnCore mitral annuloplasty ring is poorly appreciated (A,C). With 3D TEE, the ring's semicircular structure can be clearly demonstrated with en-face left atrial views during systole (B) and diastole (D) and is comparable to the actual appearance of the Medtronic Duran AnCore mitral annuloplasty ring (E).

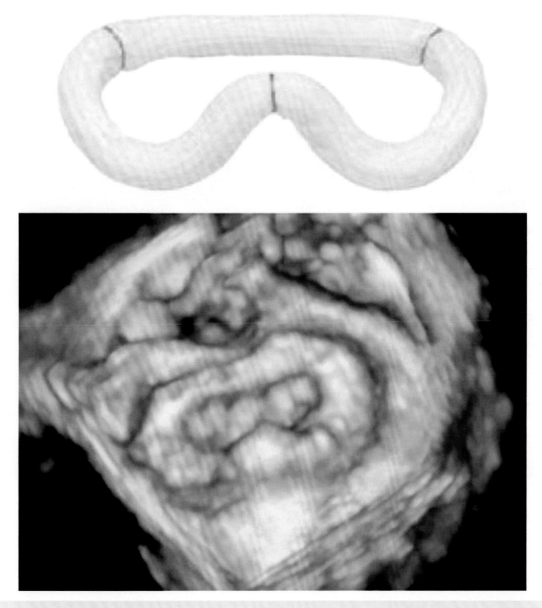

Figure 8-19. **Normal Edwards Geoform ring.** The top image demonstrates the actual appearance of an Edwards Geoform ring. The bottom picture is a 3D transesophageal echocardiographic image using zoomed mode of the Geoform ring implanted in the mitral valve position as viewed from the left atrial perspective. Accompanying Video 8-19 corresponds to the lower 3D echocardiographic image. This ring is used in patients with ischemic mitral regurgitation in an attempt to restore the saddle shape of the mitral valve.

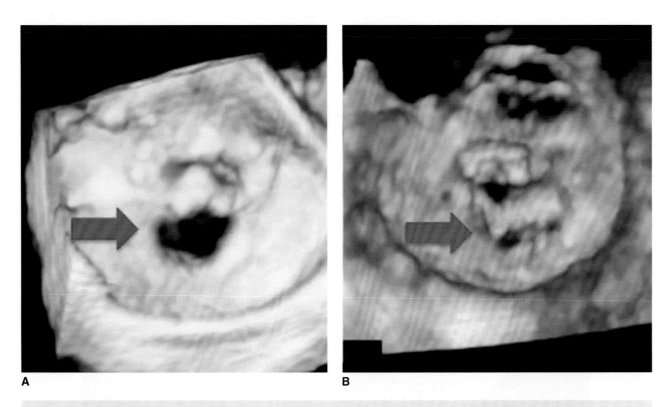

A B

Figure 8-20. **Dehiscence of a mitral valve annuloplasty ring.** Mitral valve annuloplasty rings typically experience dehiscence in the posterior portion of the annulus. This is due to four possible reasons: (1) poor visualization of this region by the surgeon due to its distal location in the surgical field leading to poor suturing, (2) cautious suturing by the surgeon to avoid of the circumflex artery, (3) poor suturing due to the propensity to develop calcification in this region, and (4) pulling of the posterior portion of the annulus by the anterior portion, which is restricted in motion after being sewn into the inflexible mitral fibrosa. On 3D TEE, the size and location of the dehiscence can be demonstrated with en-face views from the left atrial (A) and left ventricular (B) views.

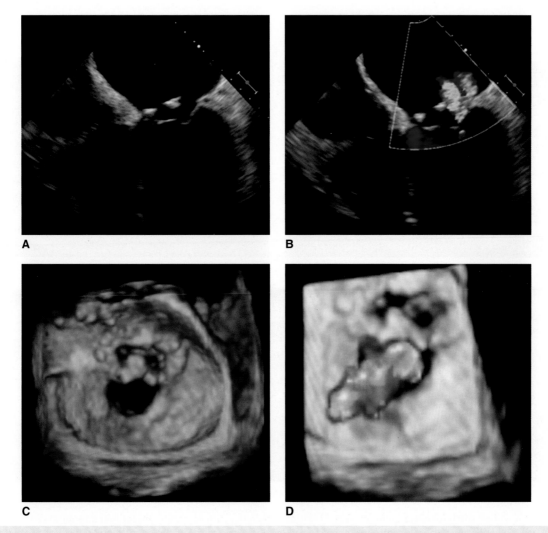

A   B

C   D

Figure 8-21. Two- and three-dimensional echocardiography of a dehisced Geoform mitral annuloplasty ring. Dehiscence of a 2D TEE can demonstrate the location of an Edwards Geoform mitral annuloplasty ring dehiscence (A) and with the use of color, the amount of regurgitation (B). However, with 3D TEE, the entire region can be presented en face from the left atrium in the "surgeon's view" for ease of communication (C). Color imaging with 3D TEE allows the entire regurgitant jet to be assessed in a single image and avoids missing other dehiscence sites (D). Accompanying Video 8-21 corresponds to Panels C and D.

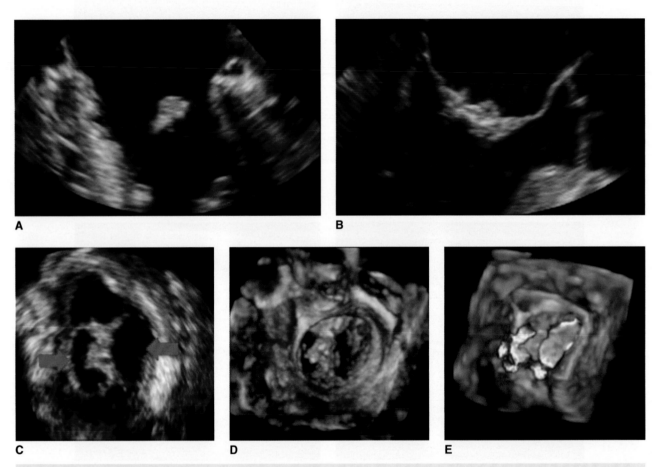

Figure 8-22. **Alfieri stitch for mitral regurgitation.** The Alfieri stitch is a surgical treatment for mitral regurgitation where the anterior and posterior mitral valve leaflets are sutured together to improve mitral leaflet coaptation during systole thus reducing regurgitation through the valve. As a consequence of this procedure, during diastole, the mitral valve has two orifices, one on either side of the stitch. From a 3D transesophageal echocardiographic dataset, planar views of the valve demonstrate the stitch during diastole in a two-chamber (A) and long-axis view (B). From a derived en-face plane, the two orifices can be seen (C, *red arrows*). On a zoomed 3D transesophageal echocardiographic image, the two orifices are easily visualized (D), and with the addition of color, blood flow through the valve can be visualized (E).

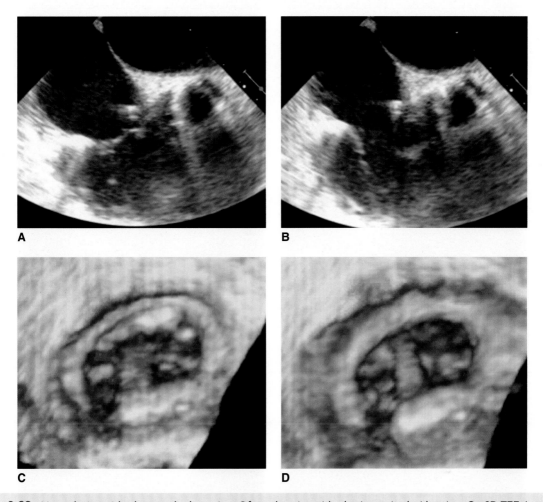

Figure 8-23. **Normal tricuspid valve annuloplasty ring.** Often, the tricuspid valve is repaired with a ring. On 2D TEE, imaging of the entire ring in systole (A) and diastole (B) is difficult due to the distance between the probe and the tricuspid valve. With zoomed mode acquisition on 3D TEE, an en-face image of the entire ring as seen from the right atrium can be displayed for assessment in systole (C) and diastole (D). Note that the tricuspid valve leaflets are difficult to visualize in their entirety during systole.

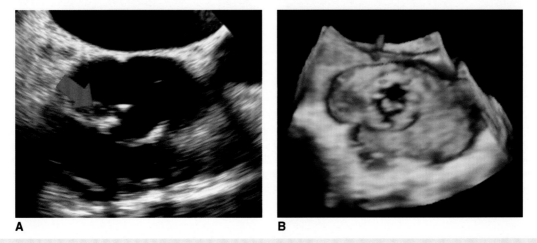

Figure 8-24. **Normal bioprosthetic tricuspid valve.** When a bioprosthetic valve is placed in the tricuspid valve position, the ring of the valve is easily visible on 2D TEE (A) and can be visualized en face from the right atrium with 3D TEE (B).

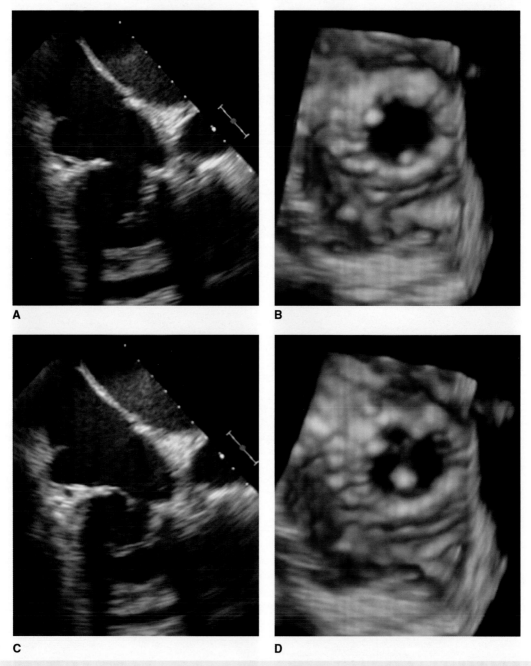

Figure 8-25. Two- and three-dimensional echocardiography of a normal bioprosthetic tricuspid valve These 2D transesophageal echocardiographic images demonstrate the presence of a bioprosthetic valve in the tricuspid position with normal function during diastole (A) and systole (B). The zoomed mode on 3D TEE allows the entire bioprosthetic tricuspid valve structure to be visualized en face from the right atrial perspective during diastole (C) and systole (D). While the ring is clearly seen in these images, the leaflets of the bioprosthetic valve may be difficult to visualize in their entirety during systole.

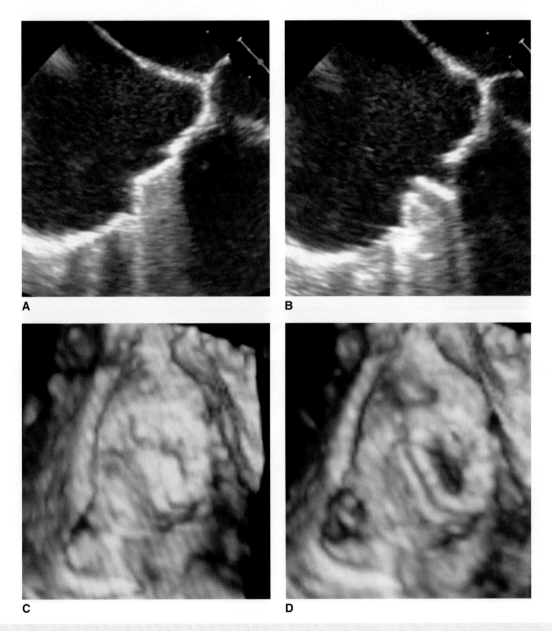

Figure 8-26. Normal bileaflet mechanical tricuspid valve. On 2D TEE, the leaflet motion in systole (A) and diastole (B) of a bileaflet mechanical valve placed in the tricuspid valve position can be visualized. With 3D TEE using zoomed mode, the en-face image of the prosthetic valve from the right atrium can be obtained showing the entire structure during systole (C) and diastole (D).

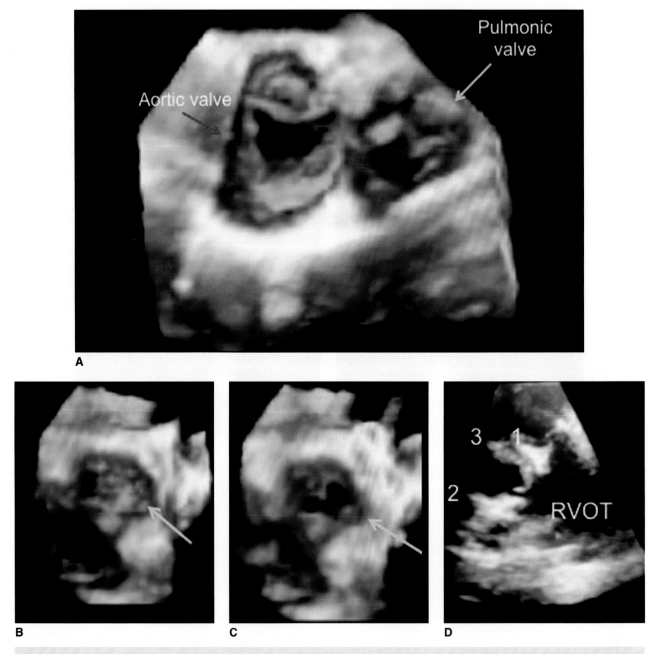

Figure 8-27. Normal bioprosthetic pulmonic valve. Due to the location of the pulmonic valve, image acquisition is challenging. Often, the prosthetic valve ring and struts can be visualized, while the leaflets are more difficult to image. Zoomed 3D transthoracic echocardiographic image demonstrating the proximity of the bioprosthetic pulmonic valve to the aortic valve (A). The bioprosthetic leaflets can be visualized during diastole (B) and systole (C) from the pulmonary artery perspective. As previously described, often, the three struts of the bioprosthetic pulmonic valve can be visualized with 3D transthoracic echocardiography (D). RVOT—right ventricular outflow tract.

References

1. Lang RM, Tsang W, Weinert L, et al. Valvular heart disease. The value of 3-dimensional echocardiography. *J Am Coll Cardiol*. 2011;58(19):1933–1944.

2. Lang RM, Badano LP, Tsang W, et al. EAE/ASE recommendations for image acquisition and display using three-dimensional echocardiography. *J Am Soc Echocardiogr*. 2012;25(1):3–46.

3. Sugeng L, Shernan SK, Weinert L, et al. Real-time three-dimensional transesophageal echocardiography in valve disease: comparison with surgical findings and evaluation of prosthetic valves. *J Am Soc Echocardiogr*. 2008;21(12):1348–1354.

4. Tsang W, Weinert L, Kronzon I, et al. Three-dimensional echocardiography in the assessment of prosthetic valves. *Rev Esp Cardiol*. 2011;64(1):1–7.

5. Sugeng L, Shernan SK, Salgo IS, et al. Live 3-dimensional transesophageal echocardiography initial experience using the fully-sampled matrix array probe. *J Am Coll Cardiol*. 2008;52(6):446–449.

6. Singh P, Manda J, Hsiung MC, et al. Live/real time three-dimensional transesophageal echocardiographic evaluation of mitral and aortic valve prosthetic paravalvular regurgitation. *Echocardiography*. 2009;26(8):980–987.

7. Kort S. Real-time 3-dimensional echocardiography for prosthetic valve endocarditis: initial experience. *J Am Soc Echocardiogr*. 2006;19(2):130–139.

8. Naqvi TZ, Rafie R, Ghalichi M. Real-time 3D TEE for the diagnosis of right-sided endocarditis in patients with prosthetic devices. *JACC Cardiovasc Imaging*. 2010;3(3):325–327.

9. Ruiz CE, Jelnin V, Kronzon I, et al. Clinical outcomes in patients undergoing percutaneous closure of periprosthetic paravalvular leaks. *J Am Coll Cardiol*. 2011;58(21):2210–2217.

10. Furukawa K, Kamohara K, Itoh M, et al. Real-time three-dimensional transesophageal echocardiography is useful for the localization of a small mitral paravalvular leak. *Ann Thorac Surg*. 2011;91(5):e72–e73.

11. Anayiotos AS, Smith BK, Kolda M, et al. Morphological evaluation of a regurgitant orifice by 3-D echocardiography: applications in the quantification of valvular regurgitation. *Ultrasound Med Biol*. 1999;25(2):209–223.

12. Chandra S, Salgo IS, Sugeng L, et al. A three-dimensional insight into the complexity of flow convergence in mitral regurgitation: adjunctive benefit of anatomic regurgitant orifice area. *Am J Physiol Heart Circ Physiol*. 2011;301(3):H1015–H1024.

13. Kronzon I, Sugeng L, Perk G, et al. Real-time 3-dimensional transesophageal echocardiography in the evaluation of post-operative mitral annuloplasty ring and prosthetic valve dehiscence. *J Am Coll Cardiol*. 2009;53(17):1543–1547.

14. Perk G, Lang RM, Garcia-Fernandez MA, et al. Use of real time three-dimensional transesophageal echocardiography in intracardiac catheter based interventions. *J Am Soc Echocardiogr*. 2009;22(8):865–882.

15. Lee AP, Lam YY, Yip GW, et al. Role of real time three-dimensional transesophageal echocardiography in guidance of interventional procedures in cardiology. *Heart*. 2010;96(18):1485–1493.

AORTIC VALVE

Gila Perk, Itzhak Kronzon, Muhamed Saric

ANATOMY

The aortic valve separates the left ventricular outflow tract (LVOT) and the aortic root. It forms the center part of the fibrous skeleton of the heart and is in close proximity with the other cardiac valves; the pulmonic valve is anterior to the aortic valve, the mitral valve (MV) posterolateral, and the tricuspid valve posteromedial to the aortic valve (Fig. 9-1). The components of the aortic valve include the annulus, cusps (or leaflets), commissures, and the interleaflet triangles. The nomenclatures used in the anatomical, surgical, and echocardiographic literature vary a little; we use the terminology that corresponds to the echocardiographic imaging of the aortic valve.

The aortic annulus is a fibrous structure extending from the junction of the aortic valve and the left ventricle up to the aortic root sinuses. The annulus is crown shaped and provides mechanical support to the valve complex. On echocardiography, the annulus size is measured at the junction of the valve and the left ventricle, at the nadir of the aortic valve, on the ventricular side of the valve.[1,2]

There are three cusps to the aortic valve, each semilunar (or crescent) shaped. The cusps are connected to the aortic root at their rim, which is somewhat thicker than the body of the cusps. The rims of adjacent cusps are slightly superimposed, providing more structural support to the valve. The free edges of the cusps come together during valve closure and form the coaptation zone of the valve. There is a small fibrous nodule at the center of the free edge of each cusp at the contact point with the other cusps. These nodules are named the nodule of Arantius. A mild dilatation of the aortic root at each of the cusps is noted. These areas form the sinuses of Valsalva. The sinuses are named according to the coronary artery originating from each of them: right, left, and noncoronary sinuses (Fig. 9-2 and Video 9-2-1 and 9-2-2).

The commissures are the small spaces between the attachment points of the cusps and the aortic root, and since they are composed of fibrous tissue extending radially into the aortic wall media, they contribute to the structural support of the MV. Between the commissures, small extensions of ventricular tissue stretch toward the sinotubular junction, forming the interleaflet triangles.

THREE-DIMENSIONAL IMAGING OF THE AORTIC VALVE

Due to anatomic considerations, the aortic valve is less well imaged by three-dimensional (3D) transesophageal echocardiography (TEE) as compared to the MV.[3] Some of the reasons for these apparent difficulties include the following:

1. The aortic valve leaflets are thinner as compared to the MV leaflets, such that when the gain is reduced to eliminate noise, dropout artifacts are seen in the aortic valve leaflets. These should not be confused with leaflet perforation; color Doppler imaging can be used to confirm lack of flow through the apparent "missing" tissue.

2. The more anterior position of the aortic valve makes its distance from the transducer greater than that of the MV.

3. In many imaging planes, the aortic valve plane is oblique to the ultrasound beam.

CONGENITAL ANOMALIES

Several anatomical variants of the aortic valve have been described. The most common one is a bicuspid aortic valve, resulting from fusion of two out of the three cusps, essentially creating a bileaflet valve (Fig. 9-3 and Video 9-3-1). The most common form of bicuspid aortic valve involves fusion of the right coronary cusp (RCC) and the left coronary cusp (LCC), creating a large anterior and a small posterior leaflet. This form accounts of approximately 80% of bicuspid aortic valve. Fusion of the right and the noncoronary cusps (resulting in a large RCC and smaller LCC) accounts for almost all the rest of the 20% of bicuspid aortic valve. The least common form involves fusion of the left and the noncoronary cusps, accounting for <1% of cases of bicuspid aortic valves.[4,5]

Other anomalies involving an abnormal number of aortic valve cusps have been described, including quadricuspid and unicuspid aortic valve (Fig. 9-4 and Videos 9-4-1 and 9-4-2).

Echocardiography plays a major role in diagnosing these anatomical variants and assessing their functional significance (e.g., creating aortic stenosis [AS], regurgitation, or both).

AORTIC VALVE DISEASE

AORTIC STENOSIS

The most common etiologies for valvular AS in developed countries include bicuspid aortic valve with superimposed aortic valve calcification and senile calcific AS on a trileaflet valve. Rheumatic disease accounts for only few cases of AS in Europe and the USA; however, worldwide, it is still a very common cause for AS.[6,7] Echocardiography plays a central role in the diagnosis and management of AS. Anatomic imaging allows for identification of the cause for the valvular dysfunction (e.g., bicuspid vs. tricuspid valve, Fig. 9-5 and Video 9-5-1), whereas Doppler echocardiography allows for the measurement of gradients across the valve, calculation of valve area, and assessment for the presence of concomitant aortic insufficiency. Current guidelines recommend the use of echocardiography for determination of the presence and severity of AS, management decisions (e.g., timing of surgical intervention) with use of invasive data only when inconsistent results are obtained by echocardiography.[8]

AS is most commonly treated surgically with aortic valve replacement. Choice of prosthetic valve (bioprosthesis vs. mechanical prosthesis) depends on patient characteristics including age, coexisting illnesses, preference, and technical considerations. Other treatment options include valve repair and balloon valvuloplasty. Valve repair is utilized in only a minority of patients who have relatively preserved leaflet mobility, which may be seen in patients with a stenotic bicuspid valve with only minimal calcification. Balloon valvuloplasty is utilized mainly as a temporizing measure in preparation for a more definitive treatment, or in patients at unacceptable risk for surgery who are unresponsive to medical therapy. Unfortunately, balloon valvuloplasty provides only short-term, minimal improvement for patients with AS.[9–11]

An important advancement of the past several years is the introduction of percutaneous treatment of AS, with catheter-based valve replacement. These procedures offer a new treatment modality for patients who are at high risk for conventional open heart surgery.[12,13] It is important to note that these procedures rely heavily on echocardiography (2D and 3D) for proper patient selection, intraprocedural guidance, and postprocedural surveillance.[14,15] The preprocedure echocardiographic assessment involves verifying the presence and severity of AS as well as confirming anatomic suitability for the procedure. Anatomic suitability mainly relies on accurate measurement of the aortic annulus and left ventricular (LV) outflow tract sizes (Fig. 9-6). Also, pre- or intraprocedural TEE is utilized to rule out severe aortic arch plaque, which can impact the approach to the aortic valve. During the procedure, 2D as well as 3D TEE, fluoroscopy, and computed tomography are utilized to facilitate catheter manipulations in the heart, guidance of the preimplant balloon valvuloplasty, and real-time evaluation of proper valve deployment and presence of any acute complications (e.g., paravalvular aortic insufficiency, pericardial effusion) (Figs. 9-7 and 9-8 and Videos 9-7-1 and 9-7-2).

AORTIC REGURGITATION

Aortic regurgitation (AR) can result from intrinsic valvular pathology or from aortic root pathology. Rheumatic heart disease, bicuspid aortic valve, infective endocarditis, subaortic membrane, ventricular septal defects, systemic lupus erythematosus, and ankylosing spondylitis are some of the diseases that can affect the aortic valve and result in AR. Dilatation of the aortic root with disruption of the normal valve anatomy interfering with proper co-optation of the leaflets is a common cause of progressive AR (Fig. 9-9 and Video 9-9-1). Dilatation of the aortic root can be seen in patients with Marfan's syndrome, cystic medial necrosis of the root, aortic aneurysm and dissection, systemic hypertension, syphilitic aortitis, and in a myriad of autoimmune disease with large-vessel involvement (e.g., giant cell arteritis). Like the case in AS, echocardiography plays a major role in the diagnosis of AR and in management decisions. Anatomic imaging can often identify the cause for the AR, as well as provide information regarding chamber sizes, overall LV function, and associated abnormalities (Fig. 9-10 and Video 9-10-1). Doppler echocardiography is helpful in quantifying the degree of AR, defining its severity, and assessing the hemodynamic consequences of the valvular pathology. Management decisions, in both the symptomatic and asymptomatic patients, rely heavily on echocardiographic assessment, which also aids in deciding about appropriate surgical intervention (e.g., valve replacement vs. valve sparing intervention).[16]

AORTIC VALVE MASSES

Masses seen on the aortic valve have a wide differential diagnosis. This includes tumors (most commonly fibroelastoma), strands, clots, and vegetations (both infectious and noninfectious). TEE with 3D imaging can help delineate the exact anatomic location, characteristics of the mass (heterogeneous vs. homogenous, shaggy, mobile, etc.), and the effect it has on the valve function (Fig. 9-11 and Video 9-11-1). For exact determination of the nature of aortic valve masses, clinical, laboratory, and occasionally pathologic data may be required.

PROSTHETIC AORTIC VALVES

Since aortic valve disease is very common, prosthetic aortic valves are encountered commonly in echocardiography practice. There are many types of prosthetic valves that are utilized in the aortic position: bioprosthetic valves, mechanical valves, and root conduits. Similar to native valves, anatomic considerations make the 3D TEE imaging of aortic prosthetic valves suboptimal as compared to that of mitral prosthetic valve. The aortic valve plane is often parallel or oblique to the ultrasound beam, making the anatomical imaging of the prosthetic valve challenging. However, despite these difficulties, TEE with 3D imaging often allows for adequate assessment of prosthetic valve morphology and function (Figs. 9-12 and 9-13 and Video 9-12-1). Real-time 3D (RT3D) imaging also plays a central role for diagnosis and occasionally treatment of prosthetic valve pathology. Over the past several years, percutaneous treatment of paravalvular leaks has become available, utilizing RT3D TEE imaging for guidance of the procedures (Fig. 9-14 and Video 9-14-1). In selected cases, percutaneous procedures are an attractive alternative for repeat open heart surgery, which by definition involves increased risk for the patient.[17]

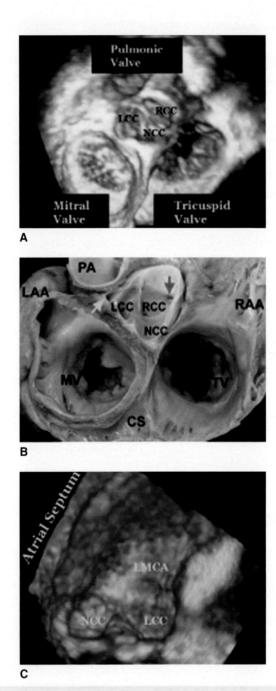

Figure 9-1. **Aortic valve view. A.** Four-valve view–RT3D transesophageal imaging allows for the acquisition of this unique view where all four valves and the fibrous skeleton of the heart can be visualized. **B.** Pathology correlate of the short-axis view of the base of the heart viewed from above looking downward. It shows the normal relationship of the tricuspid (TV), mitral (MV), and aortic valves. The noncoronary cusp (NCC) is in closest approximation to the tricuspid valve. The right coronary artery (RCA) (*red arrow*) arises from the RCC and the left coronary artery (*yellow arrow*) from the LCC. **C.** Spatial relationship of the aortic valve and the interatrial septum can be assessed by 3D echocardiography. The border between the interatrial septum and the aortic valve can be visualized and examined, for example, for suitability for percutaneous closure of atrial septal defects. Note the close proximity of the NCC of the aortic valve to the atrial septum (see also Chapter 11, Fig. 11-4). CS, coronary sinus; LAA, left atrial appendage; LCC, RCC, NCC, left, right, and noncoronary cusps of the aortic valve, respectively; LMCA, left main coronary artery; PA, pulmonary artery; RAA, right atrial appendage. Accompanying Video 9-1-1 corresponds to C.

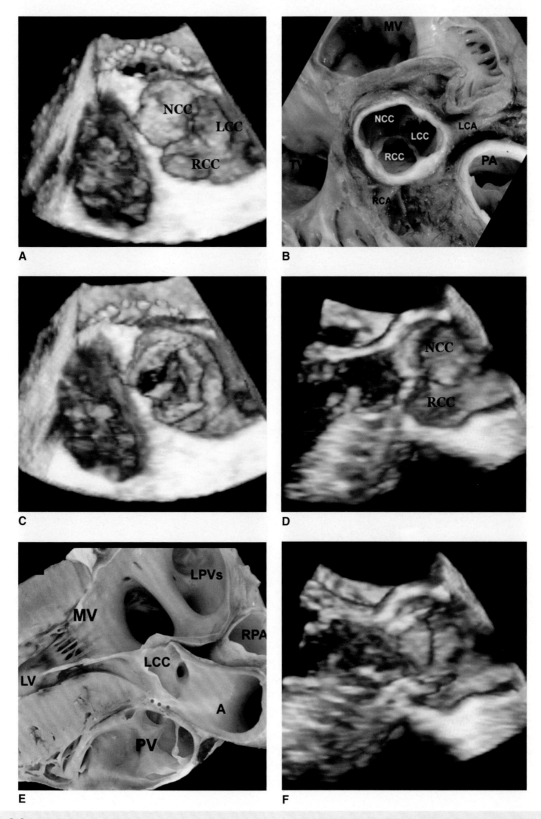

Figure 9-2. **Normal aortic valve. A–C.** Normal aortic valve as seen en face from the aortic root perspective (on RT3D echo-cardiography and a pathologic correlate) in diastole (A, B) and systole (C). **D–F.** Normal aortic valve as seen on long axis (on RT3D echocardiography and a pathologic correlate) in diastole (D, E) and systole (F). LCC, NCC, RCC, left, non-, and right coronary cusps, respectively; LPV, left pulmonary veins; RPA, right pulmonary artery; PA, main pulmonary artery. Accompanying Videos 9-2-1 and 9-2-2 correspond to A and C, respectively.

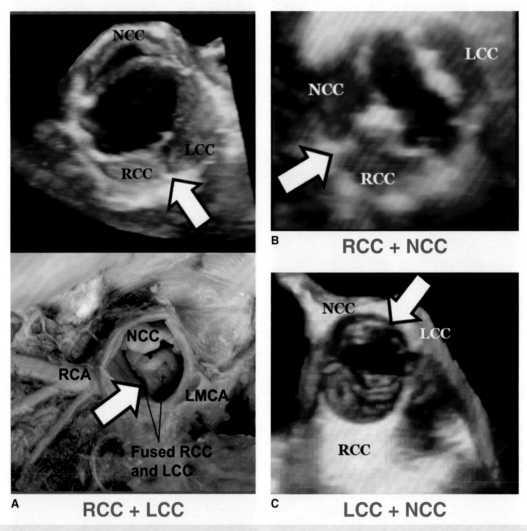

Figure 9-3. Bicuspid aortic valve variants. In general, bicuspid aortic valves are characterized by a fusion line (raphe) between two cusps. Each panel shows the 3D TEE zoom view of the aortic valve in its short axis. A. RT3D TEE zoom view and pathologic correlate of a raphe (*arrow*) between the RCC and the LCC. This is the most common type of bicuspid aortic valve; it accounts for approximately 80% of all bicuspid valves. B. Raphe (*arrow*) between the RCC and the NCC. This is the next most common type; it accounts for approximately 20% of all bicuspid aortic valves. Video 9-3-1 corresponds to B. C. Raphe (*arrow*) between NCC and LCC. This is a very rare type of bicuspid aortic valve. Accompanying Video 9-3-1 corresponds to B.

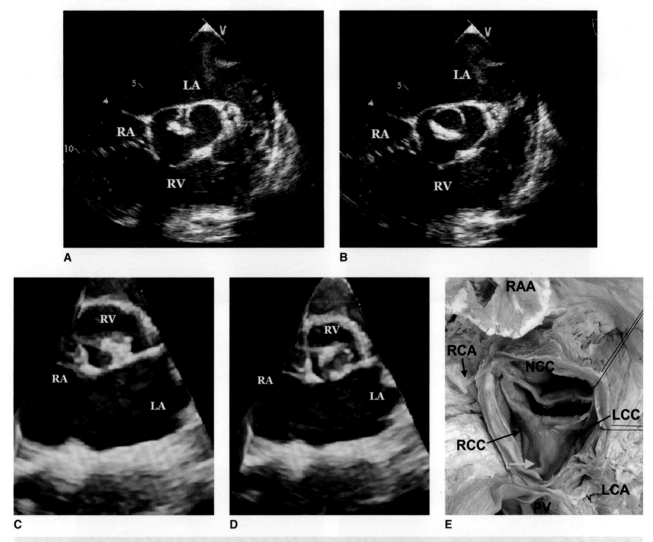

Figure 9-4. **Unicuspid aortic valve.** A rare congenital variant of aortic valve is a unicuspid valve. A and B show a unicuspid valve as seen en face from a TEE, in diastole and systole, respectively. C and D show a 3D, en-face view, from a transthoracic echocardiogram of the same patient. E shows a pathologic correlate of a unicuspid aortic valve viewed from the ascending aorta looking down. The leaflets are thickened; the orifice has an eccentric location within the aortic root. There is a single commissure marked with the *yellow arrow.* The RCA arises in the usual fashion. The left coronary orifice can be seen within a dilated aortic sinus. PA, pulmonary artery; RAA, right atrial appendage. Accompanying Videos 9-4-1 and 9-4-2 correspond to A and C, respectively. Courtesy of Dr. J. Mohan, All India Institute of Medicine.

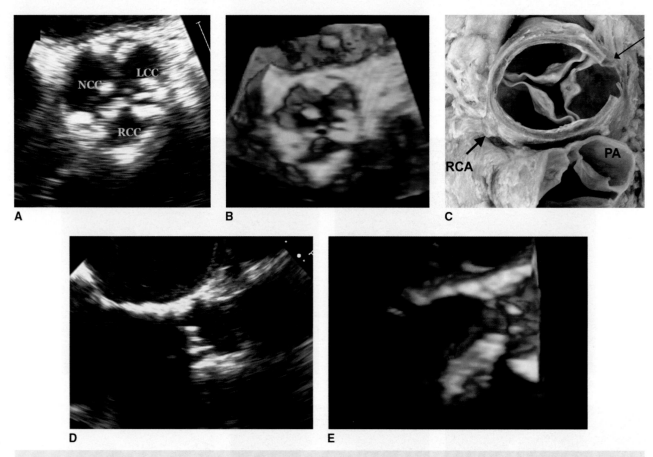

Figure 9-5. **Calcific aortic stenosis.** Trileaflet aortic valve with severe calcific aortic stenosis as seen on 2D (A, D) and 3D (B, E) TEE, as well as pathologic correlate. A and B and C show en-face view of the aortic valve from the aortic root perspective. D and E show a long-axis view of the aortic valve obtained at 120 degrees. LCC, NCC, RCC, left, non-, and right coronary cusps, PA, pulmonary artery, RCA, right coronary artery. Accompanying Video 9-5-1 corresponds to D.

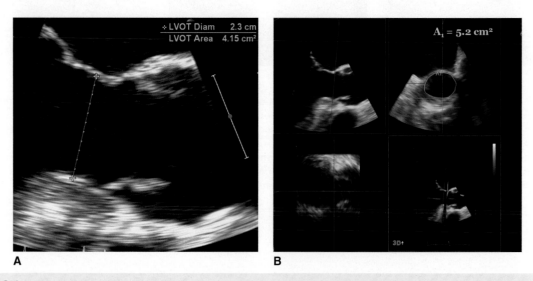

Figure 9-6. **Valve, LVOT, and root measurements.** Accurate measurements of the LVOT, aortic annulus, aortic root (at sinuses and sinotubular junction) can be of utmost significance. Postprocessing with 3D guided planimetry allows for direct measurement of these variables without the need for any geometrical assumptions. A shows a measurement of the LVOT as obtained on 2D TEE. Utilizing this measurement, the LVOT area is calculated to be 4.2 cm^2. B shows 3D guided direct planimetry of the LVOT area. Tracing of the LVOT shows an area of 5.2 cm^2.

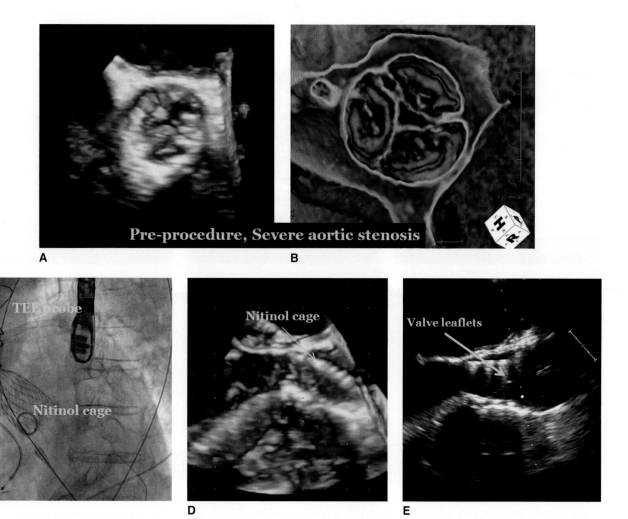

A   B

C   D   E

Figure 9-7. Multimodality imaging in percutaneous aortic valve replacement. A and B. Preprocedure assessment of aortic valve stenosis by RT3D TEE (A) and by computed tomography (B). C–E. Images obtained during deployment of percutaneous aortic valve prosthesis. C shows the fluoroscopic image during deployment of the valve. Note that the valve is only partially expanded. D shows 3D long-axis view of the aortic valve. E shows a 2D long-axis image of the aortic valve. Note that the thin leaflets within the nitinol cage can be visualized. Accompanying Video 9-7-1 corresponds to D, accompanying Video 9-7-2 corresponds to E.

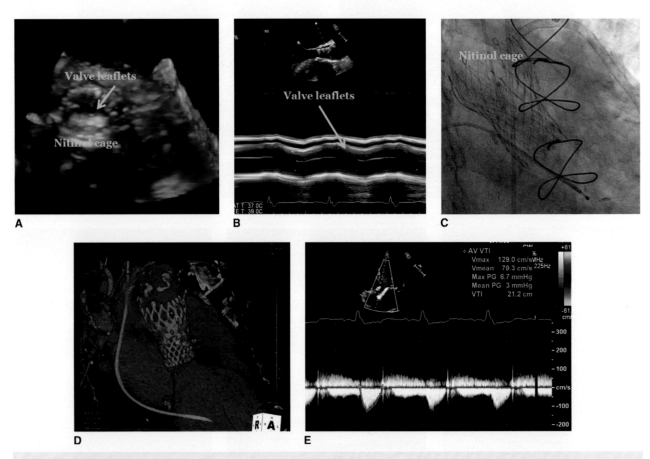

Figure 9-8. Multimodality imaging in percutaneous aortic valve replacement—cont. A. RT3D image showing the prosthetic valve as seen en face from the aortic root perspective. Note that the thin leaflets can be seen within the nitinol cage. B. M-mode image of the new prosthetic aortic valve showing clear delineation of the motion of the aortic valve leaflets with a typical "box on a string" appearance as seen in native aortic valves. C. Fluoroscopic image of the fully expanded aortic prosthesis. D. Computed tomography image of the prosthetic valve in good position in the LVOT and aortic root across the native aortic valve. E. Continuous wave Doppler obtained from a five-chamber view on a follow-up transthoracic echocardiogram showing no residual gradient across the aortic valve.

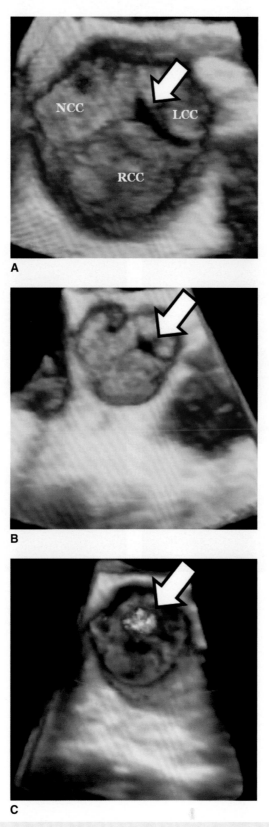

Figure 9-9. AR due to noncoapting leaflets. A. Three-dimensional TEE zoom view of the short axis of the aortic valve. A regurgitant orifice (*arrow*) arises because of underdevelopment and partial retraction of the LCC. NCC, noncoronary cusp; RCC, right coronary cusp. B. The so-called live 3D TEE view of the same aortic valve seen in A. Arrow points to the regurgitant orifice. C. Short-axis color Doppler view in the same patient demonstrating the aortic regurgitant jet (*arrow*). Accompanying Video 9-9-1 corresponds to A, B, and C.

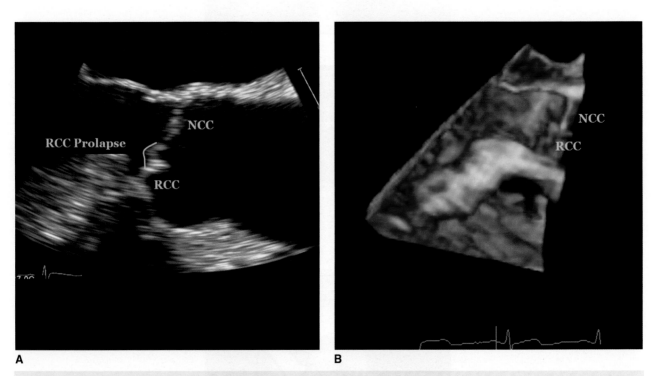

A   **B**

Figure 9-10. Aortic valve prolapse. Aortic valve prolapse can occasionally be found, which may or may not cause AR. Prolapse is defined as displacement of a part of a cusp below the attachment line of the aortic leaflets. In the example shown, prolapse of the RCC is seen on the long-axis view (both on 2D TEE [A] and 3D imaging [B]). The central part of the cusp can be seen reaching behind the leaflet closure line. RCC, NCC, right, and noncoronary cusps, respectively. Accompanying Video 9-10-1 corresponds to B.

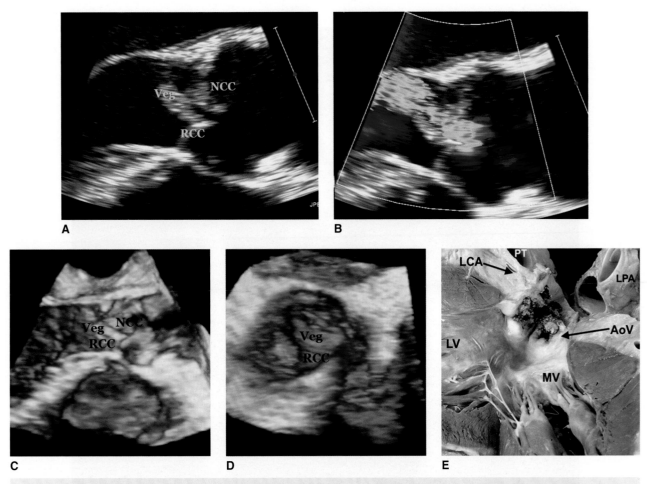

A

B

C

D

E

Figure 9-11. **Aortic valve vegetation.** Endocarditis can affect any one of the cardiac valves. In this example, a vegetation can be seen on the right coronary cusp of the aortic valve (A), causing severe AR (B). The mass can be also easily identified on 3D imaging, both on the long-axis view (C) and the en-face view (D). The key echocardiographic feature, typical of a vegetation, is that it has motion independent of the valve leaflet motion, which can be seen on accompanying video. Note on the video the vegetation prolapsing in and out of the aortic root and LVOT, as well as the independent oscillating notion of it. E shows a pathologic specimen obtained from a case of aortic valve endocarditis. The viewing perspective is from the apex into the LV outflow tract. The MV is thickened, with fused chordae tendinae. There is a calcified vegetation on the aortic valve (AoV). This vegetation involves all three aortic leaflets and causes severe stenosis. LCA, left coronary artery; LPA, left pulmonary artery. Accompanying Video 9-11-1 corresponds to C.

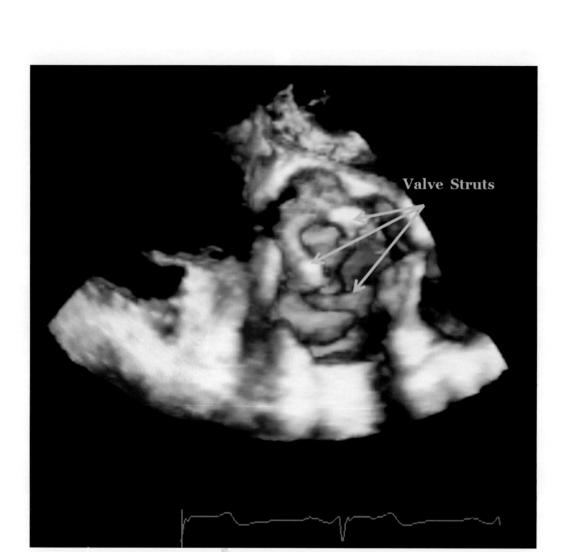

Figure 9-12. Aortic bioprosthesis. As explained in the text, the aortic valve is less optimally visualized by RT3D echocardiography as compared to the MV. In this figure, a normal bioprosthetic aortic valve is shown en face from the aortic root perspective. The valve struts are seen well pointing toward the aortic root; however, the leaflets are less well visualized. Nonetheless, RT3D imaging can be used to supplement assessment of aortic prosthetic valves. Accompanying Video 9-12-1 corresponds to the figure.

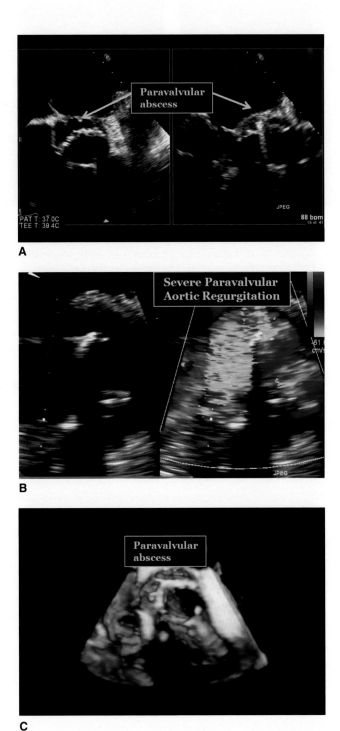

Figure 9-13. Paravalvular abscess. Endocarditis of a prosthetic valve can be complicated by development of paravalvular abscess. A. 2D transesophageal biplane view showing the aortic valve en face (left) and on long axis (right). Note the abscess cavity seen as a heterogeneous space around the posterior aspect of the aortic prosthesis. B. Due to the paravalvular abscess, severe paravalvular AR developed. C. RT3D image of the aortic bioprosthesis and paravalvular abscess seen en face from the aortic root perspective.

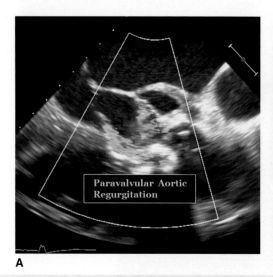
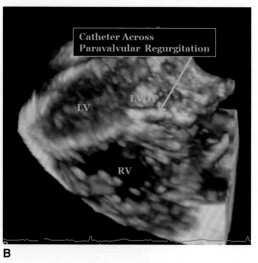

A   B

Figure 9-14. Percutaneous closure of paravalvular AR. Prosthetic valve endocarditis can be complicated by valve dehiscence and development of paravalvular AR. A. Paravalvular AR around an aortic bioprosthetic valve. The regurgitation jet can be seen in the anterior aspect of the prosthetic valve. B. The patient underwent a percutaneous closure procedure of the paravalvular AR. A catheter was introduced via a retrograde arterial approach and advanced into the left ventricle thorough the anterior paravalvular leak site, such that a closure device could be placed in the dehisced segment. Accompanying Video 9-14-1 corresponds to A.

References

1. David TE. An anatomic and physiologic approach to acquired heart disease. 8th annual meeting of the European Cardio-thoracic Association, The Hague, Netherlands, September 25–28, 1994. *Eur J Cardiothorac Surg.* 1995;9(4):175–180.

2. Sutton JP III, Ho SY, Anderson RH. The forgotten interleaflet triangles: are view of the surgical anatomy of the aortic valve. *Ann Thorac Surg.* 1995;59(2):419–427.

3. Faletra FF, DeCastro S, Pandian NG, et al. *Atlas of Real Time 3S Transesophageal Echocardiography.* 1st ed. Springer-Verlag London Limited; 2010:47.

4. Roberts WC. The congenitally bicuspid aortic valve. A study of 85 autopsy cases. *Am J Cardiol.* 1970;26(1):72–83.

5. Siu SC, Silversides CK. Bicuspid aortic valve disease. *J Am Coll Cardiol.* 2010;55(25):2789–2800 [Review].

6. Rajamannan NM, Evans FJ, Aikawa E, et al. Calcific aortic valve disease: not simply a degenerative process: a review and agenda for research from the National Heart and Lung and Blood Institute Aortic Stenosis Working Group. Executive summary: calcific aortic valve disease-2011 update. *Circulation.* 2011;124(16):1783–1791.

7. Kurtz CE, Otto CM. Aortic stenosis: clinical aspects of diagnosis and management, with 10 illustrative case reports from a 25-year experience. *Medicine (Baltimore).* 2010;89(6):349–379 [Review].

8. Baumgartner H, Hung J, Bermejo J, et al; American Society of Echocardiography; European Association of Echocardiography. Echocardiographic assessment of valve stenosis: EAE/ASE recommendations for clinical practice. *J Am Soc Echocardiogr.* 2009;22(1):1–23; quiz 101–102. Erratum in: *J Am Soc Echocardiogr.* 2009;22(5):442.

9. Otto CM, Mickel MC, Kennedy JW, et al. Three-year outcome after balloon aortic valvuloplasty. Insights into prognosis of valvular aortic stenosis. *Circulation.* 1994;89:642–650.

10. Safian RD, Berman AD, Diver DJ, et al. Balloon aortic valvuloplasty in 170 consecutive patients. *N Engl J Med.* 1988;319:125–130.

11. Percutaneous balloon aortic valvuloplasty. Acute and 30-day follow-up results in 674 patients from the NHLBI Balloon Valvuloplasty Registry. Circulation 1991;84:2383–2397.

12. Leon MB, Smith CR, Mack M, Miller DC, et al; PARTNER Trial Investigators. Transcatheter aortic-valve implantation for aortic stenosis in patients who cannot undergo surgery. *N Engl J Med.* 2010;363(17):1597–1607.

13. Smith CR, Leon MB, Mack MJ, et al; PARTNER Trial Investigators. Transcatheter versus surgical aortic-valve replacement in high-risk patients. *N Engl J Med.* 2011;364(23):2187–2198.

14. Chin D. Echocardiography for transcatheter aortic valve implantation. *Eur J Echocardiogr.* 2009;10(1):i21–i29.

15. Jayasuriya C, Moss RR, Munt B. Transcatheter aortic valve implantation in aortic stenosis: the role of echocardiography. *J Am Soc Echocardiogr*. 2011;24(1):15–27.

16. Zoghbi WA, Enriquez-Sarano M, Foster E, et al; American Society of Echocardiography. Recommendations for evaluation of the severity of native valvular regurgitation with two-dimensional and Doppler echocardiography. *J Am Soc Echocardiogr*. 2003;16(7):777–802.

17. Ruiz CE, Jelnin V, Kronzon I, et al. Clinical outcomes in patients undergoing percutaneous closure of periprosthetic paravalvular leaks. *J Am Coll Cardiol*. 2011;58(21):2210–2217.

Stephane Lambert, Mark S. Hynes

ANATOMIC CONSIDERATIONS

Often neglected because it is usually less affected by disease, the tricuspid valve (TV) operates in the lower pressure environment of the right ventricle (RV). As a result, it is not as prone to mechanical stress as the mitral valve (MV), but consequently, it is very sensitive to changes in pulmonary pressure and RV volume status. The TV is usually made up of three leaflets: the septal (S), anterior (A), and posterior (P) leaflets, but autopsy studies have demonstrated that there are frequent variants, with 30% of patients having only two leaflets, while 8% have four leaflets.[1] The number of papillary muscles and their attachment to the tricuspid leaflets is also highly variable. The TV is located more anteriorly and more apically than the MV and also has a larger surface area.[2]

The tricuspid annulus is not as well defined as its mitral counterpart, but it is dynamic and plays an equally important role in the function of the valve. Geometrically, magnetic resonance imaging (MRI) suggests that it is oval shaped and its surface area decreases by 39% during systole.[3] The tricuspid annulus also descends significantly toward the ventricular apex during systole, which is an important echocardiographic indicator of overall RV function.

PATHOLOGIC CONSIDERATIONS

Mild tricuspid regurgitation (TR) is extremely common, and it is usually asymptomatic. Significant TR is almost always *functional* in nature, as a result of some other pathologic process in the heart or pulmonary vasculature. Chronic MV or aortic valve (AV) disease, dilated cardiomyopathy, and chronic intracardiac shunt are common causes. Pulmonary hypertension from chronic lung disease can also result in significant TR. Regardless of the initial cause, the final common pathway is usually pressure and/or volume overload of the RV, which leads to ventricular dilatation, tricuspid annular dilatation, apical tethering of leaflets, and TR. Organic TR is less frequent and includes leaflet prolapse from myxomatous disease, ruptured *chordae tendinae* secondary to trauma or infection, leaflet disruption from endocarditis, tethering due to pacemaker wires or other transvalvar catheters, primary rheumatic disease, and congenital disease including Ebstein's anomaly and other congenital dysplasias.

Tricuspid stenosis (TS), on the other hand, is almost always rheumatic in origin, but the TV is involved much less frequently than the AV or MV. Other rare causes of TS include carcinoid syndrome, which usually causes a mix of TS and TR, and congenital heart disease.

ORIENTATION OF THE VALVE AND CARDIAC LANDMARKS

Echocardiographically, the standard two-dimensional transesophageal echocardiography (2D-TEE) views of the TV include the midesophageal (ME)-four-chamber view (Fig. 10-1), the ME-RV inflow/outflow view, and the transgastric (TG)-RV inflow view, which displays the TV and its subvalvular apparatus in long axis. Finally, a modified TG-RV view, which is orthogonal to the long-axis view, reveals a cross-section of the valve (Fig. 10-2), allowing an appreciation of the tricuspid leaflet anatomy. Given the variability between patients and the degree of rotation/distortion of the heart by pathology, the specific TV leaflets seen in each of these various planes can vary greatly. It is important to remember these standard two-dimensional (2D) cross-sections of the TV, because they are the same "vantage points" from which three-dimensional (3D) images are generated.

The standard 2D-TEE measurement of the tricuspid annular diameter is routinely taken in the ME-four-chamber view (Fig. 10-3). This is a transesophageal echocardiography (TEE) application of the widely accepted transthoracic measurement in the apical four-chamber view. In this imaging plane, the normal tricuspid annulus measures 28 mm ± 10 mm, with an upper limit of normal of 40 mm, or 16 mm/m^2 ± 6 mm^2.[4] Unfortunately, this measurement corresponds neither to the true short nor to the true long axis of the valve. Using 3D reconstructions, one study of 63 patients suggested that the normal tricuspid *long-axis* diameter is 40 mm ± 7 mm.[5] Real-time 3D-TEE promises to improve our ability to accurately evaluate the tricuspid annulus in the operating room (Fig. 10-4).

TECHNICAL CONSIDERATIONS FOR 3D IMAGING

Compared to other valves, the body of literature on three-dimensional transesophageal echocardiography (3D TEE) of the TV is relatively limited. This stems from the fact that the TV is not as easy to image as the MV or AV, although this may change quickly with improving technology.[6] Because the TV sits relatively far from the TEE transducer, it is sometimes difficult to achieve optimal gain. Even if enough gain is applied to visualize the thin leaflets well, the image can be "polluted" by artifact. If the gain is turned down to eliminate the artifact, the tricuspid leaflets often disappear also. The operator must decide which of these suboptimal conditions has the least impact on the valve being studied and how to adjust the settings accordingly.

As with any other cardiac structure, 3D echocardiography offers three main modalities to examine the TV: (1) *full volume and 3D-zoom*, (2) *multiplanar reconstruction*, and (3) *full-volume color flow Doppler views*. A *full volume or 3D-zoom image* (Figs. 10-4 and 10-5) displays a pyramidal volume of data that can be rotated or cropped in any direction in order to identify a relevant structural question pertaining to leaflet prolapse, ruptured chordae tendinae, or valve stenosis. By cropping or slicing the dataset volume in planes similar to standard 2D-TEE views, a more comprehensive understanding of the valve and its surrounding structures can be obtained (Fig. 10-6). Technically, highly resolved and detailed en-face views of the TV are often hard to obtain from the transesophageal position, because the valve is relatively far from the transducer. The echogenicity of the valve leaflets also tends to be relatively low compared to the surrounding tissues, making optimal gain settings difficult. By contrast, en-face views of the TV are relatively easy to obtain from the TG position, where the valve is closer to the transducer (Fig. 10-7). The challenge from this vantage point is to include the entire valve in a single sector scan in order to analyze valve structures, especially the annulus.

Multiplane reconstruction (MPR) views (Figs. 10-8A and 10-8B). Paradoxically, these allow a "deconstruction" of cardiac structures into three simultaneous orthogonal 2D axes. In the case of the TV, this proves much more useful than other 3D modes for quantitative analysis. First, the MPR technique facilitates the precise recognition of the various leaflets, by allowing cross-referencing of each view in other planes. Second, it demonstrates the coaptation between each pair of leaflets (A-P, A-S, and P-S) in a way that is not possible with 2D-TEE. Finally, MPR allows for measurement of the TV annulus.

Color Doppler 3D (Fig. 10-9) displays a real-time 3D reconstruction of blood flow, which in everyday practice provides a qualitative visual estimation of TR severity, and may also help to provide a clue to the etiology and mechanism. In addition, 2D planimetry of the *vena contracta* area promises to provide a more reliable quantitative assessment of TR than the currently used, 2D *vena contracta* diameter (Fig. 10-10).

Simultaneous orthogonal 2D views are unique to a 3D matrix transducer and allow the real-time display of two 2D perpendicular planes across a structure including the TV (Fig. 10-11). Like MPR, simultaneous orthogonal 2D views are useful to cross-reference the position of the scanning plane and to facilitate the identification of leaflets and lesions in the longitudinal planes.

FUTURE DIRECTIONS

Future research will likely focus on standardizing 3D images of the TV and validating specific measurements against other imaging techniques. The ability of 3D echocardiography to ascertain TV annular dimensions will be particularly important (Fig. 10-12). Finally, the current guidelines on the management of tricuspid annular dilatation at the time of MV surgery may be updated, based on new 3D information.

UTILITY OF 3D ECHOCARDIOGRAPHY FOR EVALUATING TV PATHOLOGY

Three dimensional echocardiographic techniques enable comprehensive analysis of the spectrum of encountered TV pathology (Figs. 10-13 through 10-22).

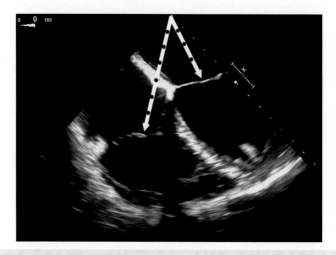

Figure 10-1. **Two-dimensional TEE, ME-four-chamber view.** Note that the TV is almost twice as far from the TEE transducer as the MV. Under most circumstances, the tricuspid leaflets are very thin and difficult to visualize in detail. Note the difference in echogenicity of the tricuspid leaflets compared to the surrounding structures. This makes proper gain adjustment difficult, in both 2D and 3D imaging. See Video 10-1.

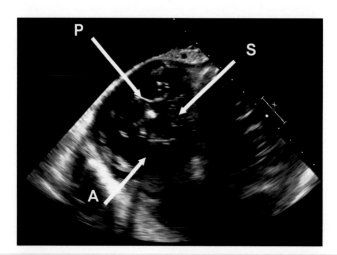

Figure 10-2. **Two-dimensional TEE image of a TG short axis of the TV.** This view can easily be obtained from the TG-RV inflow view, by rotating the transducer to about 40 to 60 degrees. The three leaflets are indicated by *arrows*: S, septal; A, anterior; and P, posterior. Note that in the TG position, the valve is much closer to the TEE transducer. Consequently, the leaflets are brighter and better defined. However, because the probe is close to the TV, it is sometimes difficult to include the entire tricuspid annulus in a single sector, making its measurement difficult. The bright artifact in the center of the valve is a pulmonary artery catheter. See Video 10-2.

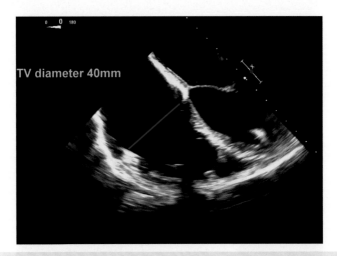

Figure 10-3. Tricuspid annular measurement by 2D-TEE. Tricuspid annular dilatation is usually associated with pulmonary hypertension and RV dilatation and is the most common cause of TR. It is important to measure the tricuspid annulus at the time of MV surgery because it may have an impact on the intraoperative management. A dilated tricuspid annulus associated with moderate to severe TR should be repaired at the time of MV surgery,[7,8] since patients who later develop severe TR have a poor prognosis.[9,10] The generally accepted measurement of the TV annulus by 2D-TEE is done in the ME-four-chamber view. Unfortunately, this diameter corresponds neither to the true long nor to the true short axis of the oval-shaped TV.

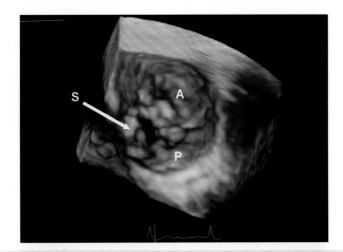

Figure 10-4. This full-volume 3D TEE en-face view of the TV is displayed from the right atrial (RA) perspective. In this view, the observer is located in the right atrium looking "down" at the TV. Note that the normal TV is not round. Because of the distance between the valve and the transducer, the gain may be difficult to adjust. The leaflets are labeled S, septal; A, anterior; and P, posterior. See Video 10-4.

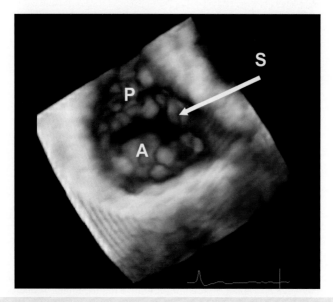

Figure 10-5. This full-volume 3D TEE en-face view of the TV is displayed from the RV perspective. In this view, the observer is located in the RV looking "up" at the TV to visualize the ventricular aspect of the leaflets. The leaflets are labeled S, septal; A, anterior; and P, posterior. See Video 10-5.

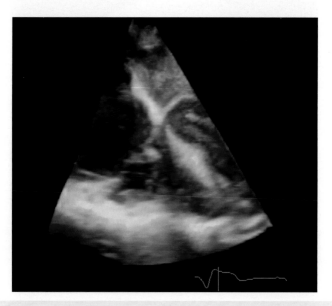

Figure 10-6. A full-volume 3D TEE view of the TV cropped to mimic a ME-four-chamber view. Once a pyramidal dataset is acquired, it can be sliced in any desired way to demonstrate a specific cardiac structure. In this view, the anterior wall of the RV and the anterior tricuspid annulus are removed to display a ME-four-chamber view equivalent, with added depth perception. The cropping plane can be adjusted anywhere through the TV. The image can also be rotated, and the posterior wall of the heart can be removed to reveal the anterior leaflet of the valve. See Video 10-6.

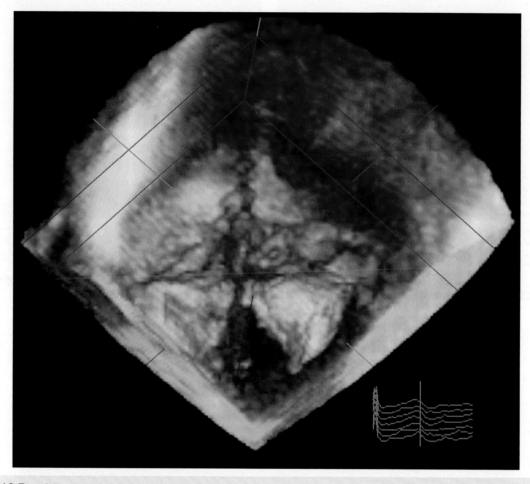

Figure 10-7. A full-volume 3D TEE reconstruction of the TV obtained from the TG position. This is a multibeat reconstruction image, as evidenced by the gated-ECG signal at the bottom of the screen. Also, this is not an en-face view. Rather, the image was tilted to demonstrate the leaflet texture and part of the subvalvular apparatus. In this view, the observer is "sitting" on the posterior leaflet, looking anteriorly: The septal leaflet is deep and to the left of the image, while the anterior leaflet is deep and to the center-right of the image. Note how clear and detailed the leaflets and subvalvular apparatus appear in this view when the image is obtained from the TG position because of the closer proximity to the transducer. The artifact in the center of the valve is a pulmonary artery catheter. See Video 10-7.

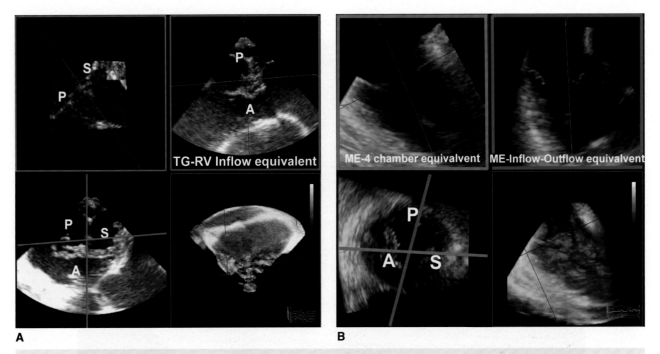

A

B

Figure 10-8A and 10-8B. MPR of the TV. Because 3D acquires a "pyramidal volume" of data rather than a single plane of data, simultaneously multiple planes of the same structure can be displayed. In MPR mode, three orthogonal planes are displayed in three boxes. Adjusting the plane in one box causes a change to the corresponding image in the other two boxes according to a color code (*blue line corresponds to blue box, red line to red box, and green line to green box*). When the TV is set in the middle of these three planes, this powerful tool facilitates the precise recognition of the valve structures, by allowing cross-referencing of each view in the other two planes. In this example, the reference image in the blue box (**lower left**) is adjusted to show a perfect transverse plane across the base of the valve. This allows easy identification of the three leaflets (labeled S, septal; A, anterior; P, posterior). By placing the green line across the posterior and septal leaflets, the green box (**top left**) displays the same leaflets in an anteroposterior cross-section. Similarly, the red box (**top right**) displays the third orthogonal plane, in an axis determined by the position of the red line. See Videos 10-8A and 10-8B.

Figure 10-8A and Video 10-8A were obtained with the TEE probe in the TG position, as evidenced by the position of the apex of the scan. The image in the top right box (*red*) corresponds to the scanning plane defined by the red line in the bottom left box. Note how in a typical TG-RV inflow view the imaging plane usually cuts through the posterior and anterior leaflets. Note also that the dilated tricuspid annulus cannot be seen in its entirety in this view, which would preclude accurate measurement in this image.

Figure 10-8B and Video 10-8B were obtained with the probe in the transesophageal position. The green plane was adjusted to produce a typical ME-four-chamber view in the top left box (*green*) and a typical ME-inflow/outflow view in the top right (*red*) box. This technique clearly demonstrates that in the ME-four-chamber view, the scanning plane typically cuts through the septal and anterior leaflets. In the ME-RV inflow/outflow view, the scanning plane usually cuts through the anterior and posterior leaflets although this could change depending on the degree of probe and transducer rotation.

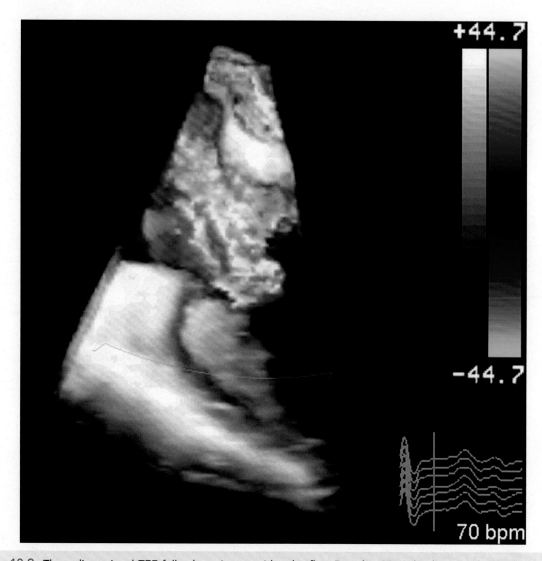

Figure 10-9. **Three-dimensional TEE full-volume image with color flow Doppler.** 3D technology can be applied not only to cardiac structures but also to blood flow. In this example, a severe TR jet was captured in 3D and is cropped to mimic a ME-four-chamber view. Rotating the image allows a better appreciation of the size of the jet, its precise origin (i.e., center of the valve vs. commissure), and direction (i.e., central vs. eccentric). Note from the position of the apex of the scan that this image was obtained in the ME position. Some jets may be seen better when the probe is in the TG position. This mode provides mostly a qualitative and semiquantitative analysis of a regurgitant jet. See Video 10-9.

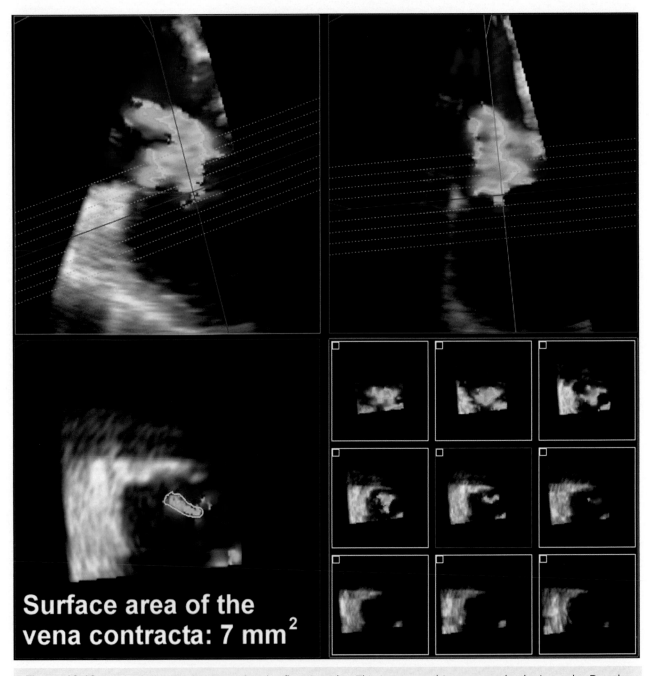

Surface area of the
vena contracta: 7 mm²

Figure 10-10. **Three-dimensional MPR, with color flow Doppler.** This image combines two technologies: color Doppler and MPR. Once a color Doppler jet is captured in 3D, it can be cropped or "sliced" just like any other 3D structure. The regurgitant jet is perfectly aligned in the red and green axes (*red line in the top left box and green line in top right box*). This technique provides a series of perfectly transverse cuts through the jet (*multiple blue lines*). The number and thickness of the blue planes are set by the operator. Each blue plane is displayed in one of the multiple boxes at the bottom right of the screen. The vena contracta is defined as the narrowest point of the jet. Thus, the plane with the smallest aliasing jet is used to perform planimetry of the vena contracta area. In this example, the measurement is 7 mm², consistent with severe TR. This technique promises to be more reliable than the simple diameter measurement in 2D, because most regurgitant jets are not perfectly circular. See Video 10-10.

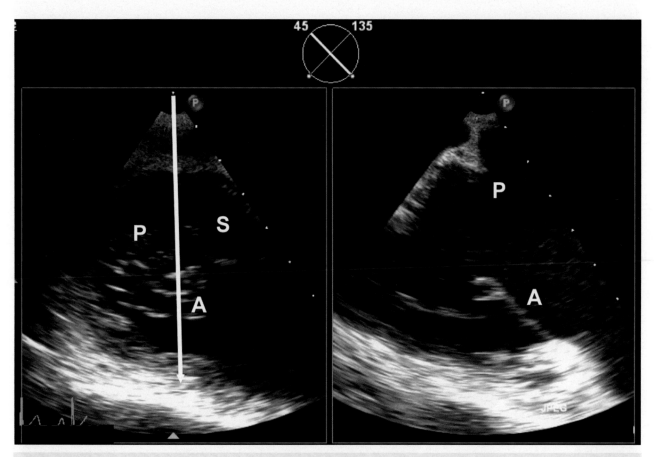

Figure 10-11. Simultaneous orthogonal cross-sections, with the probe in the TG position, allow the simultaneous real-time display of two 2D perpendicular planes across a structure. The cursor in the left image can be adjusted to modify the scanning plane in the right image. This is similar to MPR, but it only displays two perpendicular planes. However, simultaneous orthogonal cross-sections can be displayed in real time and can be more efficient. Like MPR, this technique is useful to cross-reference the position of the scanning plane and to facilitate the identification of leaflets and lesions in the longitudinal planes. This image of the TV is displayed in short axis on the left with its three leaflets, S, septal; A, anterior; and P, posterior. The white cursor line on the left defines the scanning plane on the right-hand side and cuts through edge of the posterior near the annulus and across most of the anterior leaflet. These structures are clearly seen in the image on the right. See Video 10-11.

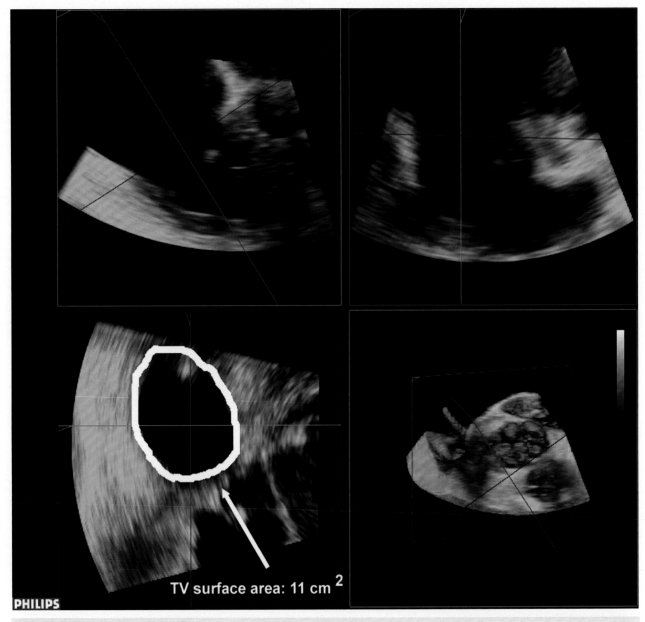

Figure 10-12. Planimetry of the TV annulus using MPR. After aligning the valve in two orthogonal axes (*red line in top left box and green line in the top right box*), the third plane (*blue*) is set across the TV annulus in both of the top boxes. This technique produces a perfectly transverse cut through the tricuspid annulus. The annulus is then measured by planimetry to obtain its surface area. Specific diameters can also be measured in both the long and short axes. Note that the plane defined by the green line in the bottom left box corresponds to a typical ME-four-chamber view (*displayed in the top left box*). Note how this plane cuts the valve annulus obliquely (*bottom left box*), reflecting neither the true short axis nor the true long axis of the valve.

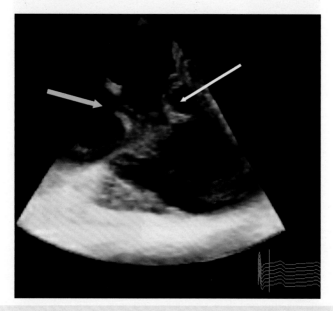

Figure 10-13. Three-dimensional TEE image of a flail TV. This image is a 3D full-volume view of the TV, which has been cropped to mimic a ME-four-chamber view. The image is taken in midsystole. The *yellow arrow* demonstrates a flail anterior tricuspid leaflet, while the *white arrow* points to the septal leaflet, which is redundant and slightly prolapsed. Note that in the standard 2D, ME-four-chamber view, the leaflet seen on the left-hand side can be either the anterior or the posterior leaflet, depending on the patient's anatomy, the position of the probe and the degree of ante-/retroflexion. Likewise, in this image, the leaflet seen on the left-hand side could be the anterior or the posterior leaflet. Progressive cropping of the image from front to back would allow for clear identification of each leaflet. Note also the brown artifact in the center of the valve. In order to display the leaflets correctly, one must often accept a certain degree of "gain artifact." Eliminating the gain artifact may also result in the loss of part of the leaflet structure. See Video 10-13.

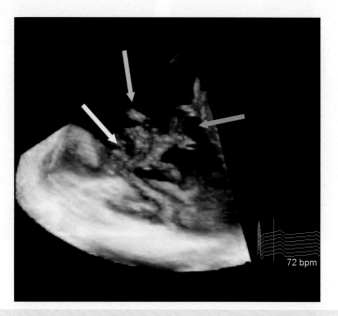

Figure 10-14. Three-dimensional TEE image of a flail TV. This is the same image as in Figure 10-13, but the image is slightly tilted between a standard en-face top view and a four-chamber equivalent in a nonstandard, modified view. The cropping plane was also moved slightly anteriorly, just anterior to the flail segment of the anterior leaflet. Note the billowing septal leaflet (*blue arrow*), the posterior leaflet (*white arrow*), and the flail segment of anterior leaflet (*yellow arrow*). The bulk of the anterior leaflet is cropped out of the picture. The gain in this image is also decreased compared to Figure 10-13. As a result, note the multiple small apparent "drop-out" artifacts in the posterior and septal leaflets. See Video 10-14.

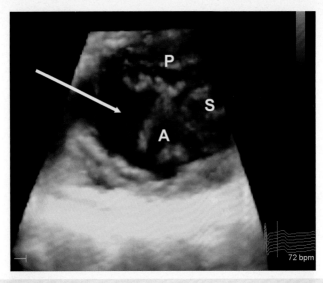

Figure 10-15. Three-dimensional TEE image of a flail TV. This full-volume en-face view of the TV is displayed, from the RV perspective, in the same patient as in Figures 10-13 and 10-14. In this image, the TEE transducer is in the TG position, and the valve is seen from the RV apex, much like in a CT scan or cardiac MRI. Note the three tricuspid leaflets, labeled S, septal; A, anterior; and P, posterior. The *white arrow* points to an apparent missing segment of anterior leaflet. This is not an artifact, nor an effect of inadequate gain. The apparent defect is the flail segment of the anterior tricuspid leaflet. In this image, the viewer is positioned in the RV, looking up at the TV. In systole, the flail segment is positioned in the right atrium, resulting in an apparent defect in the valve. See Video 10-15.

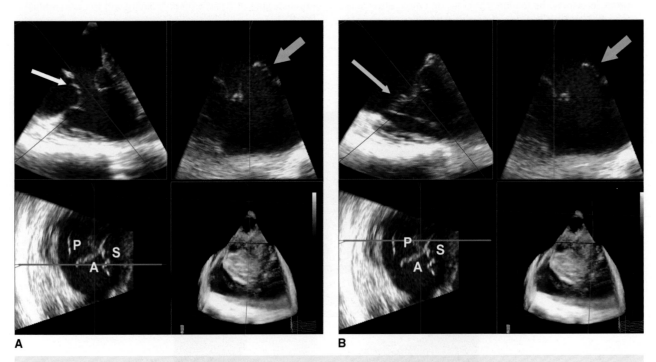

A

B

Figure 10-16A, B. Three-dimensional TEE image of a flail TV. This is an MPR of the TV, in the same patient as Figures 10-13–10-15. By aligning two planes (*red line in the top left box and green line in the top right box*), a perfectly transverse cut through the base of the valve in the third plane (*bottom left box*) can be obtained. By adjusting the position of the *green* and *red* lines in the bottom left box, the cross sections displayed can be changed in the corresponding boxes at the top. This powerful technology allows precise localization of any valve lesion, as described below:

A. When the green line is set across the anterior leaflet, the flail is obvious in both the top left (*white arrow*) and top right boxes (*blue arrow*). See Video 10-16.

B. When the green line is moved back to the posterior leaflet, the flail disappears from the top left box (*yellow arrow*). However, since the red line has not moved, the top right box still displays the flail segment in the anterior leaflet (*blue arrow*). See Video 10-16.

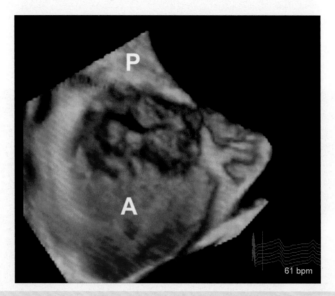

Figure 10-17. Three-dimensional TEE image of a rheumatic TV. This is a full-volume en-face view of the TV from the RA perspective. The orientation of the image (not the leaflets) is indicated in the figure. A, anterior of the patient; P, posterior of the patient. Note the thickened, fibrosed leaflet edges and the partial commissural fusion, creating in effect a "bicuspidization" of the TV with mild TS and severe regurgitation (TR). The incidence of primary rheumatic TV involvement detected by 2D echocardiography has been reported in 6% of patients with rheumatic MV disease.[11] Although patients may have mixed disease, TR is more common than TS. Autopsy studies suggest a higher incidence, which may imply that the ability of standard 2D echocardiography to detect subtle changes in TV morphology may be limited. However, in a report of 22 patients who underwent 3D TEE during mitral surgery for rheumatic disease, all patients with severe TR had abnormal valve morphology, which was more often detected and better characterized using 3D TEE than 2D TEE.[12] See Video 10-17.

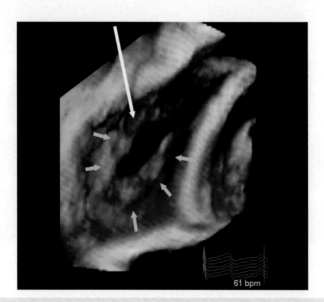

Figure 10-18. Three-dimensional TEE image of a rheumatic TV. This is the same valve as in Figure 10-17 and Video 10-17. The image is a full-volume en-face view of the TV but from the RV perspective. Note the thickened tricuspid leaflets marked by the *yellow arrows*. Note also the mobile brown structures in the middle of the image. These are not artifacts. Rather, they represent thickened chordae tendinae—the largest one is designated by the *white arrow*. The TV area can be estimated in this view by freezing the image in diastole and measuring the orifice by planimetry. However, depth perception is poor in an en-face view, because the screen is flat and it is difficult to establish the level at which the orifice is the narrowest from this perspective. For that reason, planimetry should ideally be performed using MPR. See Video 10-18.

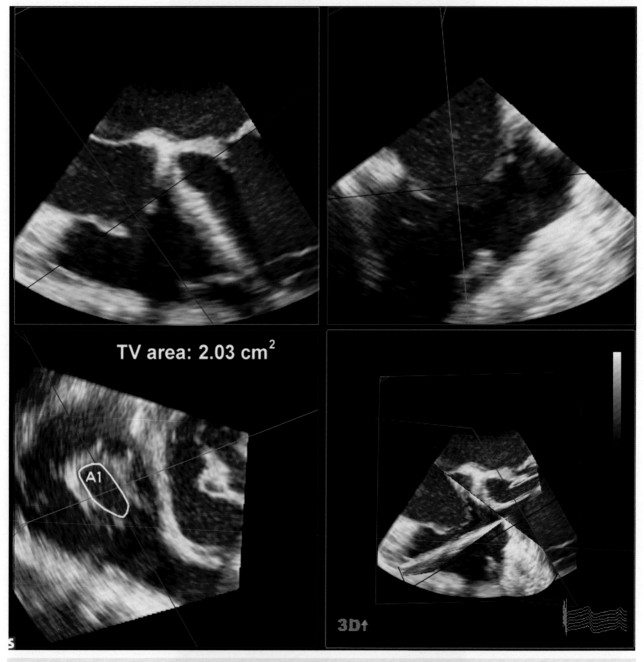

Figure 10-19. MPR of a stenotic TV, with the transducer in the ME position, demonstrating planimetry of the stenotic orifice. The various planes are adjusted to obtain a perfectly transverse section across the valve. In this example, the transverse plane (*blue line*) is moved to the narrowest point of the valve, at the tip of the leaflets. Note that depending on the disease process, the narrowest point of the stenotic valve could be anywhere between the midportion of the leaflets and the subvalvular apparatus. The orifice is then measured by planimetry (bottom left box). See Video 10-19.

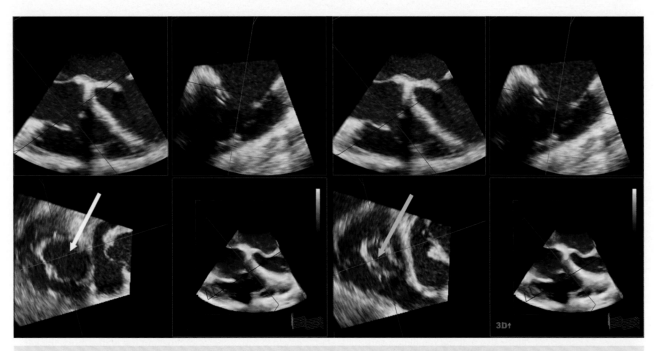

Figure 10-20. Planimetry of a rheumatic TV using MPR. This image is taken from the same patient as Figure 10-19 and demonstrates one of the pitfalls associated with planimetry of a stenotic orifice. If the measurement is not taken at the narrowest point of the valve, the degree of stenosis may be underestimated. In this example, after properly aligning the valve in the top boxes, the short axis of the valve is displayed in the bottom left corner. Moving the blue plane in the top left box by just a few millimeters has a dramatic effect on the apparent valve area in the bottom left box. The *white arrow* on the left side shows a falsely large apparent valve area, while the *yellow arrow* on the right demonstrates the real valve orifice. Compare the level of the blue line in the top left box in each example. Correct plane alignment and orientation are particularly important in a disease like rheumatic valvular stenosis, where the disease can not only affect the leaflets but also the subvalvular apparatus.

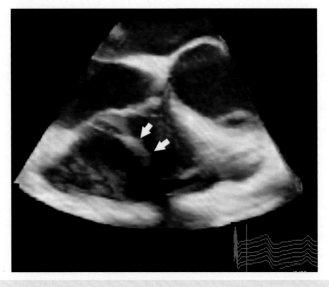

Figure 10-21. Three-dimensional TEE image of a rheumatic TV. Full-volume view of the TV cropped to mimic a ME-four-chamber view. Note from the position of the apex of the scan that the transducer is in the ME position. The image is cropped to reveal the thickened subvalvular apparatus. The *white arrows* point to a very thick chorda tendinae, the same that was marked by the large *white arrow* in Figure 10-17. See Video 10-21.

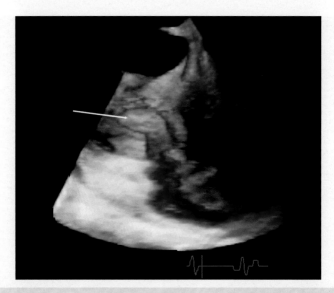

Figure 10-22. Three-dimensional TEE image of TV endocarditis. Three-dimensional full-volume loop cropped to mimic a ME-four-chamber view with the 3D TEE transducer in the ME position. This patient developed acute severe endocarditis of his TV. Note that the anterior leaflet was partially destroyed by infection, leaving a leaflet that flails into the right atrium during systole (*white arrow*). Note also that the remaining anterior leaflet is covered with vegetation, making the leaflet much thicker and echogenic than a normal leaflet. Note also that the rest of the TV is not visible. This is not a matter of inadequate gain or acoustic dropout in this case but rather represents significant destruction of the valve. See Video 10-22.

References

1. Sutton JP, Ho SY, Vogel M, et al. Is the morphologically right atrioventricular valve tricuspid? *J Heart Valve Dis.* 1995;4:571–575.

2. Tei C, Pilgrim JP, Pravin MB, et al. The tricuspid valve annulus: study of size and motion in normal subjects and in patients with tricuspid regurgitation. *Circulation.* 1982;66(3):665–671.

3. Anwar AM, Soliman OII, Nemes A, et al. Value of assessment of tricuspid annulus: real-time three-dimensional echocardiography and magnetic resonance imaging. *Int J Cardiovasc Imaging.* 2007;23:701–705.

4. Cohen GI, White ME, Sochowski RA, et al. Reference values for normal adult transesophageal echocardiographic measurements. *J Am Soc Echocardiogr.* 1995;8:221–230.

5. Anwar AM, Geleijnse ML, Soliman OII, et al. Assessment of normal tricuspid valve anatomy in adults by real-time three-dimensional echocardiography. *Int J Cardiovasc Imaging.* 2007;23:717–724.

6. Sugeng L, Shernan SK, Weinert L, et al. Real-time three-dimensional transesophageal echocardiography in valve disease: comparison with surgical findings and evaluation of prosthetic valves. *J Am Soc Echocardiogr.* 2008;21(12):1347–1354.

7. Bonow RO, Carabello, BA, Chatterjee K, et al. ACC/AHA 2006 guidelines for the management of patients with valvular heart disease: a report of the American College of Cardiology/American Heart Association Task Force on Practice Guidelines. *J Am Coll Cardiol.* 2006;48:e1–e148.

8. Vahanian A, Baumgartner H, Bax J, et al. Guidelines on the management of valvular heart disease: the Task Force on the Management of Valvular Heart Disease of the European Society of Cardiology. *Eur Heart J.* 2007;28:230–268.

9. Shiran A, Sagie A. Tricuspid regurgitation in mitral valve disease. *J Am Coll Cardiol.* 2009;53:401–408.

10. Dreyfus GD, Corbi PJ, Chan KM, et al. Secondary tricuspid regurgitation or dilatation: which should be the criteria for surgical repair? *Ann Thorac Surg.* 2005;79:127–132.

11. Daniels SJ, Mintz GS, Kotler MN. Rheumatic tricuspid valve disease: two dimensional echocardiographic, hemodynamic and angiographic correlations. *Am J Cardiol.* 1983;51;492–496.

12. Henein MY, O'Sullivan CA, Li W, et al. Evidence for rheumatic valve disease in patients with severe tricuspid regurgitation long after mitral valve surgery: the role of 3D echo reconstruction. *J Heart Valve Dis.* 2003;12:566–572.

CATHETER-BASED PROCEDURES TO REPAIR STRUCTURAL HEART DISEASES

11

Muhamed Saric, Gila Perk, Carlos Ruiz, Itzhak Kronzon

Catheter-based procedures to repair structural heart defects are performed in cardiac catheterization laboratories or hybrid operating rooms (Fig. 11-1) and require expertise of many medical professionals. One of the major challenges in introducing catheter-based techniques into daily practice was the fact that the details of the cardiac structures were difficult to visualize. Fluoroscopy with or without contrast could not provide a working alternative to direct visualization obtained after opening the chest and the heart during surgery. The introduction of two-dimensional (2D) transsthoracic, transesophageal, and intracardiac echocardiography was an attractive imaging alternative during these procedures. Unfortunately, the 2D tomographic nature of the images could not frequently define the accurate site, size, and shape of the lesion and could not demonstrate the entire intracardiac portion of the catheters and the devices.

The introduction of the new real-time (RT), three-dimensional (3D) transesophageal echocardiography (TEE) probe in 2008 was timely and helpful.[1] This new imaging tool can be used to better diagnose, precisely locate, and accurately assess structural heart disorders.[2,3] Even more importantly, the entire intracardiac portion of the catheters and devices could now be visualized by RT3D TEE[4] (Fig. 11-2 and Video 11-2-1). Thus, guidance and navigation of the catheters and the devices into the position required for successful repair can be obtained (Video 11-2-2). It is expected (and in many cases already proven) that with the use of 3D TEE, the catheter-based procedures will improve, and they will become safer, faster, and easier.[5]

With each catheter-based procedure, 2D and 3D echocardiographic imaging includes

- **Preprocedural assessment**: To confirm the diagnosis, evaluate hemodynamics, define whether or not the condition can be successfully repaired, plan the best approach, and assess risks

- **Procedural guidance**: To identify intracardiac wires, catheters, and devices; guide the approach to the structure which is about to be repaired; and assess the repair procedure and its immediate results

- **Postprocedural assessment**: To assess the results of the procedure and identify possible complications

The use of 2D and 3D echocardiography in specific lesions is discussed below.

CLOSURE OF PATENT FORAMEN OVALE AND SECUNDUM ATRIAL SEPTAL DEFECT[5]

The 3D anatomy of the interatrial septum can be studied with great detail by 3D TEE (Fig. 11-3).[6,7] Initially, the image obtained by the RT3D zoom modality is tilted up along its horizontal axis to provide the right atrial perspective of the atrial septum (Video 11-3-1). In this view, the inferior and superior vena cava and the aortic root can be visualized. The image can then be rotated along its vertical axis to reveal the left atrial perspective of the septum. The location of the pulmonary veins and their entry site into the atrium can also be assessed in this view.[8]

When clinically indicated, patent foramen ovale (PFO) and secundum atrial septal defect (SASD) can be repaired percutaneously with the use of closure devices.[9] At present, other types of atrial septal defects such as ostium primum or sinus venosus ASD are not amenable to catheter-based repair. Partial anomalous pulmonary venous return should always be looked for, as it cannot be treated percutaneously.[10]

Before the procedure, it is essential to identify the type, dimensions, anatomy, site, and shape of the defect.[11] This information determines the device selection and the mode of approach. The width of the tissue rim around the defect (Videos 11-4-1 and 11-4-2) is important and may define the closure device stability (Fig. 11-4). Complex SASDs may present with more than one septal defect or may have tissue strips across the defect (Fig. 11-5 and Video 11-5-1). During the procedure, the course of the wires, catheters, and devices can be demonstrated (Fig. 11-6 and Video 11-6-1). At time of deployment, 3D TEE images demonstrate the entire device (Fig. 11-7), ensure its correct position, and allow for evaluation of a residual defect (Fig. 11-8) or significant shunt (Fig. 11-9 and Videos 11-9-1 and 11-9-2).[12] Occasionally, more than one device is used to close a SASD (Fig. 11-10).

VENTRICULAR SEPTAL DEFECT CLOSURE

Three-dimensional TEE is helpful in the closure of congenital and acquired ventricular septal defects (VSDs) (Fig. 11-11). The closure of post–myocardial infarction (MI) VSD is both challenging and rewarding. Patients with post-MI VSD are frequently unstable and at high risk for surgical repair. The necrotic tissue associated with these VSDs makes the surgical suturing less effective. Three-dimensional TEE can identify the defect, including location, size, and shape. It can help guiding the catheters and the closure device into the defect while imaging the deployment from the left and from the right ventricular perspective.[13]

LEFT VENTRICULAR PSEUDOANEURYSM

Left ventricular pseudoaneurysm (PA) is another life-threatening complication of acute MI. Until recently, open heart surgery was the only mode of repair. Since most patients are unstable, mortality and morbidity are quite high, and the friable myocardial wall frequently precludes complete repair.

Transcutaneous, catheter-based techniques have been recently developed for PA repair (Fig. 11-12 and Videos 11-12-1 and 11-12-2). Using radiographic, 3D computed tomography (CT) and 3D TEE guidance, the communicating tract between the LV cavity and the PA can be entered percutaneously and obliterated by a closure device. Three-dimensional TEE was proven useful in assessing the anatomy, guiding the procedure, and assessing its results.[14]

CLOSURE OF PARAVALVULAR LEAKS

Paravalvular leak (PVL) as a result of prosthetic valve dehiscence is a common complication of valve replacement (Fig. 11-13). PVL may result in congestive heart failure and/or significant hemolysis, which may require blood transfusion. Until recently, symptomatic PVLs could only be closed by open heart surgery, which was associated with significant morbidity and mortality.[15] Catheter-based closure of left-sided PVLs is now a solid alternative.[16] Definition of the exact number, location, size, and shape of the valvular dehiscence is crucial for successful closure procedure (Video 11-13-1). The left-sided valves are presented in the "surgical view" (Fig. 11-14). The mitral valve is placed in a clock-like fashion, with the aortic valve on top of the mitral valve at 12 o'clock; the left atrial appendage (LAA) (and the lateral mitral commissure) is at 9 o'clock, and the medial commissure is at 3 o'clock. A similar approach is used for the aortic valve. These details can be obtained by 3D TEE and 3D CT (Fig. 11-15).

There are several catheter-based approaches used to deliver the device into the dehiscence site: antegrade, retrograde, and transapical (Fig. 11-16). A retrograde approach with arterial puncture can be used for the delivery of closure of the device into the aortic valve dehiscence from the aortic side. For mitral valve dehiscence, the catheter and the device it carries may be delivered retrogradely from the aorta into the left ventricle and then across the dehiscence into the left atrium. Alternatively, the antegrade approach may be used; it involves puncturing a large systemic vein and advancing the catheter and the device it carries across the interatrial septum into the dehiscence site (Fig. 11-17 and Video 11-17-1). Finally, the apical approach starts with direct left ventricular puncture through the chest wall with the catheter[17]; the device is then carried antegrade across an aortic valve dehiscence or retrograde across a mitral valve dehiscence.

RT3D TEE is important in guiding the wires, catheter, and the device into the dehiscence and avoiding the prosthetic valve orifice (Fig. 11-18 and Video 11-18-1, and Fig. 11-19 and Videos 11-19-1, 11-19-2, 11-19-3). RT3D TEE, supplemented by color Doppler, is used to pinpoint the dehiscence location and to ascertain complete PVL closure (Fig. 11-20 and Videos 11-20-1 and 11-20-2). Residual leak may require a closure with a larger device or with an additional device. Complications, such as interference with valve motion leading to prosthetic stenosis or insufficiency, can be identified by color and spectral Doppler (Fig. 11-21 and Video 11-21-1).[18]

TRANSCATHETER MITRAL VALVE REPAIR PROCEDURES

MITRAL BALLOON VALVULOPLASTY

Three-dimensional echocardiography is considered the technique of choice in the evaluation of the severity of mitral stenosis (Fig. 11-22 and Video 11-22-1).[19,20] Three-dimensional TEE is useful during the transseptal puncture by guiding the operator to the optimal crossing point, which will eventually permit an easy approach to the valve orifice. The location and the position of the balloon can be evaluated before, during, and after balloon inflation (Fig. 11-23 and Video 11-23-1). Views from the left atrial and from the ventricular perspectives can define the degree of commissural separation produced by the inflation, measure the newly created mitral valve orifice, and assess the possibility of leaflet tear and the origin of new mitral regurgitation (Video 11-23-2).[21]

MITRAL VALVE REPAIR

Several technologies of transcatheter mitral valve repair for the treatment of mitral regurgitation are currently at different levels of development and stages of clinical trials (Fig. 11-24). The MitraClip valve repair system made by Abbott Laboratories, Abbott Park, IL, USA, delivers a clip via a large peripheral vein to the right atrium and then across the interatrial septum into the left atrium. In the next stage, the catheter is placed across the mitral valve (Figs. 11-25 and 11-26 and Videos 11-25-1 and 11-26-1–11-26-3). The clip wings grab the left ventricular side of the tips of scallops A2 and P2, thus creating two mitral orifices, which decreases (or even totally abolishes) the mitral regurgitant volume. Occasionally, another clip is needed (thus creating three mitral orifices). Complications such as clip dehiscence and procedure-related mitral stenosis can be identified and treated. This procedure is still experimental but has been tried on thousands of patients with very encouraging results. Three-dimensional TEE is used to guide each stage of the procedure. It has been shown to improve the results, shorten the procedure duration, and identify failures and complications.[22]

TRANSCATHETER AORTIC VALVE IMPLANTATION

This catheter-based technology is discussed in detail in Chapter 9.

OBLITERATION OF LEFT ATRIAL APPENDAGE (LAA)

Patients with chronic or paroxysmal atrial fibrillation (AF) have increased risk of left atrial clot formation and systemic thromboembolism. It is estimated that 90% clots are in nonvalvular AF are located in the LAA. LAA obliteration or amputation is often performed in patient undergoing mitral valve repair or replacement in an attempt to minimize thromboembolic complications. Recently, catheter-based techniques have been developed for LAA obliteration. It is assumed that LAA obliteration will decrease the number of embolic events. This technology is now tried on patients with AF who cannot use anticoagulation therapy. A specially designed LAA occluder (Watchman device, Atritech, Plymouth, MN; or PLAATO device, ev3 Inc., Plymouth, MN) is advanced from a peripheral vein, across the interatrial septum into the orifice (os) of the LAA.

RT3D TEE has played a crucial role during LAA procedure.[23] Preprocedure, it is used to define the shape and the dimensions of the LAA orifice, as well as the number and location of the LAA lobes (Fig. 11-27). This is essential for selecting appropriate LAA occluder device. Three-dimensional TEE guidance during LAA device deployment is crucial (Fig. 11-28). One has to ascertain that the closure device fits snugly in the LAA orifice, without any significant communication between the excluded LAA and the left atrial body (Videos 11-28-1 and 11-28-2). Such communications become evident on color and spectral Doppler imaging.

GUIDANCE OF ELECTROPHYSIOLOGY PROCEDURES

The ability to accurately define the intracardiac portion of catheters makes 3D TEE a useful tool in the electrophysiology laboratory.[24] Using 3D TEE, catheters can be navigated into ablation sites such as the atrioventricular node, right atrial isthmus, or the area around the entry of the pulmonary veins (Fig. 11-29) during pulmonary vein isolation in patients with AF (Fig. 11-30). Complications of ablation procedure such as pulmonary vein stenosis[25] can easily be identified and quantified (Fig. 11-31).

SUCTION OF INTRACARDIAC MASSES

This novel approach uses high-power vacuum (–80 mm Hg), to suck all the blood and thrombi from the right atrium (Fig. 11-32). The blood is filtered and is pumped back into the right atrium. The procedure is guided by RT3D TEE that can identify the size and location of right atrial thrombi (Video 11-32-1) as well as the presence of intracardiac tubes and their anatomic relations.[26] Using the vacuum system, the intracardiac thrombus can successfully be removed percutaneously (Video 11-32-2).

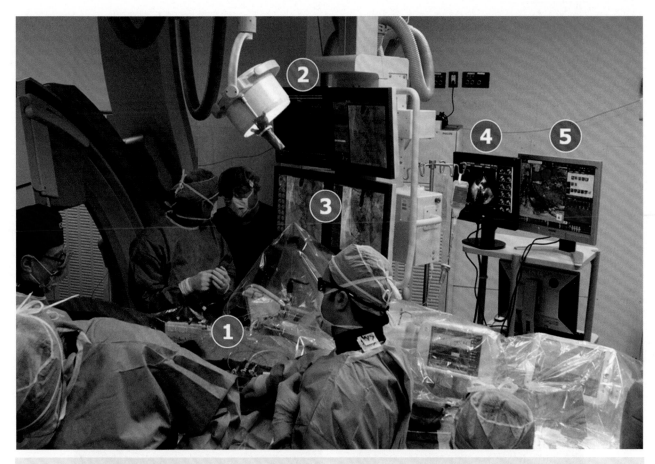

Figure 11-1. Interventional room setup. Percutaneous interventions are performed in a cardiac catheterization laboratory or in a specialized hybrid room that combines elements of a cardiac catheterization laboratory and an operating room. Monitoring of a patient (1) during percutaneous interventions includes hemodynamics tracings (2), fluoroscopy (3), transesophageal echocardiography (4), and computed tomography (5).

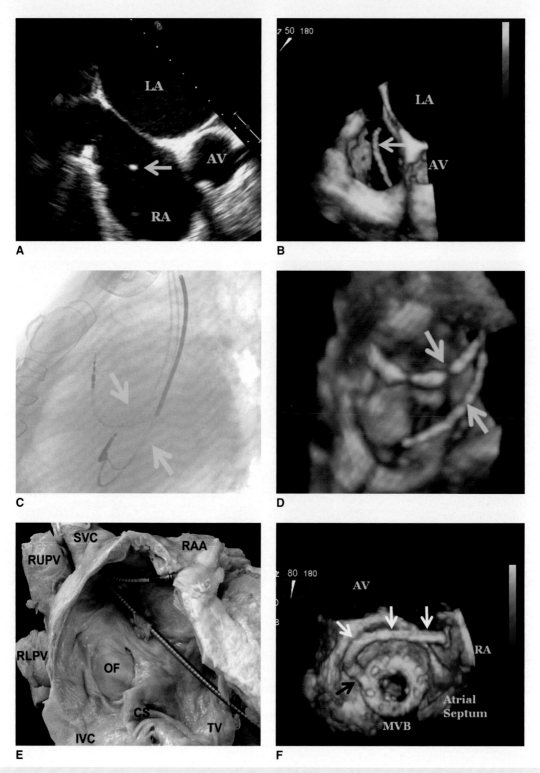

Figure 11-2. Two- and three-dimensional imaging of pacemaker wires and catheters. A. On 2D TEE, only a cross section (*arrow*) or a short length of a pacemaker lead can be seen (Video 11-2-1). B. In contrast to 2D-TEE, 3D-TEE can visualize the entire length of pacemaker leads and catheters. The *arrow* points to the entire right atrial portion of a right ventricular pace-maker lead (Video 11-2-1). C. Dual-chamber pacemaker leads (*arrows*) seen on a lateral chest radiograph. The insert shows the corresponding 3D-TEE view of two pacemaker leads in the right atrium (Video 11-2-2). D. Three-dimensional TEE view of two pacemaker leads in the right atrium that corresponds to chest radiograph in panel C (Video 11-2-2). E. Pacemaker leads in the right heart. The right atrium has been opened to reveal pacemaker leads extending from the mouth of the superior vena cava (SVC) into the atrium. One lead extends to the tip of the right atrial appendage (RAA) and the other through the tricus-pid valve (TV) orifice into the right ventricle. CS, coronary sinus; IVC, inferior vena cava; OF, oval fossa; RLPV, right lower pul-monary vein; RUPV, right upper pulmonary vein. F. The entire length of a catheter (*white arrows*) used in percutaneous closure of paravalvular mitral regurgitant orifice (*black arrow*) is seen; the catheter enters the left atrium through interatrial septum. AV, aortic valve; LA, left atrium; MVB, mitral valve bioprosthesis; RA, right atrium.

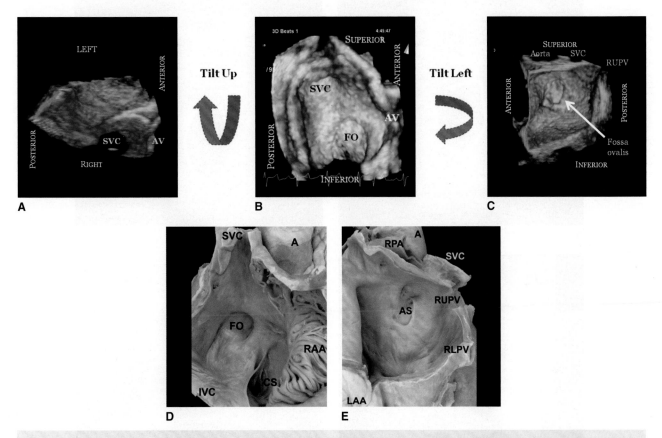

Figure 11-3. Imaging of the interatrial septum. To image the interatrial septum in anatomically correct orientation, we use the tilt-up-then-left (TUPLE) maneuver using 3D zoom technology. This example shows a patient with intact interatrial septum. A. The TUPLE maneuver in this example starts with the initial image obtained at the 0-degree TEE angle ("opening scene"). Superior vena cava (SVC) and the aortic valve (AV) are seen in short axis; the interatrial septum is foreshortened, and its left atrial side is seen in the top portion of the panel. B. In the next step, the image is tilted up along the horizontal axis to reveal the en face view of the right atrial side of the interatrial septum. Fossa ovalis is in the middle of the septum; SVC is cranial, and the aortic valve (AV) is anterior to fossa ovalis in this view. C. In the final step, the image is rotated along the vertical axis to reveal the left atrial side of the interatrial septum. RUPV, right upper pulmonary vein. In the accompanying Video 11-3-1, the TUPLE maneuver is performed in another patient who had a small secundum atrial septal defect. D. Anatomic view of the right atrial aspect of the interatrial septum that corresponds to panel B. The free wall of the right atrial appendage (RAA) has been lifted away to show the right side of the interatrial septum. A, aorta; CS, coronary sinus; FO, fossa ovalis; IVC, inferior vena cava; SVC, superior vena cava. E. Anatomic view of the left atrial aspect of the interatrial septum that corresponds to panel C. The opened left atrium reveals the intact interatrial septum (AS) and exhibits the typical horse shoe-like structure where the infolded area of the septum secundum becomes adherent to the flap valve within the oval fossa. A, aorta; LAA, left atrial appendage; RLPV, right lower pulmonary vein; RPA, right pulmonary artery; RUPV, right upper pulmonary vein; SVC, superior vena cava.

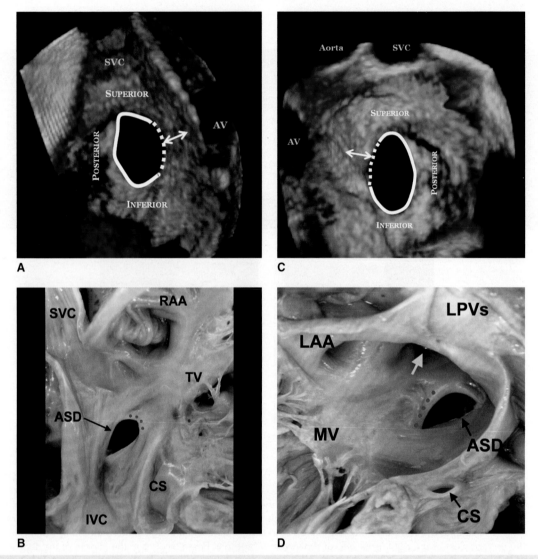

Figure 11-4. **Secundum atrial septal defect rims: preprocedural evaluation. A.** En face view of the right atrial side of the atrial septum reveals a large secundum atrial septal defect (ASD). The *dashed line* indicates the aortic valve rim of the ASD. The width of this rim is indicated by the *arrow*. The *solid line* denotes the nonaortic rims of the ASD. SVC, superior vena cava; AV, aortic valve. Accompanying videos show the right atrial side of a secundum ASD with ample (Video 11-4-1) and insufficient (Video 11-4-2) aortic rim. **B.** Anatomic view that corresponds to panel A. Secundum atrial septal defect, right atrial aspect—this anatomic view of the right atrial septal surface reveals a large atrial septal defect (ASD). The *red dots* mark the aspect of the defect that has the closest approximation to the aorta. CS, coronary sinus; IVC, inferior vena cava; RAA, right atrial appendage; SVC, superior vena cava; TV, tricuspid valve. **C.** En face view of the left atrial side of the ASD. For abbreviations, see panel A legend. **D.** Anatomic view that corresponds to panel C. Secundum atrial septal defect, left atrial aspect. This anatomic view of the left atrial septum of the same heart as shown in panel B illustrates a large atrial septal defect (ASD). The *red dots* mark the aspect of the defect that has the closest approximation to the aorta. CS, coronary sinus; LAA, left atrial appendage; LPVs, left pulmonary veins; MV, mitral valve; *yellow arrow*, right pulmonary veins.

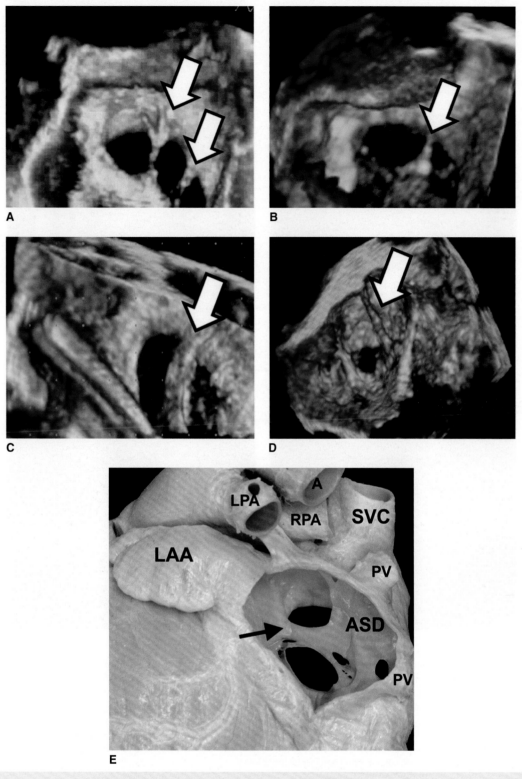

Figure 11-5. **Complex secundum ASDs.** Panels A through D show the 3D TEE en face view of complex secundum ASDs from the left atrial perspective. *Arrows* point to tissue bands across the fossa ovalis; these bands give rise to a fenestrated ASD appearance. Accompanying Video 11-5-1 corresponds to panel B. E. Anatomic view of fenestrated atrial septum from the left atrium. A window cut in the posterior wall of the left atrium reveals a fenestrated septum and a large secundum atrial septal defect (ASD) with several bands of tissue traversing the opening, the largest marked with a *black arrow*. The left pulmonary veins have been removed. The right pulmonary veins (PVs) are seen draining in the usual fashion. A, aorta; LAA, left atrial appendage; LPA, left pulmonary artery; RPA, right pulmonary artery; SVC, superior vena cava.

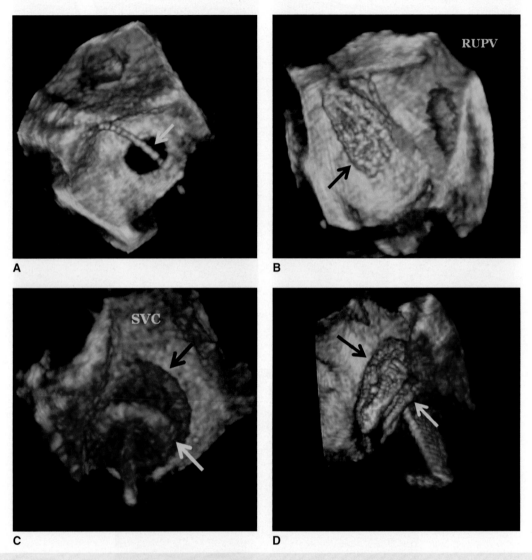

Figure 11-6. ASD closure monitoring. Three-dimensional TEE guidance is provided throughout the percutaneous ASD closure. A. Secundum ASD seen from the left atrial perspective. At the onset of ASD closure procedure, a catheter (*arrow*) is seen entering the left atrium through the ASD. The catheter is used to measure intracardiac pressures and oxygen saturation. B. In the next step, the secundum ASD, here seen from the left atrial perspective, is sized using a sizing balloon (*arrow*). RUPV, right upper pulmonary vein. C. In the final step, an appropriate ASD occluder device is deployed. In this panel the device is seen from the right atrial perspective. The *black arrow* points to the left atrial disc and the *yellow arrow* to the right atrial disc of the device. SVC, superior vena cava. D. The atrial septum is sandwiched between the left atrial disc (*black arrow*) and the right atrial disc (*yellow arrow*); see also accompanying Video 11-6-1.

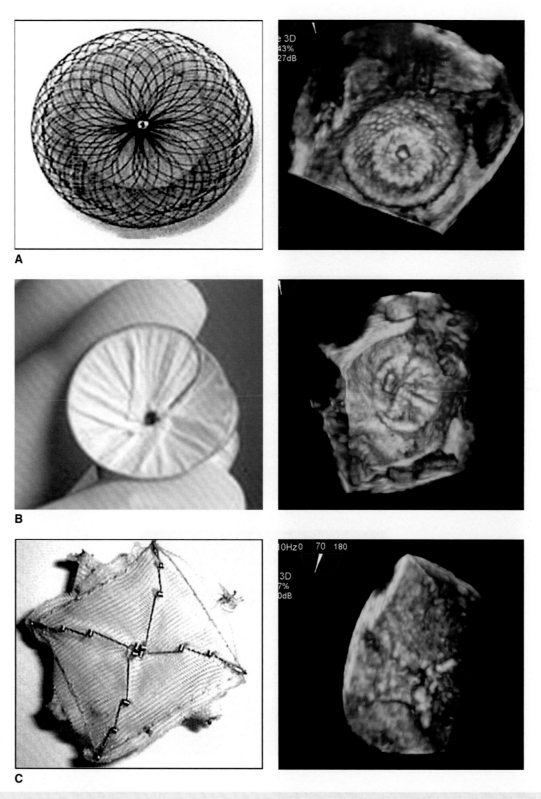

Figure 11-7. Type of ASD closure devices. Atrial septal defects (secundum ASDs and PFO) can be closed percutaneously using a variety of devices. Top row shows preimplantation photographs, and the bottom row shows implanted devices from the left atrial perspective on 3D TEE. A. Amplatzer ASD occluder (St. Jude Medical, Inc., St. Paul, MN). B. Gore-Helix ASD occluder (W.L. Gore & Associates, Inc., Flagstaff, AZ). C. CardioSeal ASD occluder (NMT Medical, Boston, MA).

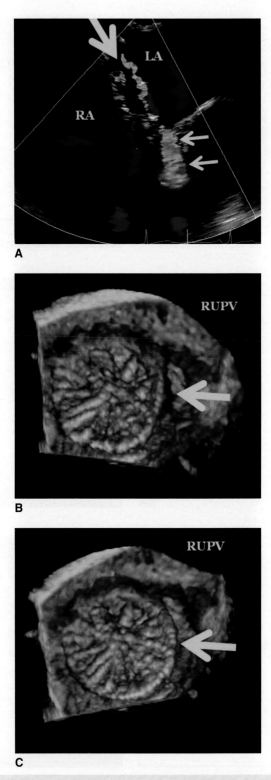

Figure 11-8. **ASD closure complications, part 1. A.** Residual left-to-right shunt (*small arrows*) adjacent to the aortic valve after percutaneous placement of an ASD occluder visualized by color Doppler on 2D TEE. RA, right atrium; LA, left atrium. **B.** Residual atrial septal defect adjacent to the right upper pulmonary vein (RUPV) not covered by the ASD occluder seen in another patient from the left atrial perspective on 3D TEE. **C.** After repositioning the ASD occluder, the residual defect seen in panel B is no longer present.

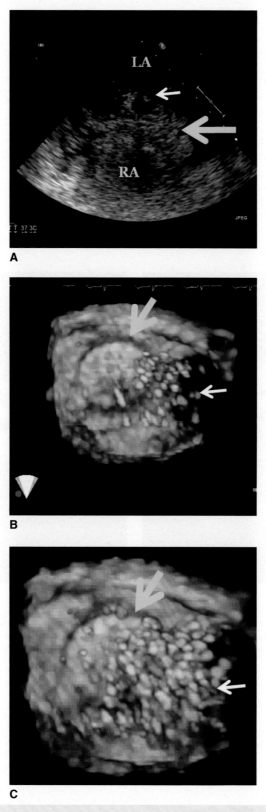

Figure 11-9. ASD closure complications, part 2. Residual right-to-left shunt across an ASD occluder (*big yellow arrow*) seen after agitated saline bubble injection. A. Bubbles (*white arrow*) are seen entering the left atrium on 2D TEE. B and C. Bubbles (*white arrow*) are seen on the left atrial side of the ASD occluder (*yellow arrow*) in the same patient. Panel C frame comes later in the cardiac cycle compared to panel B. Accompanying Videos 11-9-1 and 11-9-2 correspond to panels B and C, respectively.

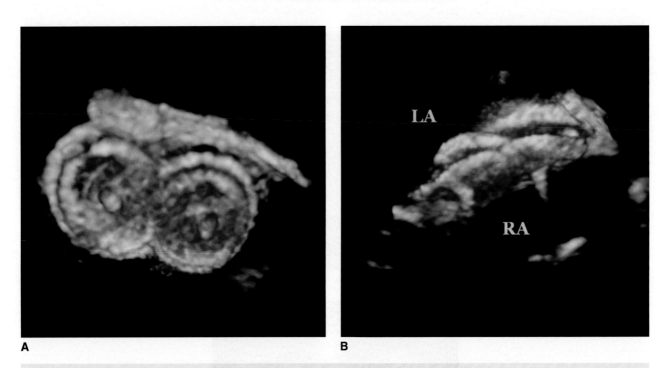

A

B

Figure 11-10. Multiple ASD closure devices. Occasionally, more than one device is needed to close a secundum ASD. In this patient, two Amplatzer ASD occluders were used and visualized by 3D TEE. A. Two ASD septal occluders seen en face from the right atrial perspective. B. Two ASD septal occluders seen sideways. LA, left atrium; RA, right atrium.

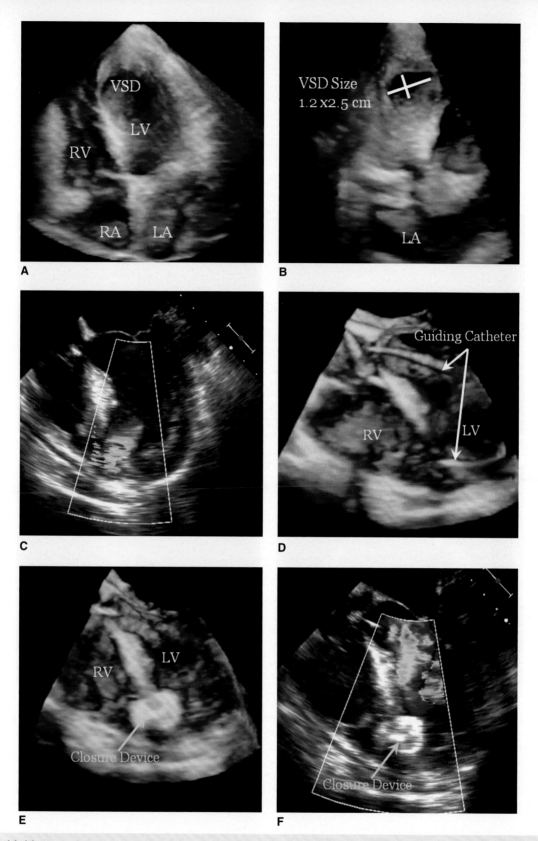

Figure 11-11. **Postinfarction ventricular septal defect.** A. Four-chamber view, acquired by transthoracic echocardiography. The VSD can be seen in the apical portion of the interventricular septum. B. Postprocessing and rotation of the image from panel A allows for en-face visualization of the VSD, which enables direct measurement and accurate assessment of the defect's size. This in turn allows for proper sizing of the required closure device. C. Color Doppler imaging during TEE demonstrating flow across the interventricular septum. D. Transesophageal echocardiographic guidance of percutaneous closure procedure. The guiding catheter, advanced via retrograde arterial approach, can be seen crossing the VSD into the right ventricle. E. Upon completion of the procedure, a closure device is occluding the VSD (obtained by TEE from the four-chamber view). Positioning of the device can be easily assessed utilizing RT3D echocardiography. This is further supplemented by color Doppler imaging, which confirmed no residual flow across the interventricular septum (F).

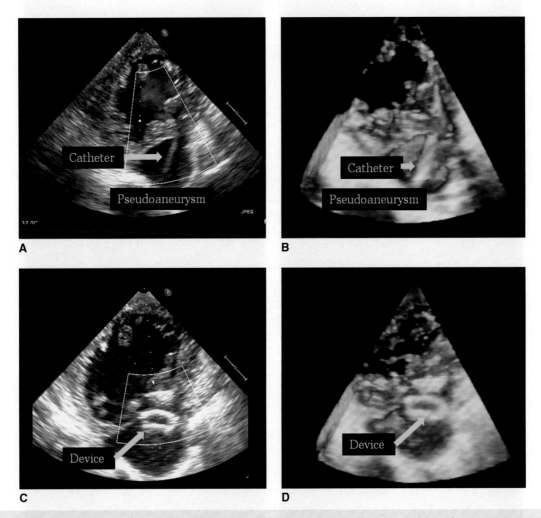

Figure 11-12. Percutaneous closure of postinfarction pseudoaneurysm. A. Transgastric view demonstrating an infarct-related PA of the left ventricular anterior wall. Color Doppler imaging demonstrates to-and-fro flow, confirming the diagnosis of a PA. Image obtained during catheter-based procedure; a percutaneous puncture of the PA was performed; note the catheter seen in the PA. B. RT3D image obtained from the transgastric view at the same time the 2D image in panel A taken. Note the catheter clearly seen in the PA and crossing its opening. C and D. Closure device successfully placed at the neck of the PA; both plates of the device are seen, one on the PA side and one in the ventricular side of the PA, achieving complete occlusion of the opening. Accompanying Video 11-12-1 corresponds to panel A, Video 11-12-2 corresponds to panel D.

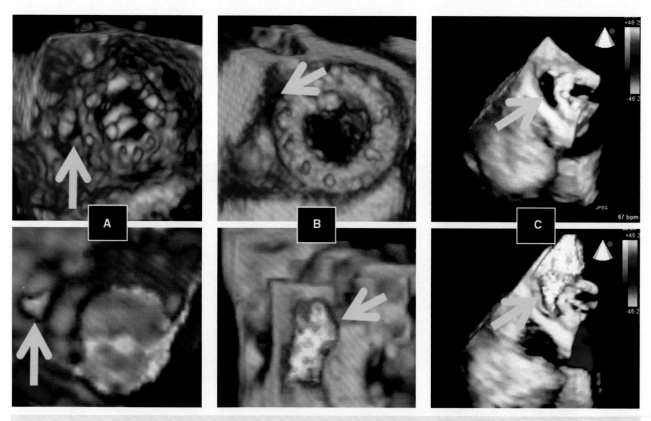

Figure 11-13. Paravalvular and para-annular leaks after mitral valve replacement or repair. Top row reveals en face 3D zoom view of the mitral valve, while the bottom row shows corresponding 3D TEE color Doppler images. A. PVL (*arrow*) at approximately 9 o'clock in a patient with a mechanical mitral valve. B. PVL (*arrow*) at approximately 10 o'clock in a patient with a bioprosthetic mitral valve. C. Para-annular leak (*arrow*) at approximately 9 o'clock in a patient with mitral annuloplasty. Accompanying Video 11-13-1 corresponds to panel C. Para-annular leaks are currently not amenable to catheter-based repair.

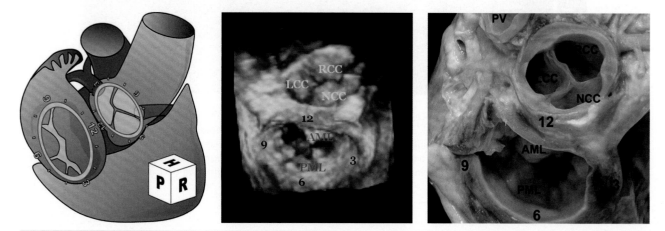

Figure 11-14. Standard "surgical" orientation of the mitral valve. For purposes of uniform definitions, communication, and accurate anatomic descriptions of mitral valve–related pathology, it is customary to position en face images of the mitral valve as seen from the atrial perspective in a standardized, "surgical" view. In this orientation, the image is rotated such that the aortic valve is positioned on the top part of the image (left panel—cartoon depiction; middle panel—RT3D echocardiographic image; right panel—pathologic correlate). Assuming a round mitral valve annulus, using a clockface numbering, the aortic valve is thus placed at the 12 o'clock position (anterior). On the left side of the image, structures that are lateral to the mitral valve are seen, while on the right side medial structures are seen. With this view, the LAA is seen at the 9 o'clock position (lateral). AML, anterior mitral leaflet; PML, posterior mitral leaflet; LCC, NCC, RCC, left, non-, and right coronary cusps, respectively.

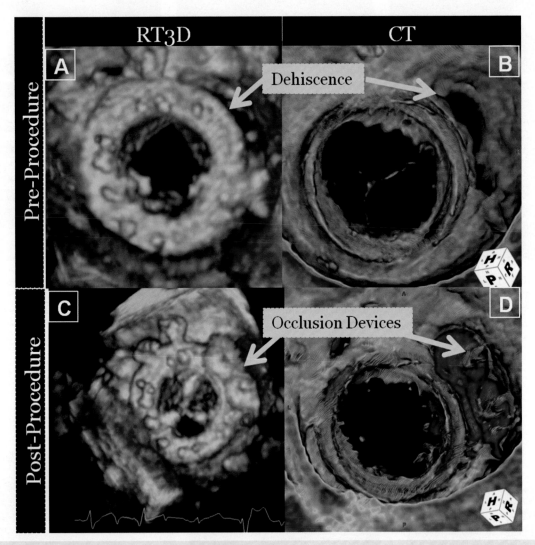

Figure 11-15. Mitral bioprosthesis PVL: 2D TEE versus CT. A and B. RT3D transesophageal echocardiographic image (A) and corresponding computed tomography (CT) image (B) showing a mitral bioprosthesis dehiscence. Both images show the mitral valve en face, from the left atrial perspective, oriented in the standard surgical view. The dehiscence is seen between 1 and 3 o'clock (anteromedial) position. C and D. RT3D transesophageal echocardiographic image (C) and corresponding computed tomography (CT) image (D) showing successful closure of the dehiscence with two occlusion devices side by side. Orientation identical to panels A and B.

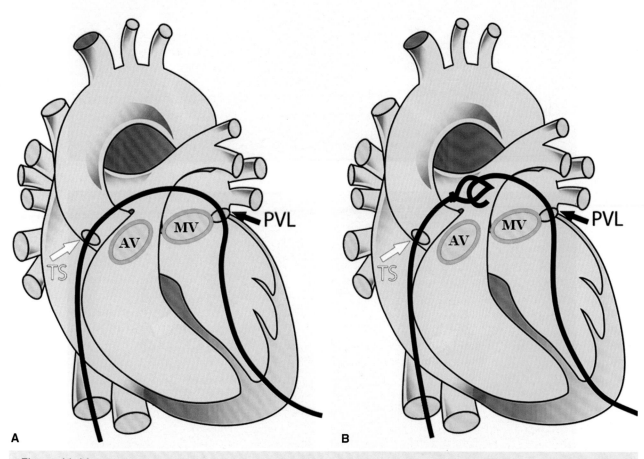

A

B

Figure 11-16. **PVL roadmap.** Access to mitral paravalvular leak (PVL) site can be accomplished via a venous approach and transseptal (TS) puncture or via a direct left ventricular apical puncture (A). Occasionally, both approaches are utilized simultaneously with snaring of the catheters and essentially creating a "rail" on which devices can be manipulated from both sides (B).

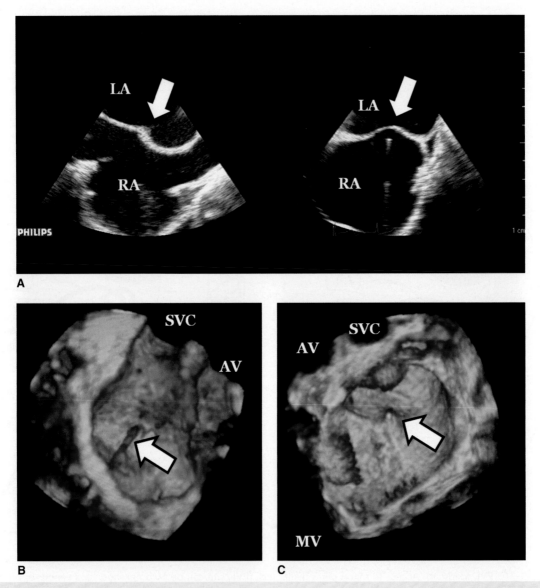

Figure 11-17. Transseptal puncture. Atrial septal puncture is often necessary to enter the left atrium during percutaneous repair of structural heart disease. A. Three-dimensional TEE biplane view demonstrates tenting (*arrow*) by the puncture needle in two orthogonal views. B. Three-dimensional TEE zoom view of the interatrial septum from the right atrial perspective shows the needle assembly (*arrow*) pushing through the superior aspect of the fossa ovalis. C. Three-dimensional TEE zoom view of the interatrial septum from the left atrial perspective demonstrates tenting (*arrow*) of the interatrial septum by the needle assembly. Accompanying Video 11-17-1 shows tenting on 3D TEE; courtesy of Dr. Francesco Faletra, Lugano Medical Center, Switzerland. AV, aortic valve; LA, left atrium; RA, right atrium; SVC, superior vena cava.

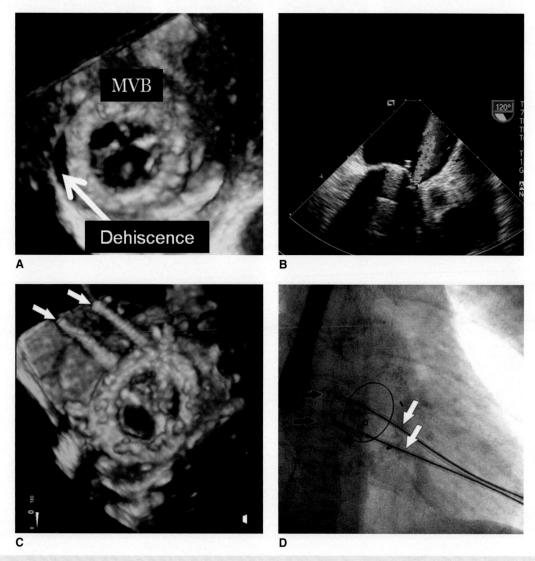

Figure 11-18. PVL (bioprosthesis) 3D TEE guidance. A and B. Preprocedure assessment of dehiscence site and severity of mitral valve bioprosthesis (MVB) paravalvular regurgitation. RT3D en face view from the atrial perspective (A) demonstrates the exact anatomic location of the dehisced segment, at the 9 o'clock (lateral) position. Color Doppler imaging (B) shows moderate paravalvular (PVL) mitral regurgitation. C and D. Images obtained during catheter advancement and manipulation during closure procedure. Catheters are introduced through a left ventricular apical puncture and viewed from the left atrial perspective. Since the dehisced site was deemed to be too large to be occluded by one closure device, two guiding catheters were introduced through the apical puncture into the PVL site (D and E). Note how clearly the path of both catheters through the dehisced site can be seen on the RT3D en face view (D), while on fluoroscopy (E), the spatial relationship of the catheters cannot be precisely discerned. Accompanying Video 11-18-1 corresponds to panel A.

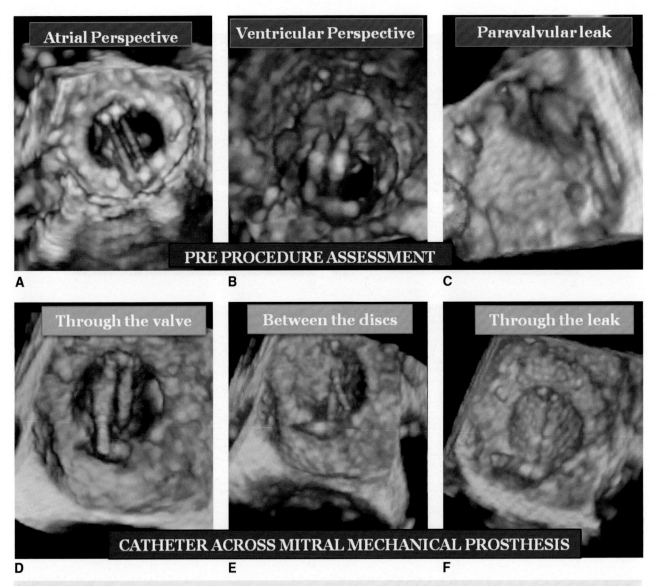

Figure 11-19. PVL (mechanical) 3D TEE guidance. A–C. Preprocedure assessment of dehiscence site and severity of a mitral mechanical prosthesis paravalvular regurgitation (St. Jude, bidisc). The valve can be seen from the atrial side (A) as well as ventricular side (B). Full-volume color acquisition (C) confirms the presence of a PVL at the 7 o'clock (posterolateral) position. D–F. Images obtained during a catheter-based closure procedure via a transapical approach; the guiding catheter is advanced from the left ventricle into the left atrium. Images show en face view of the mitral valve from the atrial perspective and allow for exact delineation of the guiding catheter position in relation to the valve discs. Panel D shows the guidewire passing through the valve, lateral to the discs, and panel E shows another attempt at passing the guidewire; however, this time it passes in between the two valve discs. Panel F shows successful advancement of the guidewire through the dehiscence site, allowing for continuation of the procedure and ultimately placement of a closure device and occlusion of the PVL. Accompanying Videos 11-19-1, 11-19-2, and 11-19-3 correspond to panels A, B, and C, respectively.

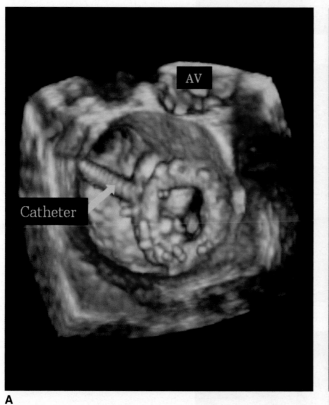

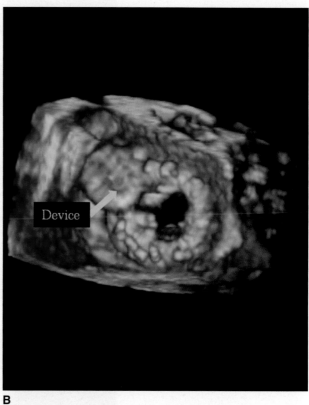

A

B

Figure 11-20. **Successful PVL closure.** A. En face view of a mitral bioprosthesis with a catheter across a PVL site, which is at 9 to 10 o'clock position. B. Closure device successfully placed at the PVL site, achieving complete occlusion and correction of the paravalvular mitral regurgitation. AV denotes aortic valve. Accompanying Videos 11-20-1 and 11-20-2 correspond to panel A and B, respectively.

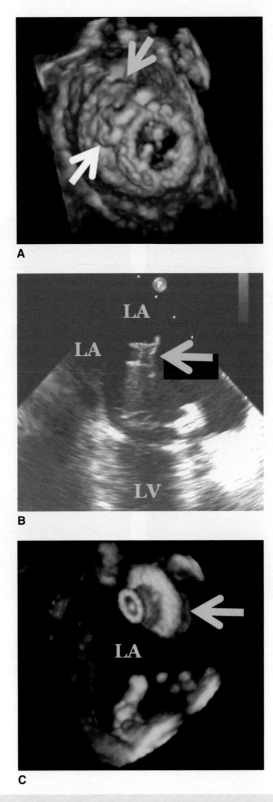

Figure 11-21. Complications of paravalvular closure. A. En face 3D TEE zoom view of a mitral bioprosthesis. PVL along the lateral aspect of the prosthetic rim necessitated the use of two occluder devices (*arrows*). B and C. Subsequently, one of the occluder devices (*arrow*) popped out into the left atrium. This was visualized by both 2D TEE (B) and 3D TEE (C). Accompanying Video 11-21-1 corresponds to panels B and C.

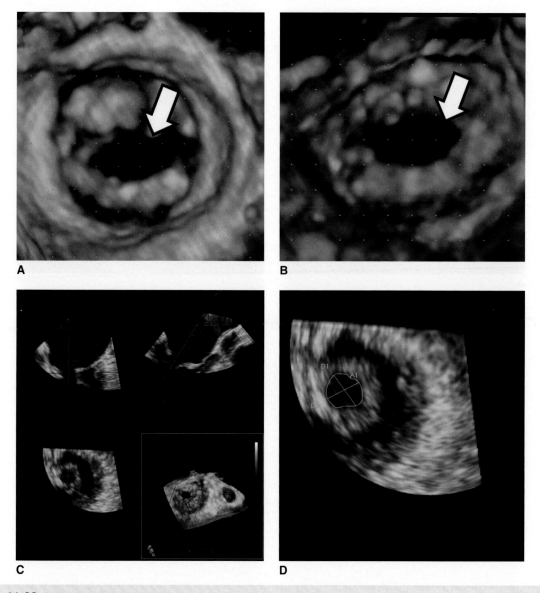

Figure 11-22. Mitral stenosis—preprocedural mitral valve area calculation. A and B. Semiquantitative sizing of the mitral valve area on 3D TEE zoom views of the mitral valve from the left atrial (A) and the left ventricular side (B). The distance between two dots on the grid overlaying the mitral valve is 5 mm. C and D. Precise measurements of the mitral valve area at leaflet tips are obtained by multiplane reconstruction techniques. In panel C, the two images in the top row show the mitral valve in its long axis, while the bottom images show the valve in its short axis. Panel D is a blown-up version of the bottom left image in panel C. By tracing the perimeter of the mitral valve at leaflet tips, one can precisely measure the mitral valve area (0.8 cm^2 in this case). Accompanying Video 11-22-1 corresponds to panels C and D.

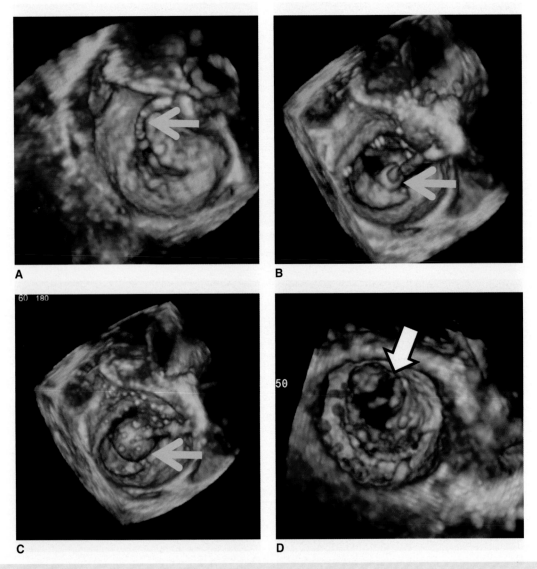

Figure 11-23. Three-dimensional TEE guidance of percutaneous mitral balloon valvuloplasty. A. Three-dimensional TEE zoom en face view of the mitral valve from the left atrial perspective shows the catheter (*arrow*) with deflated Inoue balloon being positioned at the orifice of the mitral valve. B. Partly inflated balloon is seen in the mitral orifice from the left atrial perspective. C. Fully inflated balloon in the mitral orifice from the left atrial perspective. Accompanying Video 11-23-1 corresponds to panels A, B, and C. D. Mitral valve seen from the left ventricular perspective. Percutaneous mitral balloon valvuloplasty was complicated in this patient by an anterior leaflet tear (*arrow*) and severe mitral regurgitation (not shown). Accompanying Video 11-23-2 corresponds to panel D.

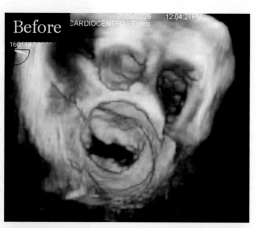

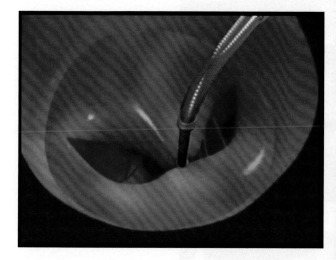

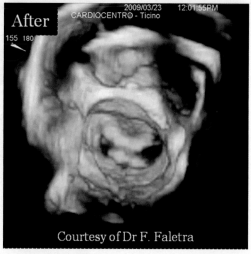

Figure 11-24. **Mitral valve clipping.** The basic principle of percutaneous treatment of mitral regurgitation utilizing the clip procedure. On the left side, a cartoon demonstrating the optimal placement of a mitral clip, in the center of the mitral valve, grasping together the two middle scallops (A2 and P2) of the mitral valve. On the right side, pre- and postclip RT3D images of the mitral valve en face from the left atrial perspective. The clip creates a double-orifice mitral valve, allowing for decreasing the mitral regurgitation effective orifice area.

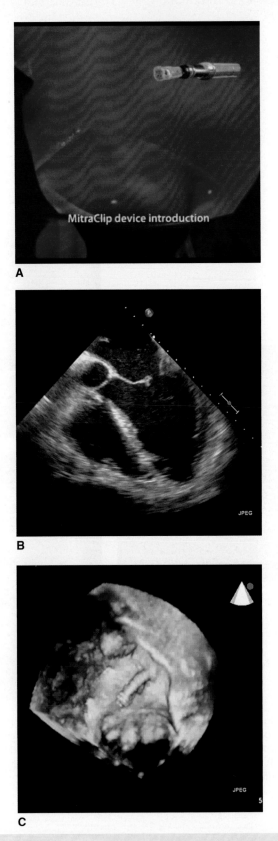

A

B

C

Figure 11-25. MV clipping cartoon versus 2D versus 3D. For percutaneous treatment of mitral regurgitation, the mitral valve is approached via a venous access and a transseptal puncture. A. Cartoon depiction of the guiding catheter as it is advanced through a transseptal puncture. B. 2D image obtained during a clipping procedure. Note how the catheter partially "disappears" in the left atrium due to the tomographic nature of 2D echocardiographic imaging. C. Simultaneously acquired 3D image of the guiding catheter as it is advanced through the transseptal puncture. Note how the entire left atrial portion of the catheter is well seen, allowing for its safe advancement. Accompanying Video 11-25-1 corresponds to panel C.

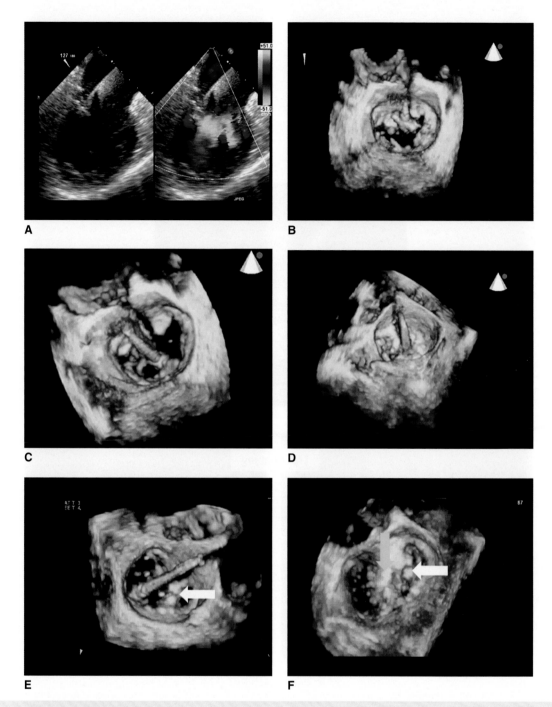

Figure 11-26. MV clipping—procedure stages. A. 2D image taken as the clip device is advanced in the left atrium. B. En face view of the mitral valve as the clip is advanced further toward the valve. Note the clear visualization of the clip arms, allowing for proper alignment of the clip such that the arms are perpendicular to the mitral valve coaptation line. C. Once the clip is aligned properly, it is further advanced across the mitral valve, into the left ventricle. The clip is then slowly pulled back, attempting to grasp the valve leaflets onto the open arms of the clip. D. Grasping attempt as viewed en face from the left atrial perspective. The valve leaflets appear to be adhered to the clip arms. E. After the clip was deployed, the severity of the remaining mitral regurgitation was assessed and found to be still significant. Anatomic evaluation of the clip position utilizing RT3D imaging demonstrated that the clip was positioned somewhat medial to the central portion of the mitral leaflets (connecting P3 and A3 rather than P2/A2). A second clip was introduced, and utilizing RT3D imaging was directed into the larger orifice that was created with the first clip. Note on this image the clear spatial relationship between the deployed clip (*white arrow*) and the newly introduced clip (still on the delivery system), which is lateral to the first one. F. Final result showing two clips well positioned in the mitral valve, creating a triple-orifice mitral valve (*white arrow* pointing to the first clip, *yellow arrow* pointing to the second, lateral clip). The mitral regurgitation was significantly improved. Accompanying Video 11-26-1 corresponds to panel B, Video 11-26-2 corresponds to panel D, and Video 11-26-3 corresponds to panel E.

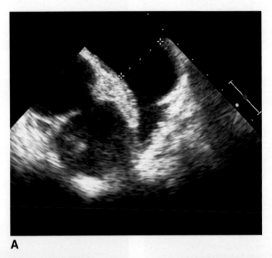

A

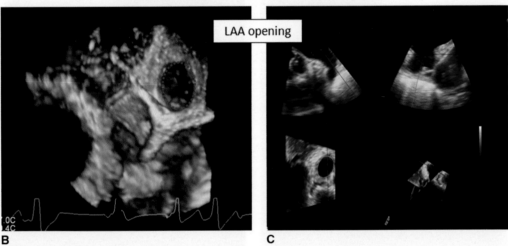

LAA opening

B   **C**

Figure 11-27. **LAA sizing.** Preprocedure assessment of suitability for percutaneous left atrial appendage (LAA) obliteration procedure. A shows 2D measurement of the LAA orifice area. Note that only one dimension of the orifice can be measured at any given angle, necessitating repeated measurements at multiple angles and "mental reconstruction" of the LAA orifice shape. B shows RT3D image of en face view of the LAA opening, allowing for direct visualization of its shape. C shows postprocessing and 3D guided direct planimetry of the LAA orifice size. This allows for accurate measurement without a need for any geometric assumptions regarding the shape of the LAA opening.

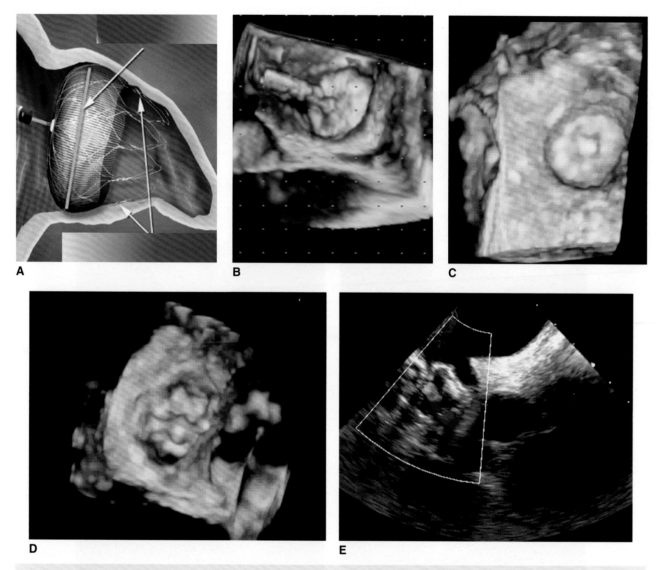

Figure 11-28. LAA occlusion procedure. A. Cartoon depiction of a closure device used to obliterate the LAA. The device is placed utilizing venous access and transseptal puncture. B. Closure device positioned at the LAA opening. Note that the anatomic position of the device can be assessed utilizing en face, RT3D view while the device is still on the delivery system. If the position is judged to be unsatisfactory, further manipulation and positioning can be done. C. Final result of successful deployment of a LAA obliteration device. Note the clear anatomic delineation of the complete occlusion of the LAA opening. D and E. Malpositioning of an obliteration device in the LAA opening. Note the easy anatomic assessment of the device position (D), not achieving complete occlusion of the LAA orifice. Color Doppler imaging (E) further confirms residual flow to and from the main left atrium, around the device. Accompanying Video 11-28-1 corresponds to panel C, Video 11-28-2 corresponds to panel E.

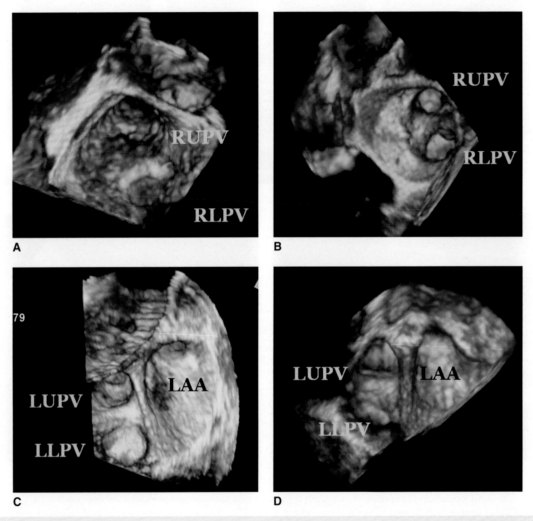

Figure 11-29. Anatomy of pulmonary veins. Three-dimensional TEE zoom view of right-sided (A and B) and left-sided pulmonary veins (C and D). Pulmonary veins can have individual ostia (A and C) or can converge to a common antrum (B and D). LAA, left atrial appendage; LLPV, left lower pulmonary vein; LUPV, left upper pulmonary vein; RLPV, right lower pulmonary vein; RUPV, right upper pulmonary vein.

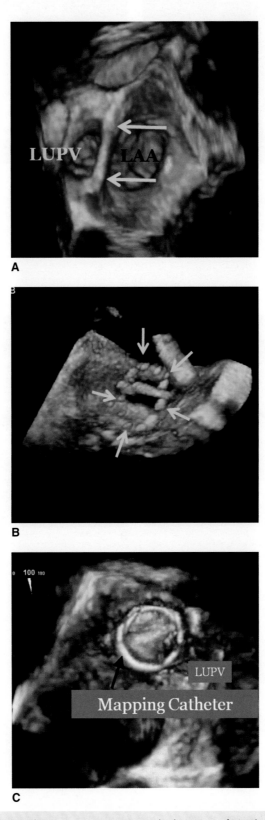

Figure 11-30. Electrophysiology procedures. A. *Arrows* point to the ligament of Marshall ("Coumadin ridge"), an important anatomic landmark for electrophysiologists, visualized by 3D TEE zoom. It separates the left atrial appendage (LAA) from the orifice of the left upper pulmonary vein (LUPV). B. The so-called lasso catheter (*arrows*) is seen in the left atrium using the 3D TEE zoom technique. Image courtesy of Drs. Scott Bernstein and Jan Purgess of the Manhattan VA Medical Center. C. Three-dimensional TEE appearance of a mapping catheter (*arrow*) adjacent to the left upper pulmonary vein (LUPV). Image courtesy of Dr. Miguel A Garcia-Fernandez, Madrid University Hospital.

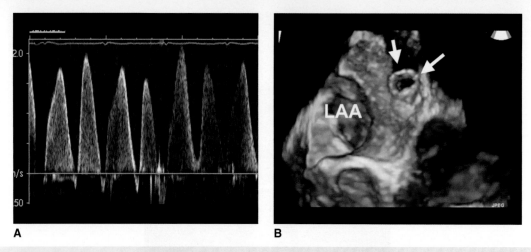

Figure 11-31. Pulmonary vein stenosis. A. Pulmonary vein spectral Doppler tracing demonstrates high-velocity antegrade flow (peak velocity 1.5 to 2.0 m/s) indicative of pulmonary vein stenosis in this patient who previously underwent pulmonary vein ablation. **B.** Three-dimensional TEE zoom image shows a stent (*arrows*) in the left upper pulmonary vein placed to relieve postablation pulmonary vein stenosis. LAA, left atrial appendage. Images courtesy of Dr. Miguel A Garcia-Fernandez, Madrid University Hospital.

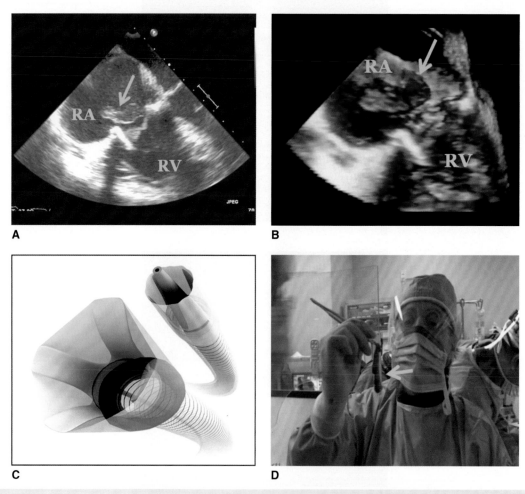

Figure 11-32. Percutaneous removal of intracardiac thrombus. A. Two-dimensional TEE image shows a large thrombus (*arrow*) floating in the right atrium. RA, right atrium; RV, right ventricle. **B.** Three-dimensional TEE image corresponding to panel A. **C.** *Schematic* depiction of the AngioVac extractor (Vortex Medical, Norwell, MA, USA) used to remove the intracardiac thrombus seen in panels A and B. **D.** A large sausage-shaped thrombus (*arrow*) held by the interventionalist after the thrombus was removed percutaneously using the vacuum extractor seen in panel C. Video 11-32-1 corresponds to panels A and B while Video 11-32-2 corresponds to panel D.

References

1. Perk G, Ruiz C, Saric M, et al. Real-time three-dimensional transesophageal echocardiography in transcutaneous, catheter-based procedures for repair of structural heart diseases. *Curr Cardiovasc Imaging Rep.* 2009;2(5):363–374.

2. Perk G, Lang RM, Garcia-Fernandez MA, et al. Use of real time three-dimensional transesophageal echocardiography in intracardiac catheter based interventions. *J Am Soc Echocardiogr.* 2009;22(8):865–882.

3. Lang RM, Badano LP, Tsang W, et al. EAE/ASE recommendations for image acquisition and display using three-dimensional echocardiography. *J Am Soc Echocardiogr.* 2012;25(1):3–46.

4. Tsang W, Lang RM, Kronzon I. Role of real-time three dimensional echocardiography in cardiovascular interventions. *Heart.* 2011;97(10):850–857.

5. Garcia-Fernandez MA, Perk G, Saric M, et al. Real-time three-dimensional transesophageal echocardiography for guidance of catheter based interventions. In: Badano LP, Lang RM, Zamorano JL, Eds. *Textbook of real-time three-dimensional echocardiography.* Chapter 12, 1st ed. Springer; 2011:121–134.

6. Skolnick A, Vavas E, Kronzon I. Optimization of ASD assessment using real time three-dimensional transesophageal echocardiography. *Echocardiography.* 2009;26(2):233–235.

7. Faletra FF, Nucifora G, Ho SY. Imaging the atrial septum using real-time three-dimensional transesophageal echocardiography: technical tips, normal anatomy, and its role in transseptal puncture. *J Am Soc Echocardiogr.* 2011;24(6):593–599.

8. Saric M, Perk G, Purgess J, et al. Imaging atrial septal defects by real-time 3D transesophageal echocardiography: step-by-step approach. *J Am Soc Echocardiogr.* 2010;23(11):1128–1135.

9. Kronzon I, Ruiz CE. Diagnosing patent foramen ovale: too little or too much? *JACC Cardiovasc Imaging.* 2010;3(4):349–351.

10. Kliger C, Jelnin V, Perk G, et al. Use of multi-modality imaging in a patient with a persistent left superior vena cava, partial anomalous pulmonary venous connection, and sinus venosus-type atrial septal defect. *Eur Heart J Cardiovasc Imaging* 2012;13(6):499.

11. Price MJ, Smith MR, Rubenson DS. Utility of on-line three-dimensional transesophageal echocardiography during percutaneous atrial septal defect closure. *Catheter Cardiovasc Interv.* 2010;75(4):570–577.

12. López AL, Palomas JL, Rubio DM, et al. Three-dimensional echocardiography-guided repair of residual shunt after percutaneous atrial septal defect closure. *Echocardiography.* 2011;28(3):E64–E67.

13. Halpern DG, Perk G, Ruiz C, et al. Percutaneous closure of a post-myocardial infarction ventricular septal defect guided by real-time three-dimensional echocardiography. *Eur J Echocardiogr.* 2009;10(4):569–571.

14. Dudiy Y, Jelnin V, Einhorn BN, et al. Percutaneous closure of left ventricular pseudoaneurysm. *Circ Cardiovasc Interv.* 2011;4(4):322–326.

15. Kronzon I, Sugeng L, Perk G, et al. Real-time 3-dimensional transesophageal echocardiography in the evaluation of post-operative mitral annuloplasty ring and prosthetic valve dehiscence. *J Am Coll Cardiol.* 2009;53(17):1543–1547.

16. Ruiz CE, Jelnin V, Kronzon I, et al. Clinical outcomes in patients undergoing percutaneous closure of periprosthetic paravalvular leaks. *J Am Coll Cardiol.* 2011;58(21):2210–2217.

17. Jelnin V, Dudiy Y, Einhorn BN, et al. Clinical experience with percutaneous left ventricular transapical access for interventions in structural heart defects a safe access and secure exit. *JACC Cardiovasc Interv.* 2011;4(8):868–874.

18. Tsang W, Weinert L, Kronzon I, et al. Three-dimensional echocardiography in the assessment of prosthetic valves. *Rev Esp Cardiol.* 2011;64(1):1–7.

19. Schlosshan D, Aggarwal G, Mathur G, et al. Real-time 3D transesophageal echocardiography for the evaluation of rheumatic mitral stenosis. *JACC Cardiovasc Imaging.* 2011;4(6):580–588.

20. Weyman AE. Assessment of mitral stenosis: role of real-time 3D TEE. *JACC Cardiovasc Imaging.* 2011;4(6):589–591.

21. Kronzon I, Saric M, Lang RM. Mitral stenosis. In: Lang RM, Vannan MA, Khanderia BK, Eds. *Dynamic echocardiography: a case-based approach.* Chapter 9, 1st ed. Springer; 2010:38–45.

22. Biner S, Perk G, Kar S, et al. Utility of combined two-dimensional and three-dimensional transesophageal imaging for catheter-based mitral valve clip repair of mitral regurgitation. *J Am Soc Echocardiogr* 2011;24(6):611–617.

23. Perk G, Biner S, Kronzon I, et al. Catheter-based left atrial appendage occlusion procedure: role of echocardiography. *Eur Heart J Cardiovasc Imaging* 2012;13(2):132–138.

24. Faletra FF, Ho SY, Auricchio A. Anatomy of right atrial structures by real-time 3D transesophageal echocardiography. *JACC Cardiovasc Imaging* 2010;3(9):966–975.

25. Levy MS, Todoran TM, Kinlay S, et al. Use of real-time 3D transesophageal echocardiography in percutaneous intervention of a flush-occluded pulmonary vein. *Circ Cardiovasc Interv* 2010;3(4):394–395.

26. Dudiy Y, Kronzon I, Cohen HA, et al. Vacuum thrombectomy of large right atrial thrombus. *Catheter Cardiovasc Interv* 2012;79(2):344–347.

3D ECHO FOR GUIDANCE OF INTERVENTION IN STRUCTURAL HEART DISEASE

12

Robert J. Siegel, Swaminatha Gurudevan, Kirsten Tolstrup, Nirmal Singh, Huai Luo, Takahiro Shiota

In the past several years, there have been significant advances in the development of transcatheter technologies to treat structural heart disease. Fluoroscopy and angiography have in the past been used to guide mitral balloon valvuloplasty and closure of patent foramen ovale (PFO), atrial septal defect (ASD), ventricular septal defect (VSD), and patent ductus arteriosus (PDA). However, 2D echocardiography with transesophageal echocardiography (TEE) or intracardiac echocardiography (ICE) has subsequently been shown to enhance the safety and efficacy of these procedures. More complex transcatheter procedures are now being done for structural heart disease and include percutaneous aortic valve replacement (AVR) for aortic stenosis (AS), pulmonic valve replacement (PVR) for pulmonic valve regurgitation (PR), placement of left atrial appendage (LAA) occlusion devices and MitraClip repair for mitral regurgitation (MR). While all of the above-mentioned procedures can be guided by 2D echo imaging—TEE and in some cases ICE—in our experience, we have found live 3D TEE enhances percutaneous atrial and VSD closures and sizing and delivery of percutaneous aortic valves (AVs). For mitral valve (MV) procedures, 3D TEE is especially useful to visualize the MV apparatus and to identify the pathoanatomy responsible for both mitral stenosis and MR. In addition, the identification of optimal candidates and exclusion of patients are greatly facilitated by 3D imaging. The advent of live 3D TEE has, in our interventional laboratory, enhanced guidance of the MitraClip catheter system and clip placement. The number of recent publications on the use of live 3D TEE for transcatheter therapy reflects its utility and the increased adoption for use during transcatheter therapy for structural heart disease.[1–7] Table 12-1 lists the types of structural heart disease cases for which we have used live 3D TEE imaging for preselection of cases as well as for guidance of device deployment and postprocedural assessment. It is expected that as innovations occur for the transcatheter as well as the percutaneous transapical treatment of structural heart diseases, 3D ultrasound imaging will continue to grow and evolve as the imaging standard for these procedures.

TRANSSEPTAL PUNCTURE OF THE ATRIAL SEPTUM

TEE has been shown to be useful in transseptal (TS) puncture, which is a prerequisite for a number of percutaneous interventions, which include MV balloon valvuloplasty, MitraClip repair, implantation of LAA occlusion devices, and repair of paravalvular leaks. Three-dimensional TEE enables the TS puncture to be performed not only safely but also precisely in the location of the interatrial septum (IAS) most optimal for the particular structural heart intervention that is being performed. Three-dimensional TEE probes have the advantage of providing simultaneous biplane imaging of the atrial septum at a range of angulations. Biplane imaging allows for assessment of the TS needle in regard to how superior or inferior it is along the IAS, as well as to how anterior or posterior the needle is positioned.[3,4] In addition, 3D TEE shows en face imaging of the IAS and is very sensitive for detecting tenting of the atrial septum by the TS needle prior to puncture.

MITRAL STENOSIS

Mitral balloon valvuloplasty has been guided by fluoroscopy with or without 2D transthoracic echo or TEE. Recent experience using 3D TEE adds additional information in the assessment of MV stenosis, valve morphology, and the potential for successful valvuloplasty. Three-dimensional imaging allows the interventional cardiologist to decide where to inflate the valvuloplasty balloon for maximum benefit while avoiding fracture of the valve in calcific areas (Table 12-2).

ATRIAL SEPTAL DEFECT

Recent 3D imaging studies have shown the value of a sequential approach for the 3D TEE assessment of ASDs. Saric et al. have demonstrated that at a 0-degree angle, the 3D image should first be tilted up to reveal the right side of the atrial septum. If the image is then rotated 180 degrees around its vertical axis, the left side of the septum and the aortic rim can be demonstrated. From this angulation, the aortic rim is to the left, the superior vena cava (SVC) is superior and the ostium of the right pulmonary vein is on the right side of the image plane[8,9] (Table 12-3).

VENTRICULAR SEPTAL DEFECT

Three-dimensional echocardiography provides excellent visualization of VSDs in patients as well as in experimentally created VSDs in animals.[10] From a left ventricular (LV) en face projection, the position, size, and shape of VSD can be accurately determined. The authors predicted that precise imaging by 3D echocardiography may be beneficial for surgical and catheter-based closure of difficult perimembranous and singular or multiple muscular VSDs. More recently, real-time 3D echocardiography has been employed for the catheter-based closure of muscular VSD.[11] We have found real-time 3D TEE useful for transcatheter and surgical closure of congenital as well as post–myocardial infarction VSDs (Table 12-3).

WATCHMAN DEVICE GUIDANCE

As with the other procedures, 3D TEE benefits deployment of the LAA occlusion device by facilitating TS puncture and guidance of the intracardiac catheter to the LAA and to the apex of the LAA. Postdeployment 3D TEE color flow Doppler is especially useful to detect and assess the severity of regurgitation around the LAA occlusion device. Unlike 2D imaging, 3D TEE uniquely permits assessment of the device and leakage around the device from a 360-degree perspective[12] (Table 12-4).

TRANSCATHETER AORTIC VALVE IMPLANTATION

Two-dimensional TEE is routinely used to assess aortic annular dimensions prior to transcatheter aortic valve implantation (TAVI). Recent studies demonstrate that the aortic annulus is frequently oval, not circular, suggesting that CT may be a better modality than echo to evaluate aortic annular dimensions.[13] However, 3D imaging whether done by CT or 3D TEE has similar results and reveals that the aortic annulus is often wider in the coronal cross section than the sagittal cross section.[3,14–16] In addition to precise multiplanar dimensional measurements, 3D imaging provides superb anatomic detail of the stenotic AV, aortic root, the subvalvular anatomy, and shape of the basal ventricular septum as well as the relationship of the AV to the anterior mitral leaflet (AML). This relationship is especially important for TAVI, as basal septal hypertrophy may impair effective transapical TAVI procedures. These cases may also be associated with elevated left ventricular outflow tract (LVOT) pressure gradients post procedure. Moreover, placement of the percutaneously delivered AV too low in the LVOT can lead to impingement on the AML. Postprocedural assessment of residual aortic regurgitation is often difficult, but 3D color flow allows more accurate assessment of the site of origin of the leak—paravalvular or transvalvular. Additionally, when there is a paravalvular leak, 3D color flow demonstrates the circumference of the leak around the valve and thus provides better detection of leak severity. Biplane imaging with the 3D system is also useful. An additional benefit of 3D imaging for TAVI is to be able to detect the distance of the coronary ostia from the aortic annulus. This can usually be done by 2D TEE for the right coronary artery (RCA); however, it is generally not possible by 2D TEE for the left main coronary artery (LMCA) annular distance. A 3D full-volume imaging with multiplanar reconstruction provides the annular to LMCA distance with imaging in the coronal plane (Table 12-5).

PARAVALVULAR LEAKS

With 2D TEE imaging, it is often difficult to determine the location, number, as well as size of prosthetic valve paravalvular leaks. The use of 3D TEE with and without color Doppler has greatly simplified the assessment of paravalvular leaks.[17] A 3D TEE allows the echocardiographer to obtain en face images of the valve prostheses and to detect the number, location, shape, and size of paravalvular defects[18–20] (Table 12-6).

ACKNOWLEDGMENTS

The authors acknowledge the excellent collaboration with our cardiac interventionalists Dr. Saibal Kar and Dr. Rajendra Makar. In addition, we appreciate their outstanding abilities in the percutaneous treatment of structural heart disease, and we have learned a great deal from their interest and expertise in structural heart disease.

TABLE 12-1 • 3D TEE–guided Percutaneous Interventions
• AVR for aortic stenosis
• PVR for severe pulmonic valve regurgitation
• Mitral balloon valvuloplasty for mitral stenosis
• Repair of paravalvular leak
• Closure of ASD and VSD
• Devices for LAA closure

TABLE 12-2 • Mitral Valve Valvuloplasty— Advantages of Live 3D TEE
• Entire intracardiac length of catheter visualized
• Guidance of transseptal puncture
• Localization of the balloon in MV orifice
• Excellent assessment of MV after valvuloplasty
• Assessment of postprocedure MR and mechanism

TABLE 12-3 • Transcatheter ASD and VSD Closure—3D TEE
• En face visualization of the defect
• Dynamic orifice
• Accurate assessment of defect size
• Accurate assessment of defect shape
• Assessment of defect rim
• Assessment of shunt flow

TABLE 12-4 • Watchman LAA Closure Device Selection

Max LAA Ostium (mm)	Device Diameter (mm)	Device Length (mm)
17–19.9	21	20.2
20–22.9	24	22.9
23–25.9	27	26.5
26–28.9	30	29.4
29–31.9	33	31.6

TABLE 12-5 • Transcatheter Closure of LAA— 3D TEE

- Monitor transseptal puncture
- Visualization of guide catheter/device
- Proper sizing
- Assessment of atypical LAA
- En face view of device at LAA orifice identifies optimal positioning
  - Color flow shows residual flow in cross section at device surface

TABLE 12-6 • Catheter-based AVR—PARTNER Clinical Trial—Role of TEE and 3D

- Measurement of aortic annulus (sizing 23 vs. 26 mm AVR)
- Coaxial delivery with LVOT and aortic root
- Position valve to be aligned with AV cusps
- Assessing AR postdeployment
- Assessing complications

TABLE 12-7 ● Percutaneous Closure of Paravalvular Leak—Advantages of Live 3D TEE
• Site, shape, size of dehisced segment
• Identify candidates for procedure
• Identify/verify catheter placement through the dehisced segment
• 3D TEE color—effective circumferential orifice and reduction in circumferential orifice length
• Real-time assessment of procedural success

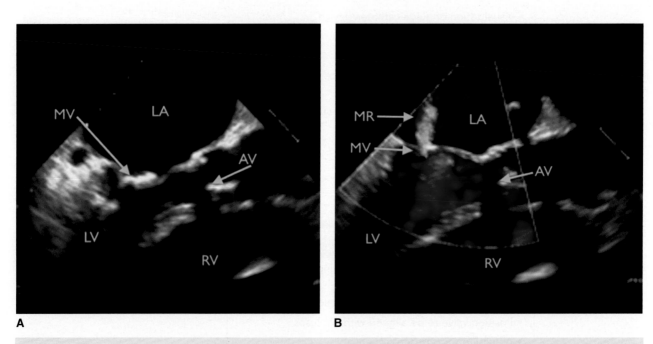

A   B

Figure 12-1. A 2D TEE of mitral stenosis prevalvuloplasty. A. 2D TEE long-axis view shows a mildly calcified, rheumatic valve labeled as MV (Video 12-8A) with spontaneous contrast seen in the left atrium (LA). B. 2D TEE long-axis view with color flow Doppler shows aliased color flow across the stenotic MV labeled as MV and trivial MR going into LA as indicated by MR (Video 12-8B).

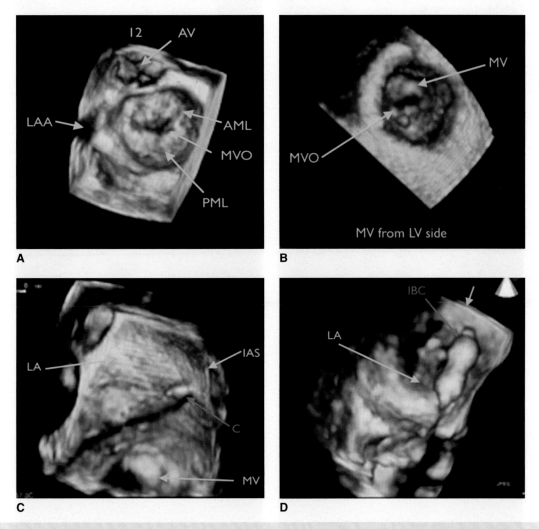

Figure 12-2. A–D. Valvuloplasty of mitral stenosis. A. This is surgical view on 3D TEE with orientation of AV anterior to MV at the "12 o'clock" position as shown in the figure. The characteristic crescent-shaped mitral valve orifice (MVO) is well appreciated in diastole. The stenotic MVO area can be measured using the grids on the image (Video 12-9A). B. The image of MV from LV side shows classical fish-mouth appearance of MVO due to rheumatic process producing commissural fusion and thickened mitral leaflets (Video 12-9B). C. Three-dimensional oblique view of the LA revealing the guide wire and catheter marked as C. The catheter is seen entering into LA after TS puncture via the IAS (Video 12-9C). D. MV balloon valvuloplasty catheter (Inoue Balloon Catheter, [IBC]) across the IAS and entering the MV orifice. The balloon catheter is clearly seen in the LA heading down toward the MV (Video 12-9D).

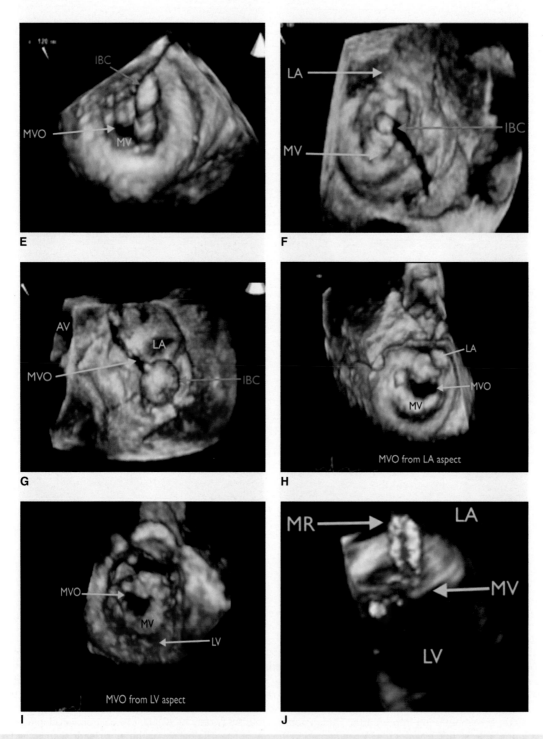

Figure 12-2. *(Continued)* 12-9E–G. Valvuloplasty of mitral stenosis. E, F. Three-dimensional views of MV balloon valvulo-plasty catheter (IBC), passing across the IAS and entering into the MVO as shown in the figure. Three-dimensional image provides detailed orientation of anatomic structures that cannot be appreciated by 2D TEE images (Videos 12-9E and 12-9F). G. Three-dimensional TEE view of the inflated IBC in the MVO (Video 12-9G). Note the detail revealed by the 3D image, which almost has the appearance of a schematic rather than an ultrasound image. H–J. Mitral stenosis postvalvuloplasty. MVO view from above, that is, left atrial aspect (H), and from below, that is, LV aspect (I), after mitral balloon valvuloplasty. The increased excursion of the mitral leaflets can be appreciated by the change in the area of MVO, which is evident in the figure (Videos 12-9H and 12-9I). J. Three-dimensional full-volume color flow Doppler image shows mild MR post mitral val-vuloplasty (Video 12-9J).

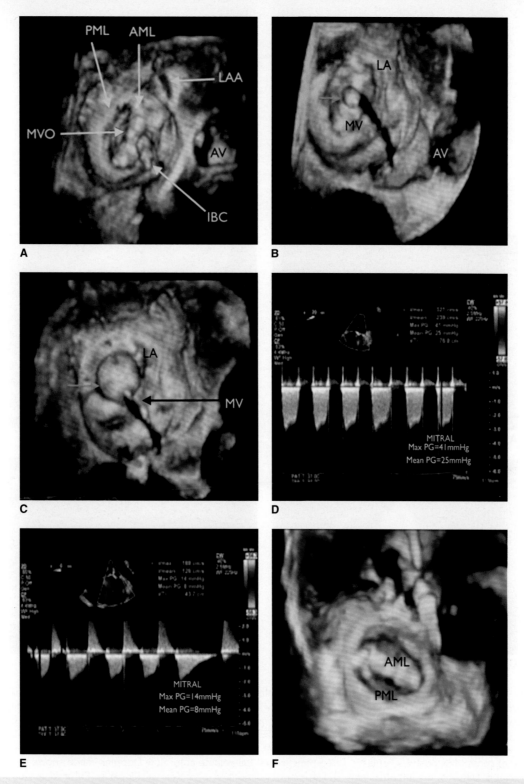

Figure 12-3. A–C. Severe calcific mitral stenosis. Three-dimensional TEE images obtained in an elderly man with critical, calcific, rheumatic MS, who had severe pulmonary hypertension, CHF, and hepatic and renal insufficiency. Note the calcific and stenotic MV hardly opens before valvuloplasty (A). The orientation of the 3D image has the AV at 3 o'clock and the LAA at 12 o'clock. The MV balloon valvuloplasty catheter is seen in the LA. This patient had been refused surgical MV repair, and valvuloplasty was undertaken despite a high Wilkins score (REF) in this valve with extensive MV calcification. Both the mitral leaflets are severely calcified, and there is critical calcific rheumatic mitral stenosis (Video 12-10A). Images obtained during mitral valvuloplasty: (B) IBC entering into the MVO before inflation and (C) inflated IBC across the MVO (Videos 12-10B and 12-10C). D, E. Transmitral gradient by Doppler before and after valvuloplasty. Continuous wave Doppler (CWD) images with a peak and mean pressure gradient across the MV: (D) peak gradient of 41 mm Hg with a mean of 25 mm Hg before balloon valvuloplasty qualifying it for severe mitral stenosis, and (E) the drop in both the peak gradient to 14 mm Hg and mean gradient to 8 mm Hg after valvuloplasty. F. Three-dimensional TEE findings after valvuloplasty. Improved excursion of the mitral leaflets after valvuloplasty as evident by the change in the mitral orifice area (Video 12-10F).

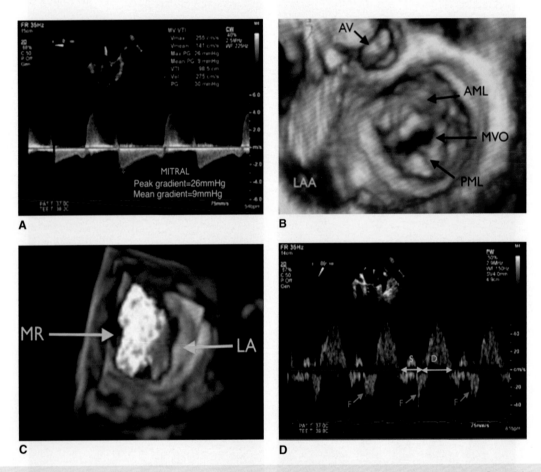

Figure 12-4. A–D. MV stenosis treated with balloon valvuloplasty. A. Middle-aged woman with significant dyspnea on exertion. Doppler gradient and color flow Doppler before valvuloplasty. CWD across the mitral inflow shows peak gradient of 26 mm Hg with a mean of 9 mm Hg indicating significant stenosis. Mild MR is also seen. B. Three-dimensional TEE of noncalcific mitral stenosis before valvuloplasty. Three-dimensional TEE image reveals characteristic mitral stenosis in surgical view with narrow MVO with commissural fusion and thickened AML and posterior mitral leaflet (PML). C. Three-dimensional TEE full volume of central MR postvalvuloplasty. Three-dimensional full-volume color flow Doppler image shows severe central regurgitant jet of MR from the left atrial view. D. Doppler of pulmonary veins after valvuloplasty. Pulse wave Doppler at left upper pulmonary vein shows flow reversal during systole confirming severe MR.

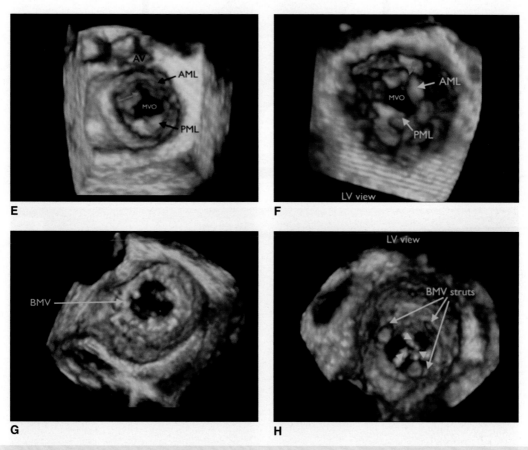

Figure 12-4. (*Continued*) E–H. MV stenosis treated with balloon valvuloplasty. Three-dimensional TEE after valvuloplasty of disrupted AML. This image is acquired after the inflation of stenosed MV. The *red arrow* indicates the tear in the AML, which caused acute severe MR correlating with images C and D. E. Image showing the torn AML from the left atrial aspect and (F) the same tear from the LV aspect. This patient was taken to the operating room for emergency surgical MV replacement with a bioprosthetic mitral valve (BMV) seen from the left atrial aspect (G) and LV aspect (H). The *arrowheads* identify the BMV leaflets while the *arrows* identify the three valve struts.

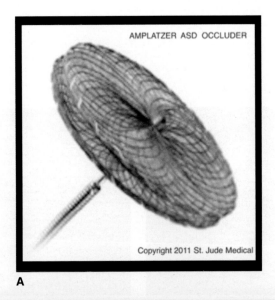

A

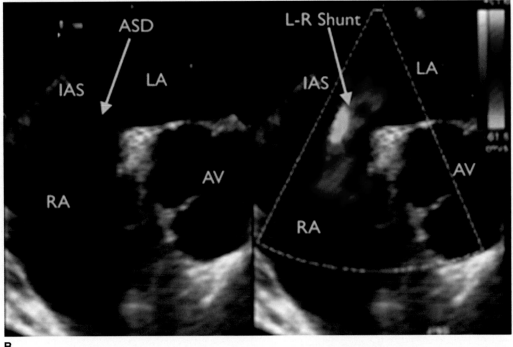

B

Figure 12-5. **Closure of secundum ASD.** A. Amplatzer ASD occluder device. B. 2D TEE showing secundum ASD and the 2D color flow image **(right)** showing left to right shunt (L-R shunt) across the ASD, which is large (>20 mm) in diameter. A prominent Eustachian valve is present. Large Eustachian valves have a propensity for being entrapped during percutaneous ASD closure. Such entrapment leads to a severe right to left shunt from the inferior vena cava (IVC) to the LA.

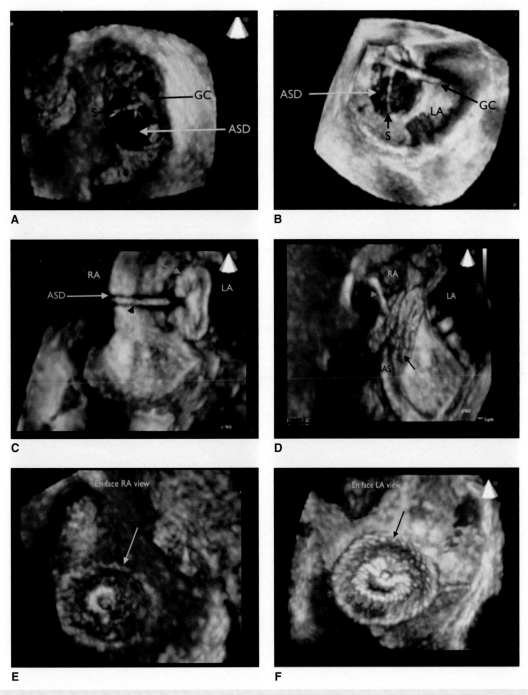

Figure 12-6. Three-dimensional TEE guidance of ASD closure. Three-dimensional TEE of secundum ASD. Detail of large ASD from right atrial side (A) and from left atrial side (B). There is a small fenestration through which the guiding catheter (GC) is traversing. A fibrous band or septation marked as S is noted traversing the ASD. C. Image showing the expanded part of left side of the Amplatzer device (*red arrow*). The catheter (*black arrowhead*) can be seen traversing across the ASD (Video 12-13C). D. Both the left and right disks of the Amplatzer device (marked with *black arrows*) are fully expanded sandwiching the IAS. E, F. En face view of the Amplatzer device from the right atrial perspective (*yellow arrow*) and left atrial perspective (*black arrow*).

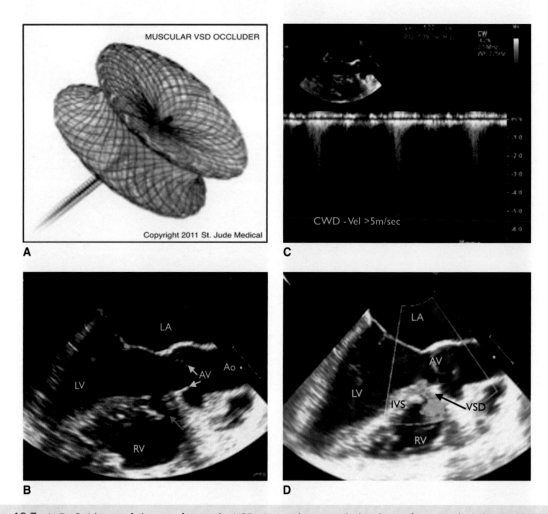

Figure 12-7. A–D. Guidance of closure of muscular VSD. A. Amplatzer occluder device for muscular VSD. B. 2D TEE long-axis view showing a congenital VSD (*red arrow*) (Video 12-14B). C. 2D TEE color flow Doppler showing the left to right shunt across the VSD (*black arrow*) (Video 12-14C). D. CWD across the VSD with a velocity >5 m/s, reflecting LV pressure exceeding RV pressure by at least 100 mm Hg.

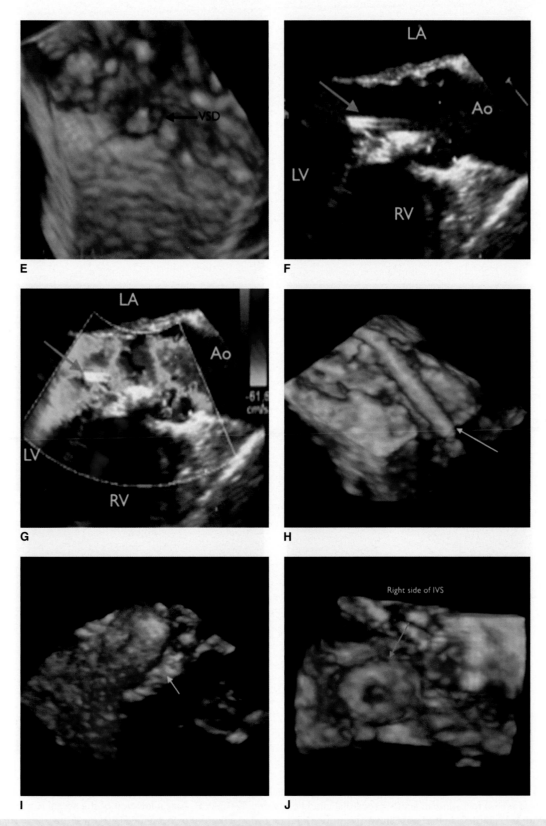

Figure 12-7. (*Continued*) E–G. Three-dimensional TEE guidance of closure of muscular VSD. E. En face view of the congenital VSD showing an almond shaped defect (*black arrow*) (Video 12-14E). F, G. Postprocedure images of the device (*red arrows*) showing no residual shunt flow across the defect by color Doppler (Video 12-14F and 12-14G). H–J. Three-dimensional TEE evaluation of congenital VSD closure. Three-dimensional TEE images during deployment (H) and after deployment (I) of an Amplatzer device for muscular VSD, revealing the left side of the device and (J) the right side of the device (Videos 12-14H, 12-14I and 12-14J).

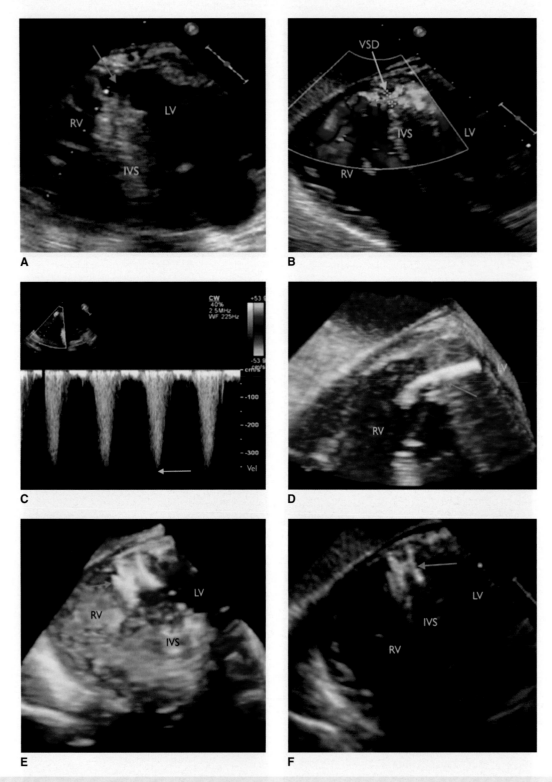

Figure 12-8. A–C. Ventricular septal rupture post myocardial infarction. A. 2D transthoracic image of a ventricular septal rupture (*red arrow*) following an acute myocardial infarction (Video 12-15A). B. Apical location of the septal rupture (*yellow arrow*) (Video 12-15B). C. Left to right shunt across the defect showing a high velocity on CWD (*yellow arrow*), consistent with LV pressure significantly exceeding RV pressure. D–F. Three- and two-dimensional TEE guidance of percutaneous closure of post–myocardial infarction VSD. D. Image taken during the percutaneous closure of ventricular septal rupture following myocardial infarction. The catheter (*red arrow*) is introduced via the right femoral artery to the aorta and then the left ventricle. Subsequently, the catheter is advanced through the defect into the right ventricle. E. Three-dimensional TEE and (F) 2D TEE image showing the occluder device (*red arrow*) (Video 12-15F).

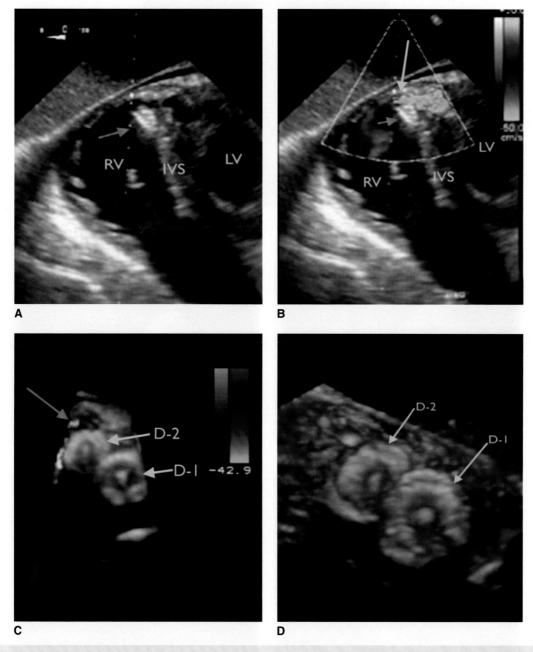

Figure 12-9. A–D. Three- and two-dimensional TEE evaluation of residual shunt and closure with echo guidance. A large residual shunt around the first device is shown by color Doppler (B). Even though the device is intact and appears to be placed in the correct position (A, *red arrow*) (Videos 12-16A and 12-16B). C. Three-dimensional image showing the placement of a second VSD occluder device (D-2) behind the first device (D-1) to close the large residual shunt. D. Full-volume color Doppler image showing two VSD occluder devices with minimal residual shunt (*arrow*).

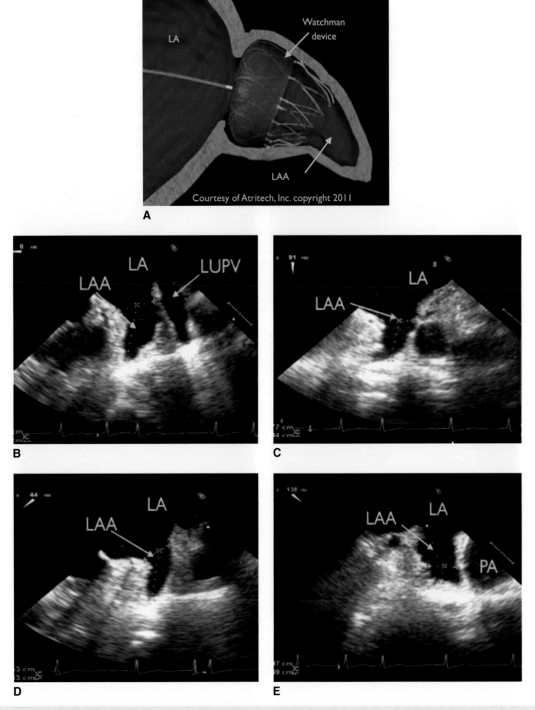

Figure 12-10. A. Schematic of an LAA with an implanted Watchman device. B–E. 2D TEE assessment of LAA shape and size. Images of the LAA evaluated at different angles, that is, 0, 45, 90, and 135 degrees. These views provide anatomic detail and help measure the dimensions of the appendage for selecting the appropriate device size. LAA, left atrial appendage; LA, left atrium; LUPV, left upper pulmonary vein; PA, pulmonary artery.

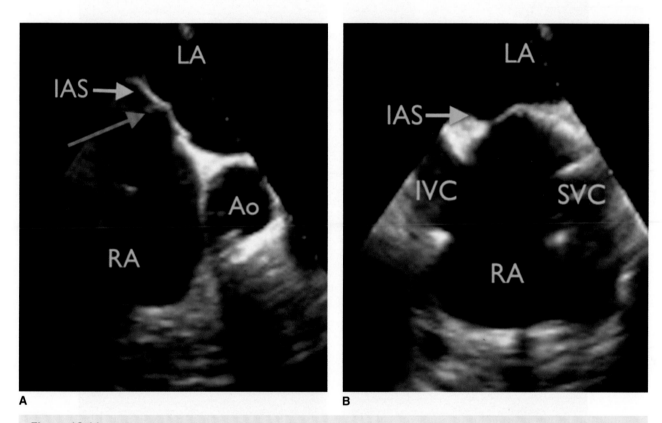

A

B

Figure 12-11. **Biplane 2D imaging and guidance of TS puncture.** An important step of the LAA closure procedure, the TS puncture, can be best guided by biplane 2D imaging. This technique helps to determine the optimal site for TS needle (*red arrow*), while avoiding important adjacent structures, such as the aorta (Videos 12-18A and 12-18B). (Reproduced from Siegel RJ, Luo H, Biner S. Transcatheter valve repair/implantation. *Int J Cardiovasc Imaging* 2011;27:1165–1177, with permission.)

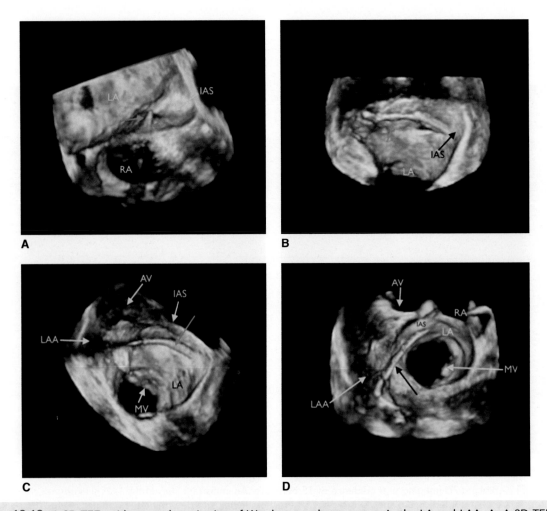

Figure 12-12. A 3D TEE guidance and monitoring of Watchman catheter system in the LA and LAA. A. A 3D TEE view from LA showing the tenting (*red arrow*) of the IAS before the TS needle (*red arrowhead*) is about to puncture the IAS (Video 12-19A). B. Precise identification of the catheter and guide wire (*red arrow*) after they have entered the LA (Video 12-19B). C, D. Three-dimensional TEE images are helpful in manipulating the catheter (*red arrow*) and deciding the exact pathway toward the LAA avoiding trauma to adjacent structures, such as the LA and the MV. In these 3D images, the catheter is oriented toward the LAA (Videos 12-19C and 12-19D). (Reproduced from Siegel RJ, Luo H, Biner S. Transcatheter valve repair/implantation. *Int J Cardiovasc Imaging* 2011;27:1165–1177, with permission.)

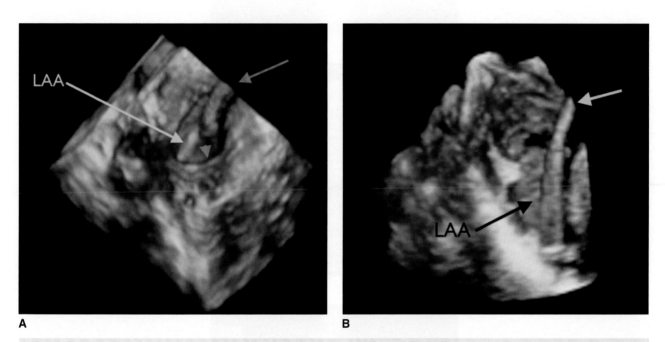

A   **B**

Figure 12-13. Guidance and monitoring of Watchman catheter system in the LA and LAA. A. Three-dimensional TEE short axis view of LAA depicting proper placement of the catheter (*red arrow*) deep into the LAA (*red arrowhead*) (Video 12-20A). B. Cross-sectional view of LAA with the catheter (*yellow arrow*) entering the LAA. Catheter tip is shown to be at the distal end of the LAA (*black arrow*) (Video 12-20B).

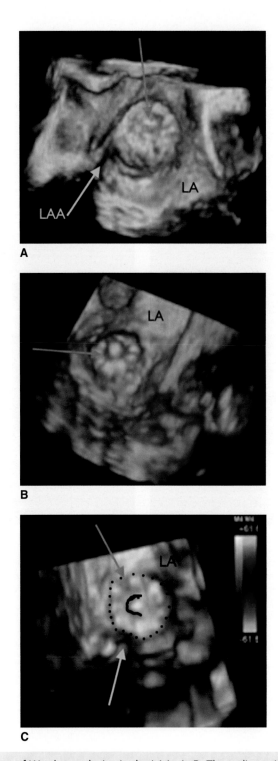

Figure 12-14. Correct placement of Watchman device in the LAA. A, B. Three-dimensional TEE images depicting correct placement of the LAA occluder device (*red arrows*) with no protrusion of the device outside the LAA boundaries (Videos 12-21A and 12-21B). C. Full-volume color Doppler TEE image showing no color flow (*yellow arrow*) coming out from the LAA around the device (*red arrow*) (Video 12-21C).

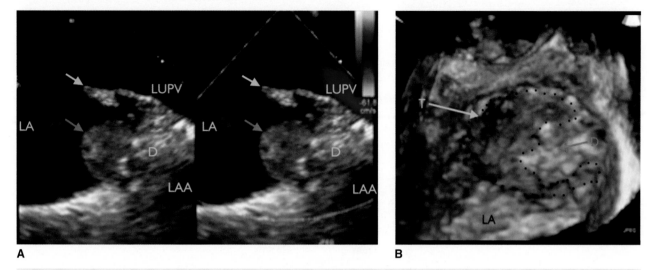

Figure 12-15. Thrombus attached to the surface of the Watchman device. A. 2D TEE images obtained several weeks after deployment of the Watchman device. These images were obtained when patient presented with intracranial bleed due to trauma. The images clearly show a large thrombus (*red arrows*) below the Coumadin ridge (*yellow arrow*) sitting firmly on the device (marked with D). B. Three-dimensional TEE image showing that most of the surface of the Watchman device (*red arrow*), which is exposed within the LA, is covered with thrombus (marked as T) (Video 12-22B).

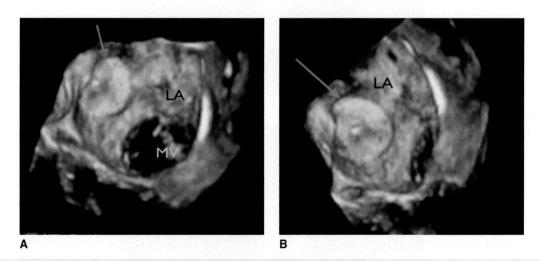

Figure 12-16. Three-dimensional images of the LAA-Amplatzer cardiac plug (ACP) device. Images demonstrating perfect deployment from two different views. This device has a relatively smooth surface (Videos 12-23A and 12-23B).

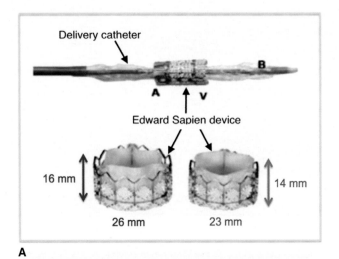

A

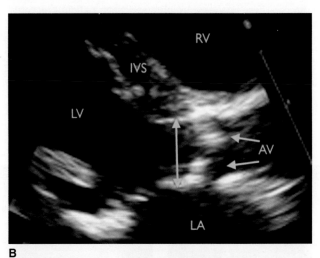

B

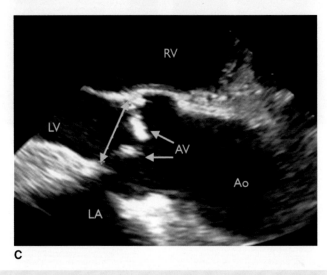

C

Figure 12-17. Edwards Sapien device crimped on the delivery catheter. A. The expanded form of devices of two different sizes (26 and 23 mm) (Reproduced from Lerakis S, Babaliaros VC, Block PC, et al. Transesophageal echocardiography to help position and deploy a transcatheter heart valve. *J Am Coll Cardiol Img.* 2010;3(2):219–221, with permission). B, C. Long-axis 2D transthoracic and transesophageal views of the AV annulus. These views are utilized to measure the AV annulus diameter to determine the size of the Sapien percutaneous AV.

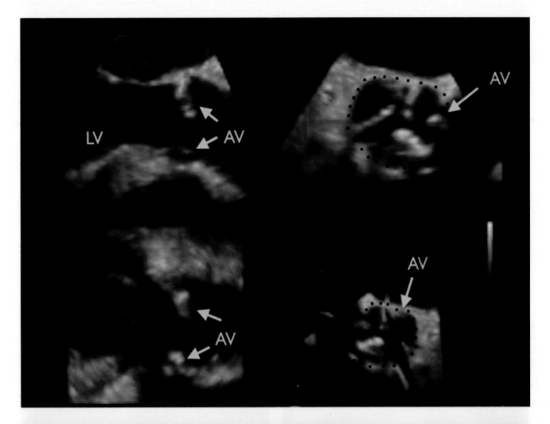

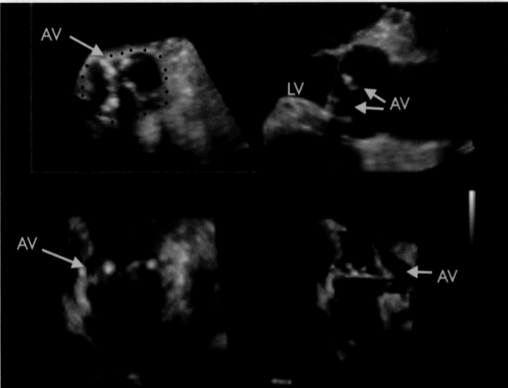

Figure 12-18. Three-dimensional TEE of the AV annulus. The AV annulus is an oval structure (marked with *black dots*), as opposed to the traditional round aortic annulus. The exact anatomy of the annulus is important to determine the right size of Sapien valve to avoid postprocedure complications such as aortic regurgitation, etc. (Video 12-25A). (Reproduced from Nguyen CT, Lee E, Luo H, et al. Echocardiographic guidance for diagnostic and therapeutic percutaneous procedures. *Cardiovasc Diagn Ther.* 2011;1(1):11–36, with permission.)

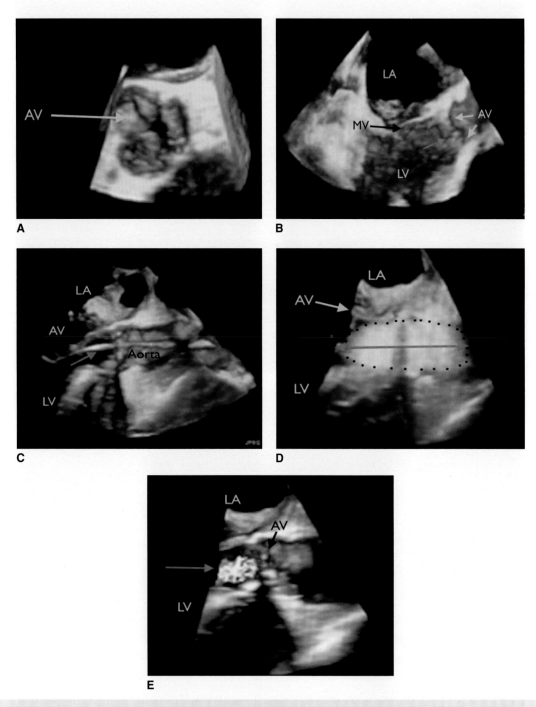

Figure 12-19. **A, B.** Three-dimensional TEE of a stenotic AV. Stenotic tricuspid AV is best appreciated in 3D TEE derived short- and long-axis views (*red arrows*) (Videos 12-26A and 12-26B). **C–E.** Balloon valvuloplasty of a stenotic AV. **C.** Three-dimensional TEE long-axis view showing a catheter (*red arrow*) across the stenotic AV (Video 12-26C). **D.** Three-dimensional TEE imaging of balloon valvuloplasty (*red arrow* closed at both sides) during rapid right ventricular pacing. This modality yields precise details regarding the location of the catheter across AV (Video 12-26D). **E.** Postvalvuloplasty 3D TEE full-volume color Doppler flow image depicting significant aortic regurgitation (*red arrow*), which is increased after balloon inflation (Video 12-26E) (Reproduced from Siegel RJ, Luo H, Biner S. Transcatheter valve repair/implantation. *Int J Cardiovasc Imaging* 2011;27:1165–1177, with permission).

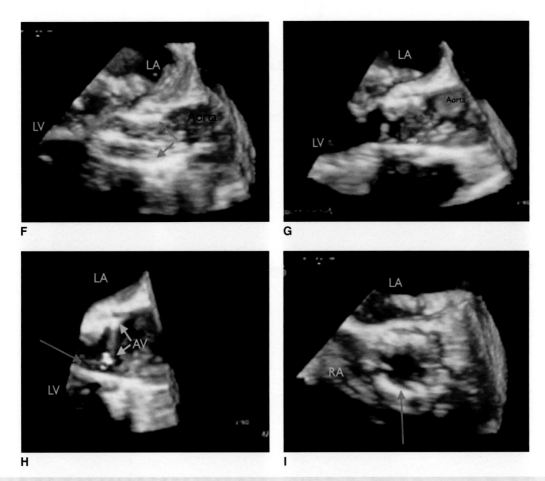

Figure 12-19. (*Continued*) F–I. Deployment of a bovine pericardial AV. The bovine pericardial stented AV is deployed during rapid right ventricular pacing. The valve sits perfectly at correct position (*red arrows*) (Videos 12-26F and 12-26G). H. Three-dimensional TEE color flow Doppler in long-axis view showing mild periprosthetic aortic regurgitation (*red arrow*) (Video 12-26H). I. A BMV is well seated at place of native AV in this 3D TEE short axis view (Video 12-26I). (Reproduced from Siegel RJ, Luo H, Biner S. Transcatheter valve repair/implantation. *Int J Cardiovasc Imaging* 2011;27:1165–1177, with permission.)

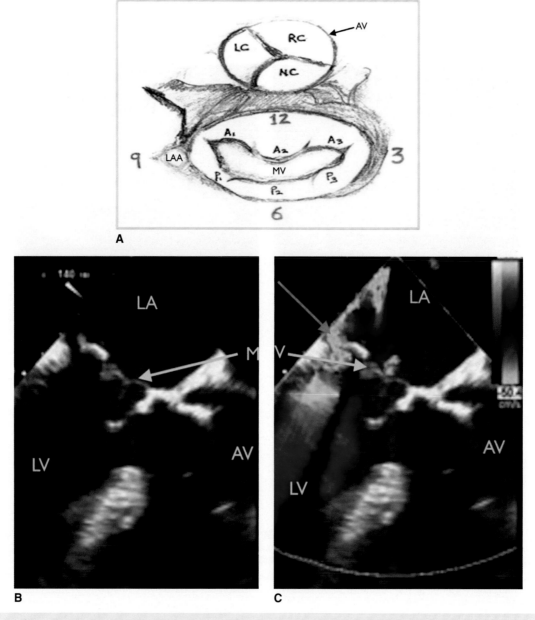

Figure 12-20. A. Schematic of the surgical view of the mitral and AVs and surrounding structures. The AV is seen at 12 o'clock position, while the LAA is at the 9 o'clock position. This schematic serves as a reference to guide interventions. B, C. BMV paravalvular leak. 2D TEE long-axis view shows the presence of paravalvular leak by color flow Doppler (*red arrow*). It can be easily differentiated from the MR by noting the site of the origin of the regurgitant jet (Videos 12-27B and 12-27C).

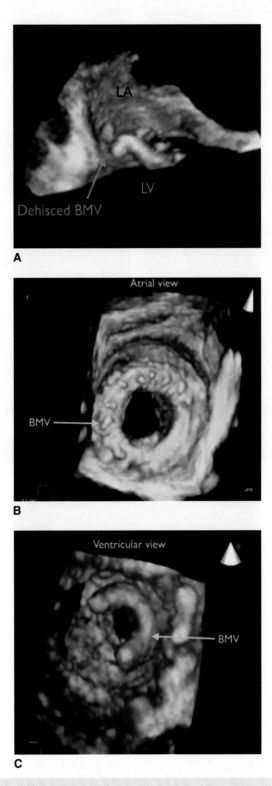

Figure 12-21. A–C. Dehisced BMV. A 3D TEE image at the level of the MV showing the dehisced BMV (A, *red arrow*). It shows increased mobility of the prosthesis. The same dehisced valve imaged from left atrial side (B) and from LV perspective (C) to identify the size and shape of the dehiscence. The 3D images provide better details and help in decision making regarding the feasibility of transcatheter closure using an Amplatzer device (Videos 12-28A, 12-28B, 12-28C).

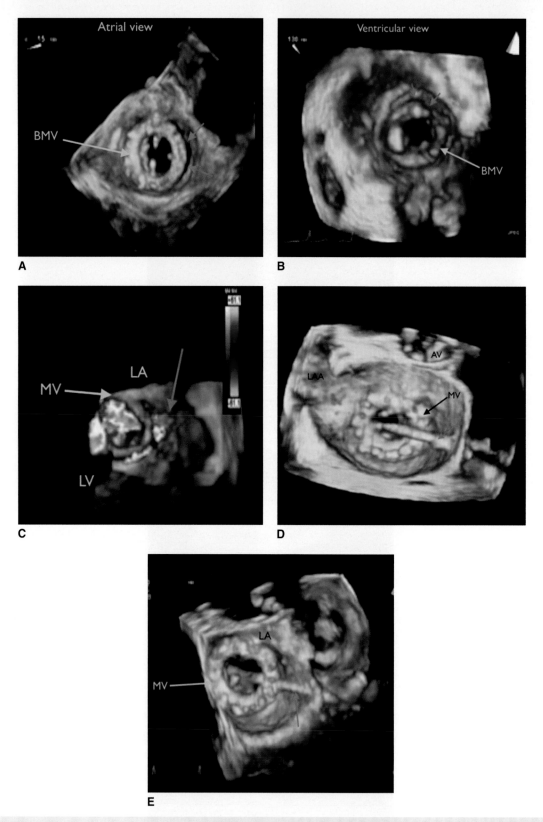

Figure 12-22. A. BMV with paravalvular leak. A BMV is seen from the left atrial perspective. The site of the paravalvular leak is identified by *red arrows* on the right side of the BMV, between 1 and 5 o'clock (Video 12-29A). B. Ventricular view of the BMV showing the MV struts. The site of the paravalvular leak (*red arrows*) (Video 12-29B). C. Three-dimensional TEE full-volume color flow Doppler image depicting the site and severity of the paravalvular leak (*red arrow*) from the left atrial view (Video 12-29C). D, E. Guidance of the paravalvular leak closure. Three-dimensional TEE is used to guide the catheter across the paravalvular leak, confirm its positioning, deploy the Amplatzer occluder device and assess the residual paravalvular leak. It is imperative to place the catheter across the defect so that the occluder device can be deployed to seal off the leak. The catheter is seen across the orifice of BMV (D, *red arrow*). Accordingly, the catheter is manipulated toward the defect and is then advanced across the leak (E). (Videos 12-29D and 12-29E).

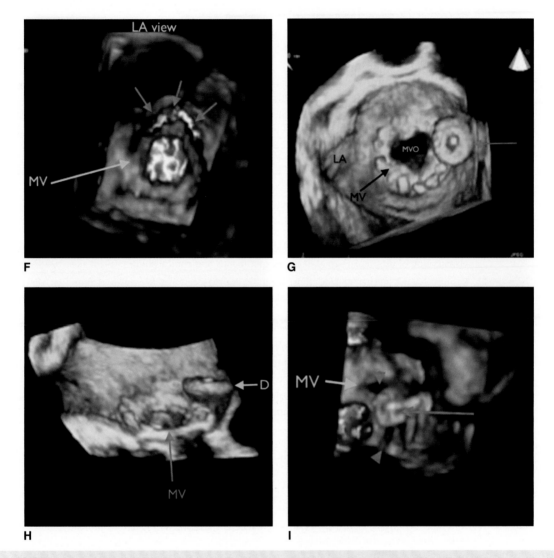

Figure 12-22. (*Continued*) F. Guidance of the paravalvular leak closure. Once the catheter is across the paravalvular leak (defect), the position of the catheter is confirmed by 3D color flow Doppler as shown in this image. Catheter can be seen in the jet of paravalvular leak (*middle red arrow*) before the final deployment of the occluder device (Video 12-29F). G–I. Guidance of the paravalvular leak closure. G. After confirming that the catheter is across the defect by color flow Doppler, the device is deployed. This view from the left atrial perspective shows the MVO and the occluder device at a 3 o'clock position (Video 12-29G). H. Cross-sectional view of the LA confirming the correct placement of the Amplatzer occluder device (*yellow arrow*) (Video 12-29H). I. Three-dimensional TEE full-volume color flow Doppler image taken after the final deployment of the occluder device (*red arrow*) showing trivial residual regurgitation (Video 12-29I).

References

1. Lang RM, Mor-Avi V, Sugeng L, et al. Three-dimensional echocardiography. The benefits of the additional dimension. *J Am Coll Cardiol.* 2006;48:2053–2069.

2. Perk G, Lang RM, Garcia-Fernandez MA, et al. Use of real time three-dimensional transesophageal echocardiography in intracardiac catheter based interventions. *J Am Soc Echocardiogr.* 2009;22:865–882.

3. Nguyen CT, Lee E, Luo H, et al. Echocardiographic guidance for diagnostic and therapeutic percutaneous procedures. *Cardiovasc Diagn Ther.* 2011;1(1):11–36.

4. Sugeng L, Shernan SK, Salgo IS, et al. Real-time three-dimensional transesophageal echocardiography in valve disease: comparison with surgical findings and evaluation of prosthetic valves. *J Am Soc Echocardiogr.* 2008;21:1347–1354.

5. Lee AP, Lam YY, Yip GW, et al. Role of real time three-dimensional transesophageal echocardiography in guidance of interventional procedures in cardiology. *Heart.* 2010;96:1485–1493.

6. Siegel RJ, Luo H, Biner S. Transcatheter valve repair/implantation. *Int J Cardiovasc Imaging.* 2011;27:1165–1177.

7. Zamorano JL, Badano LP, Bruce C, et al. EAE/ASE recommendations for the use of echocardiography in new transcatheter interventions for valvular heart disease. *Eur J Echocardiogr.* 2011;12(8):557–584.

8. Saric M, Perk G, Purgess JR, et al. Imaging atrial septal defects by real-time three-dimensional transesophageal echocardiography: step-by-step approach. *J Am Soc Echocardiogr.* 2010;23:1128–1135.

9. Taniguchi M, Akagi T, Watanabe N, et al. Application of real-time three-dimensional transesophageal echocardiography using a matrix array probe for transcatheter closure of atrial septal defect. *J Am Soc Echocardiogr.* 2009;22:1114–1120.

10. Kardon RE, Cao QL, Masani N, et al. New insights and observations in three-dimensional echocardiographic visualization of ventricular septal defects: experimental and clinical studies. *Circulation.* 1998;98:1307–1314.

11. Vasilyev NV, Melnychenko I, Kitahori K, et al. Beating-heart patch closure of muscular ventricular septal defects under real-time three-dimensional echocardiographic guidance: a preclinical study. *J Thorac Cardiovasc Surg.* 2008;135:603–609.

12. Perk G, Biner S, Kronzon I, et al. Catheter-based left appendage occlusion procedure: role of echocardiography. *Eur Heart J Cardiovasc Imaging.* 2012;13(2):132–138.

13. Shah SJ, Bardo DM, Sugeng L, et al. Real-time three-dimensional transesophageal echocardiography of the left atrial appendage: initial experience in the clinical setting. *J Am Soc Echocardiogr.* 2008;21:1362–1368.

14. Nucifora G, Faletra FF, Regoli F, et al. Evaluation of the left atrial appendage with real-time three-dimensional transesophageal echocardiography: implications for catheter-based left atrial appendage closure. *Circ Cardiovasc Imaging.* 2011;4(5):514–523.

15. Altiok E, Koos R, Schröder J, et al. Comparison of two-dimensional and three-dimensional imaging techniques for measurement of aortic annulus diameters before transcatheter aortic valve implantation. *Heart.* 2011;97(19):1578–1584.

16. Siegel RJ, Makkar, R, Domanian A, et al. Transcatheter aortic valve implantation three-dimensional echo monitoring and guidance. *Curr Cardiovasc Imaging Rep.* 2011;4:335–348.

17. Kim MS, Casserly IP, Garcia JA, et al. Percutaneous transcatheter closure of prosthetic mitral paravalvular leaks. *J Am Coll Cardiol.* 2009;2:81–90.

18. Biner S, Kar S, Siegel RJ, et al. Value of color Doppler three-dimensional transesophageal echocardiography in the percutaneous closure of mitral prosthesis paravalvular leak. *Am J Cardiol.* 2010;105:984–989.

19. Garcia-Fernandez MA, Cortes Z, Garcia-Robles, et al. Utility of real-time three-dimensional transesophageal echocardiography in evaluating the success of percutaneous transcatheter closure of mitral paravalvular leaks. *J Am Soc Echocardiogr.* 2010;23:26–32.

20. Kronzon I, Sugeng L, Perk G, et al. Real-time 3-dimensional transesophageal echocardiography in evaluation of post-operative mitral annuloplasty ring and prosthetic valve dehiscence. *J Am Coll Cardiol.* 2009;53:1543–1547.

3D ECHOCARDIOGRAPHY OF ATRIAL AND VENTRICULAR SEPTAL DEFECTS

13

David A. Roberson, Vivian Wei Cui

There have been several important developments in three-dimensional echocardiography image acquisition, cropping, and display over the last few years.[1-4] High-quality and useful images of atrial[5-13] and ventricular[14-25] septal defects can be obtained in the majority of patients. In this chapter, we describe 3D acquisition modes and cropping methods. We also present a collection of representative 3D echocardiograms of the various types of atrial and ventricular septal defects (VSDs). Both transthoracic and transesophageal 3D images of congenital and acquired defects in cardiac septation are illustrated.

ACQUISITION MODES

Three-dimensional anatomic image acquisition modes include live 3D, 3D zoom, full-volume 3D, and X-plane imaging. All four of the 3D anatomic imaging modes are available for both 3D transthoracic echocardiography and 3D transesophageal echocardiogram. In addition, 3D color Doppler flow mapping is available in both live and 3D full-volume modes (Table 13-1).

Live 3D mode is real-time live imaging with a wedge-shaped 3D echo volume adjustable from approximately 20 to 60 degrees wide. This mode requires real-time continuous manual transducer steering analogous to 2D echocardiographic transducer manipulation. In order to achieve the maximum 3D echocardiographic capabilities, the structure of interest is positioned in the middle to far field, where the 3D sector is of sufficient volume. Live 3D echo has a rapid volume rate when the sector is small, but a slow volume rate when the sector is large. It does not require EKG or respiratory gating and is void of stitch artifact. Therefore, it is ideal for those with faster heart and respiratory rates. It is also quite useful for structures with extensive and rapid motion over the cardiac cycle such as the aortic valve leaflets.

The 3D zoom mode consists of live real-time 3D imaging in which the sonographer defines the size of a truncated pyramid-shaped 3D sample volume by adjusting sample volume position, length, width, and height. Live beating heart images can be rotated and cropped to view from the optimal perspective. Unfortunately, the volume rate is slow, ranging from 5 to 18 volumes/s. This mode is very useful for demonstrating atrial septal defect (ASD) during device closure.

The 3D full-volume mode consists of either a single beat or multiple beat acquisitions. A newly developed single beat acquisition mode is available; however, the volume rate is quite slow, sometimes being <10 volumes/s. Multiple beat acquisitions involve two to four live 3D contiguous sample volumes that are stitched together sequentially beat by beat over two to four heartbeats. The most recent software version has an electronically buffered continuous loop, which reduces somewhat the appearance of stitch artifact. The result is a large, wide-angled, pyramid-shaped 3D sample volume. A 3D sample volume must be acquired, stored, and cropped according to the particular structure of interest. The volume rate is rapid but prone to stitch artifact due to rapid heart rate or respiratory motion.

X-plane imaging consists of simultaneous live biplane 2D echocardiography. The standard reference image is displayed on the left side of the screen. The plane of dissection of the reference image and the relative rotation of the variable biplane image is adjustable through 180 degrees and simultaneously displayed live on the right side of the screen.

All 3D anatomic modes have many adjustable parameters including gain, contrast, smoothing, image processing algorithms, color adjustments, color depth shading adjustments, rotation of images throughout 180 degrees in orthogonal planes, and others. Image manipulation, cropping, and quantification can be performed on the ultrasound platform, on the digital review station, or on a personal computer with the appropriate software.

Three-dimensional color Doppler flow mapping has been available for full-volume 3D for some time, and recently, it has been added to the live 3D echo mode as well.

CROPPING MODES

Cropping the 3D image is an essential procedure to provide optimal 3D images of the structure of interest. It is in part but not entirely dependent upon the mode of acquisition being live versus digitally stored 3D full-volume datasets. Current cropping modes include 3D zoom, icrop, xyz plane cropping, and adjustable plane cropping (Table 13-2).

The 3D zoom mode cropping is performed on live images and involves adjusting the length, width, and height of a truncated pyramidal-shaped echo volume on X-plane images.

In the newly developed iCrop method of cropping, the 3D echo sample volume is box shaped. Cropping adjustment is performed from any or all of the six sides of a sample volume enclosed in a box. The sonographer or reviewer selects one of the six sides of the box from which the heart is viewed.

Adjustable plane cropping involves an infinitely adjustable single or multiple cropping planes across the 3D echo volume. Multiple adjustable crop planes can be used on the same image. Steering the adjustable cropping plane can be difficult at times; however, control of this has improved with more recent software versions.

GENERAL GUIDELINES

En face, right anterior oblique, and left anterior oblique views of the cardiac septa often provide the most useful qualitative and quantitative views of septal defects. Relatively low gain and compression settings in the 10% to 20% range may enhance anatomic definition of septal structures. No or low res settings likewise may accentuate pertinent details. Slight oblique angulation of the 3D image and cropping from the posterior to the anterior aspect of the image often enhances the depth shading, thereby enhancing the 3D view effect. Cropping away extraneous noisy portions and anatomic structures that are not of particular interest from the 3D sector may allow more refined adjustment of gain, compression, smoothing, and res settings. The choice of image acquisition mode involves consideration of the balance of heart rate, respiratory rate, volume rate, and the required size of the 3D echo sample volume.

DEFECTS IN CARDIAC SEPTATION

A wide variety of types and sizes of defects in cardiac septation are encountered on a daily basis when caring for patients with congenital cardiac defects, as summarized in Tables 13-3 and 13-4.

The types of ASD include secundum (Figs. 13-1 and 13-2), primum (Fig. 13-3), sinus venosus (Figs. 13-4 and 13-5), and coronary sinus types (Fig. 13-6).

VSDs may be either congenital or acquired. Congenital types of VSD include perimembranous (Figs. 13-7 through 13-9), muscular (Figs. 13-10 through 13-12), malaligned (Figs. 13-13 through 13-15), inlet (Fig. 13-16), and outlet (Fig. 13-17) types. Acquired types of VSD include myocardial infarction (Figs. 13-18 and 13-19) and traumatic types.

TABLE 13-1 • 3D Echocardiographic Modalities

3D Mode	Strengths	Limitations
Live	High volume rate Real time	Small sector size required to achieve fast volume rate
Zoom	Precropped images Good en face views Real time	Slow volume rate
Full volume	High volume rate Large sample volume	Stitch artifact Postacquisition cropping required
X-plane	Simultaneous biplane 2D echo	2D only
Color Doppler	Color Doppler flow analysis Full volume and live modes	Relatively slow volume rate Relatively small sample volume

TABLE 13-2 • 3D Echocardiographic Cropping Modalities

3D Cropping	Description
XYZ	Basic cropping modality cuts in X, Y and Z planes from any or all sides
Adjustable plane	Steerable infinitely adjustable crop plane Multiple cut planes can be used simultaneously Planes are often difficult to steer
3D zoom	Truncated pyramid–shaped sample volume Adjustable size, position, and viewing aspect Can be applied to live images
iCrop	Box-shaped sample volume Adjustable size, position, angle, and viewing aspect Can be applied to live images

TABLE 13-3 • Types of Atrial Septal Defect (ASD)	
ASD Type	**Description**
Secundum	Oval fossa defect Involves central portion of atrial septum One or more rims may be deficient Amenable to device closure
Primum	Within AV septal defect spectrum Adjacent to AV valve at inferior apical region of atrial septum
Sinus venosus	Superior type adjacent to SVC Inferior type adjacent to IVC Vena cava overrides defect Partial anomalous pulmonary veins usually present
Coronary sinus	Shunt through CS Complete or partial unroofing of CS into LA

TABLE 13-4 • Types of Ventricular Septal Defect (VSD)	
VSD Type	**Description**
Perimembranous	Deficiency of membranous septum and surrounding region Fibrous continuity of tricuspid, mitral and aortic valves
Muscular	Completely surrounded by muscle Various locations and multiple defects possible
Inlet VSD	Due to absent or deficient atrioventricular septum
Malaligned	Anterior or posterior deviation of conal septum Seen in tetralogy of Fallot, double outlet RV, interrupted aortic arch complex
Outlet	Deficient or absent outlet portion of ventricular septum Seen in truncus arteriosus and doubly committed subarterial VSD
Acquired	Myocardial infarction Traumatic

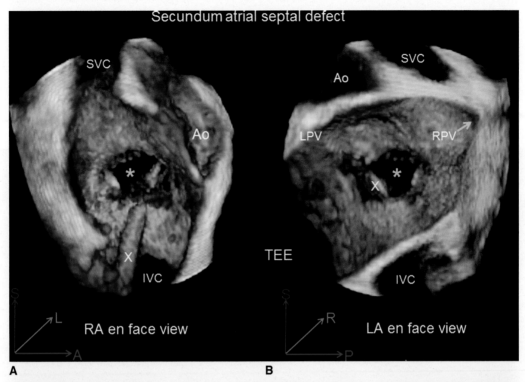

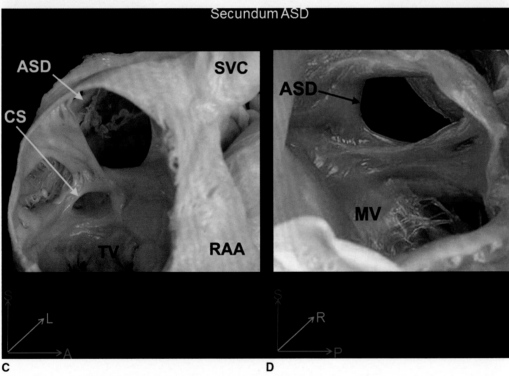

Figure 13-1. Transesophageal 3D echocardiograms of secundum atrial septal defect (ASD) and surrounding landmarks. Right- and left-sided transesophageal echocardiogram (TEE) en face views of a secundum type ASD. The ASD is located at the (*). Images were acquired using 3D zoom mode. A. The catheter (X) is seen passing through the ASD. Anatomic landmarks seen in the right side en face view from the right atrium (RA) include the aorta (Ao), inferior vena cava (IVC), and superior vena cava (SVC). B. Landmarks seen from the left side en face view from the left atrium (LA) include the left pulmonary veins (LPV) and right pulmonary veins (RPV); as well as the Ao, IVC, and SVC. Image orientation directional *arrows* are labeled A-anterior, L-left, P-posterior, R-right, S-superior. C. Companion pathology specimen to Figure 13-1A. Right atrial perspective of a secundum ASD. CS, coronary sinus; TV, tricuspid valve; RAA, right atrial appendage. D. Companion pathology specimen to Figure 13-1B. Left atrial perspective of a secundum ASD. MV, mitral valve. See accompanying Video 13-5.

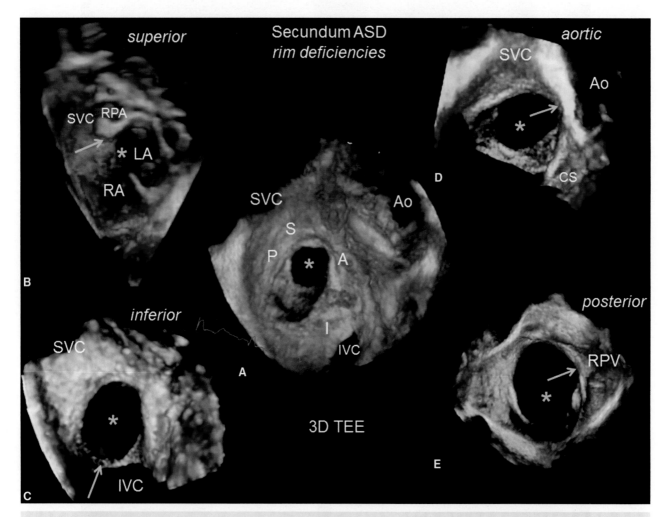

Figure 13-2. Transesophageal 3D echocardiograms of deficient secundum ASD rims. A. In the central figure, all ASD rims including anterior (A), inferior (I), posterior (P), and superior (S) are well developed, thereby making this an ideal candidate for device closure. In each of the surrounding echocardiograms, there is a deficient ASD rim (*arrows*). RPA, right pulmonary artery. B. The superior rim is deficient; this is a live 3D acquisition from the transgastric position. Images C and D are right side en face views of 3D zoom acquisitions from the midesophagus. C. The inferior rim is deficient. D. The aortic rim is deficient. E. The right pulmonary vein (RPV) rim is deficient as seen from an LA en face perspective view of a 3D zoom acquisition from the midesophagus. Other abbreviations as in Figure 13-1. See accompanying Video 13-6.

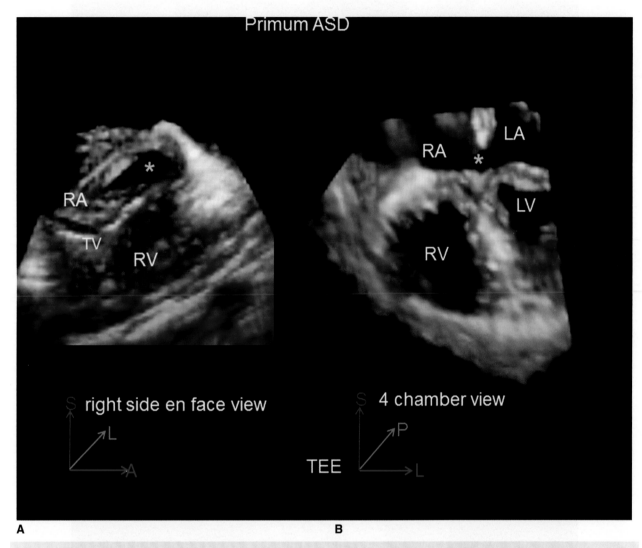

A   **B**

Figure 13-3. **Transesophageal 3D echocardiograms of ostium primum ASD.** The ostium primum ASD is located in the inferior region of the atrial septum and the inferior margin of the ASD is the atrioventricular valves. A. The right side en face view of the ostium primum ASD (*). The RA, right ventricle (RV), and TV are demonstrated. B. A four-chamber view of the ostium primum ASD (*), which includes the right heart chambers and the LA and LV. Both images were acquired with 3D full volume from the midesophagus position. See accompanying Video 13-7.

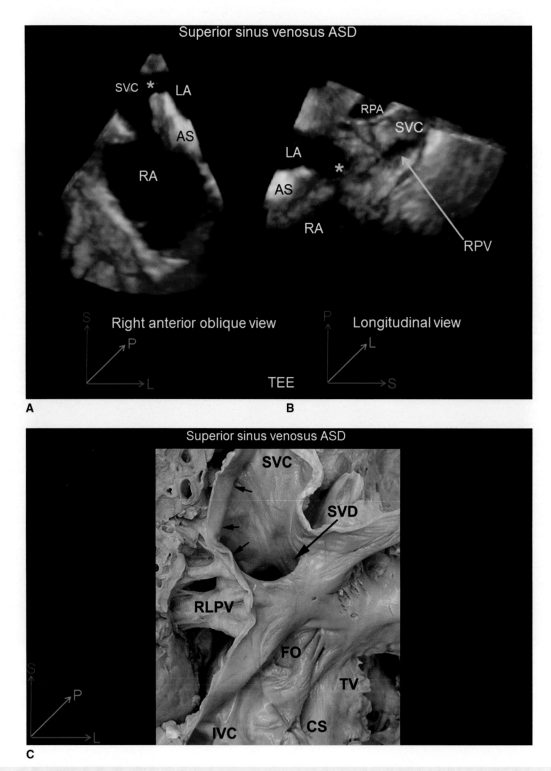

Figure 13-4. Transesophageal 3D echocardiograms of superior sinus venosus type ASD. In this type of ASD the SVC over-rides the defect at the cavoatrial junction and anomalous connection of the right pulmonary veins is typically present. A. Right anterior oblique view of the SVC overriding the ASD (*), which is located superior to the intact portion of the atrial septum (AS). B. Longitudinal view, which demonstrates the superior position of the ASD (*), the SVC override of the defect, and the RPV draining anomalously to the SVC. C. Companion pathology specimen to Figure 13-4, superior vena caval type sinus venosus ASD. The RA and TV are opened and the heart is tilted slightly forward to view the sinus venosus ASD (SVASD). This defect overrides the superior rim of the intact portion of the atrial septum. Note the anomalous pulmonary venous return of the right upper and middle pulmonary veins (small black arrows) to the SVC. The right lower pulmonary vein (RLPV) drains normally to the left atrium.

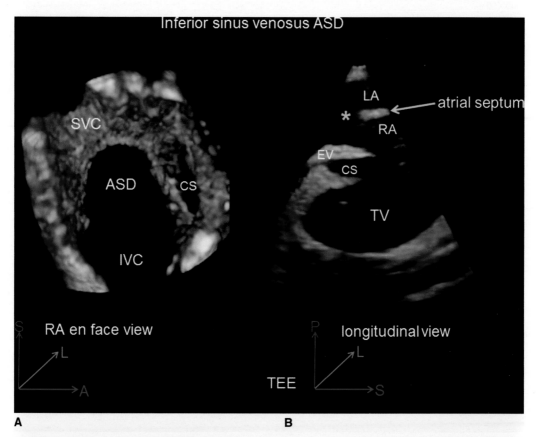

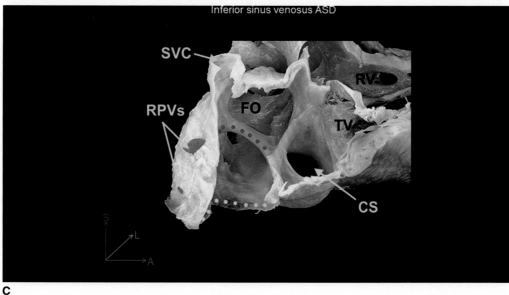

Figure 13-5. Transesophageal 3D echocardiograms of inferior sinus venosus type ASD. A. Right side en face view of a large inferior sinus venous ASD, which is confluent with a large secundum ASD. This image was acquired from the midesophagus with 3D zoom mode. B. Longitudinal view of an inferior type sinus venosus ASD (*) in which the IVC overrides the inferior portion of the atrial septum at the cavoatrial junction. The CS, eustachian valve (EV), and TV orifice are seen. This image was acquired from a midesophagus longitudinal view using full-volume 3D. C. Companion pathology specimen to Figure 13-5, inferior type sinus venosus ASD. This anterolateral view of the RA shows the interatrial communication associated with the IVC (*yellow dots* mark inferior border). There is partial anomalous pulmonary venous return involving the right middle and lower veins (RPVs). One of the left pulmonary veins (*red arrow*) can be seen through the defect, draining to the LA in the usual fashion. The inferior border (*red dots*) of the intact portion of the atrial septum forms the roof of the defect. The foramen ovale (FO) is slightly patent. The CS is large secondary to a persistent left SVC. See accompanying Video 13-9.

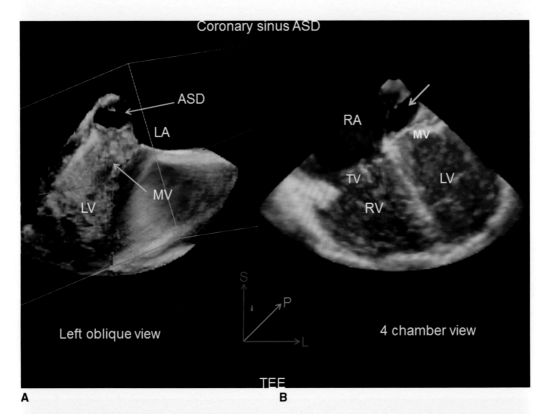

A   B

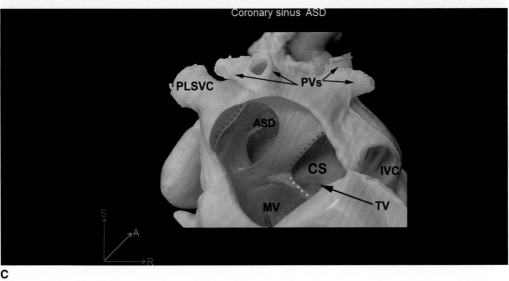

C

Figure 13-6. Transesophageal 3D echocardiograms of coronary sinus type ASD. In this rare type of ASD, the floor of the left atrium is deficient, also referred to as partial or complete unroofing of the CS into the LA, resulting in a shunt from the left atrium to the coronary sinus and subsequently to the right atrium. These images are from the midesophagus using 3D full-volume acquisition. A. Left oblique perspective. B. Anterior perspective of a four-chamber view. Note the CS type ASD is at the CS orifice near the MV and TV. C. Companion pathology specimen to Figure 13-6, CS type ASD. The LA is viewed from the posterior aspect, the heart tilted from its anatomical position with the apex pointing down. There is a persistent left superior vena cava (PLSVC). An interatrial communication is at the CS. The roof of the CS (*red dots*) is absent, allowing the PLSVC to drain directly into the left atrium. The *yellow dots* show the remaining interatrial septum. A secundum ASD is also present. PVs, pulmonary veins.

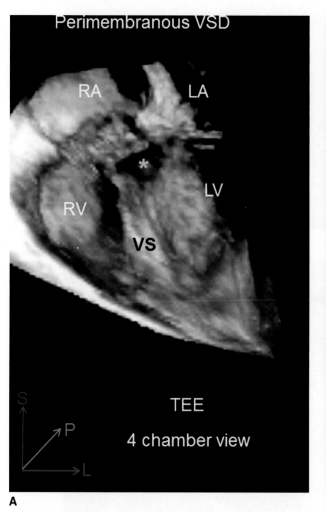

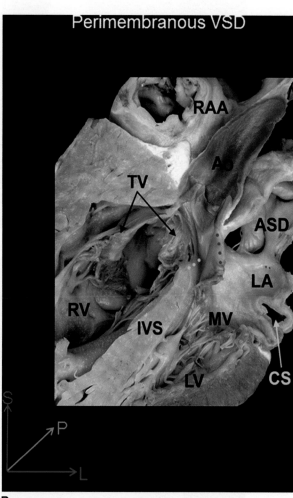

Figure 13-7. **Transesophageal 3D echocardiograms of perimembranous ventricular septal defect.** The perimembranous ventricular septal defect (VSD) involves deficiency of the membranous ventricular septum and surrounding regions, which results in fibrous continuity between tricuspid and mitral valves. A. This image is a left oblique perspective view of a large perimembranous VSD (*), which was acquired from the midesophagus four-chamber view using full-volume 3D mode. The muscular portion of the ventricular septum (VS) is intact. B. Companion pathology specimen to Figure 13-7. This long axis view shows a perimembranous ventricular septal defect (VSD) with fibrous continuity between the TV and MV. The aortic valve forms the superior margin of the VSD. The *yellow dots* mark the crest of the ventricular septum and the *red dots* the anterior leaflet of the mitral valve. See accompanying Video 13-11.

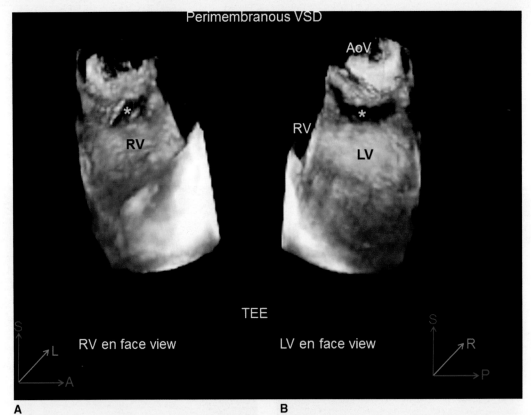

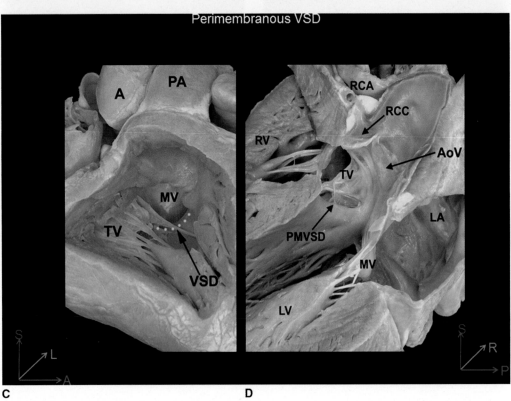

Figure 13-8. Transesophageal 3D echocardiogram en face views of large perimembranous VSD. A. Right side en face view of a large perimembranous VSD (*). B. Left side en face view of a large perimembranous VSD (*). Note the U-shaped defect is largest in the anterior to posterior plane and adjacent to the aortic valve (AoV). These images were obtained from the midesophagus four-chamber view using 3D full-volume acquisition. C. Companion pathology specimen to Figure 13-8A shows a perimembranous VSD, RV aspect. The muscular border of the VSD is demonstrated by the *yellow dots*. The MV is seen through the defect and is in fibrous continuity with the TV. A, aorta; PA, pulmonary artery. D. Companion pathology specimen to Figure 13-8B, perimembranous VSD, left ventricular aspect. The right coronary cusp (RCC) and the noncoronary cusp of the aortic valve lie along the superior border of the perimembranous ventricular septal defect (PMVSD). There is fibrous continuity between the AoV, MV, and TV. RCA, right coronary artery. See accompanying Videos 13-12A and 13-12B.

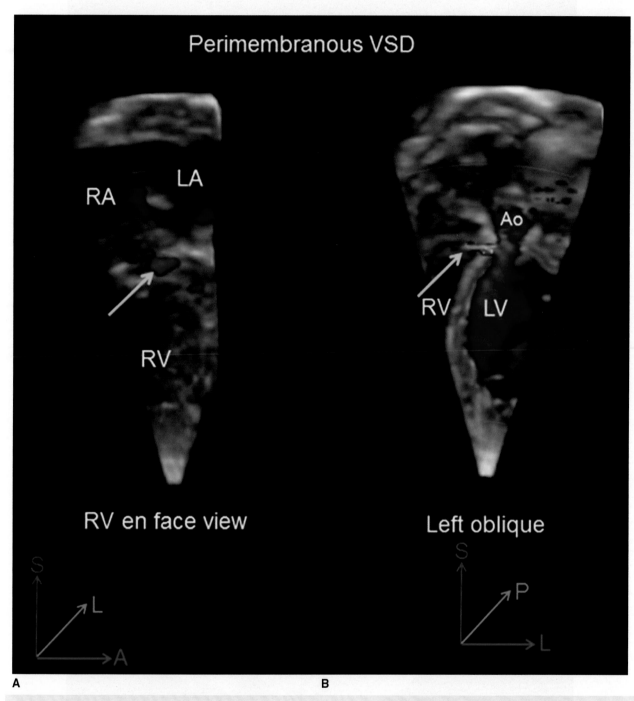

Figure 13-9. Transesophageal 3D color Doppler echocardiograms of a small perimembranous VSD. A. Right en face view. B. Left oblique view. These images were obtained from the midesophagus four-chamber view using 3D full-volume color Doppler flow acquisition mode. See accompanying Video 13-13.

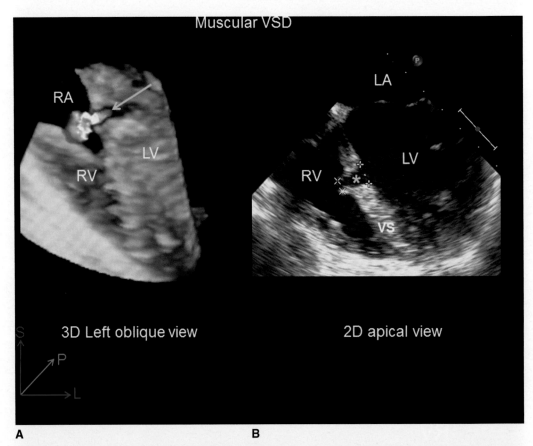

A

B

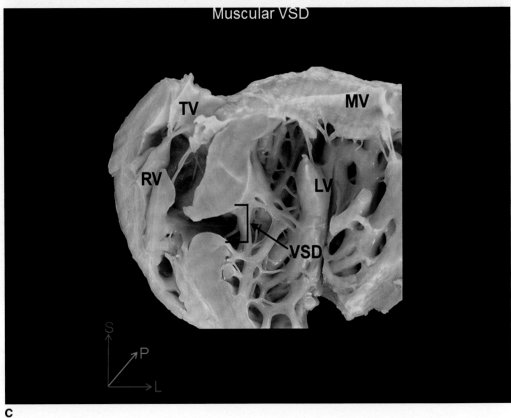

C

Figure 13-10. Transesophageal 3D and 2D echocardiogram views of small muscular VSD. Muscular VSDs are located in the muscular trabecular region of the ventricular septum. The VSD borders are completely surrounded by muscular myocardium. A. Three-dimensional color Doppler flow map viewed from a left oblique perspective, which demonstrates a small left to right shunt (*arrow*). B. The comparable 2D TEE view of the same VSD (*). Images were acquired at the midesophagus level four-chamber view. C. Pathology specimen illustrates a muscular VSD in the midportion of the ventricular septum.

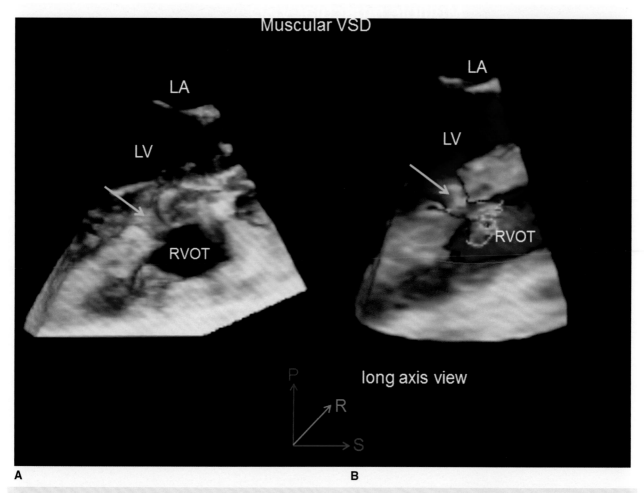

Figure 13-11. Transesophageal 3D echocardiogram longitudinal views of muscular VSD. Both images were acquired from the midesophagus longitudinal view. A. The long axis anatomic view of the muscular VSD (*arrow*). B. Three-dimensional color Doppler flow mapping of the left to right shunt, which is directed toward the right ventricular outflow tract. See accompanying Videos 13-15A and 13-15B.

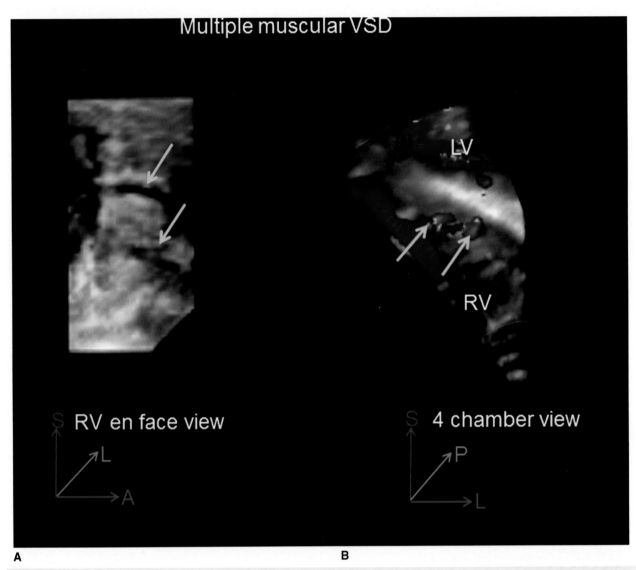

A   B

Figure 13-12. Transthoracic 3D echocardiograms from a newborn with two muscular VSDs. A. Right side en face view of two slit-like crescent-shaped muscular VSDs (*arrows*). B. Live 3D color Doppler flow map of the small left to right shunts through the VSDs. This type, size, and shape of muscular VSD are frequently seen in neonates and usually close spontaneously.

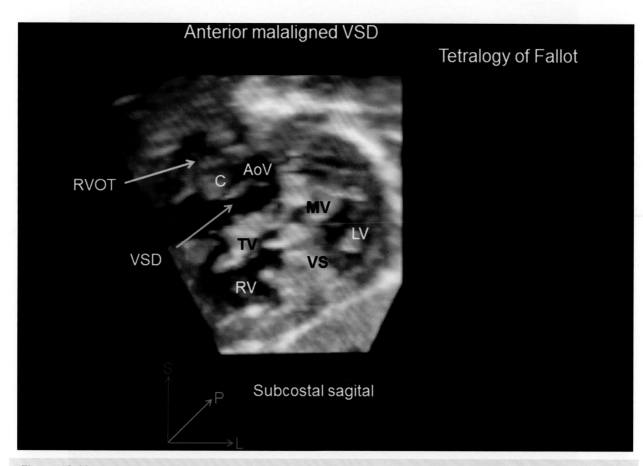

Figure 13-13. Transthoracic 3D echocardiogram of anterior malaligned VSD in tetralogy of Fallot. This image was acquired from the subcostal sagittal transducer position using full-volume 3D in a 1 month old with tetralogy of Fallot. Note the conal septum (C) is deviated anteriorly and rightward causing the right ventricular outflow tract (RVOT) to be narrow.

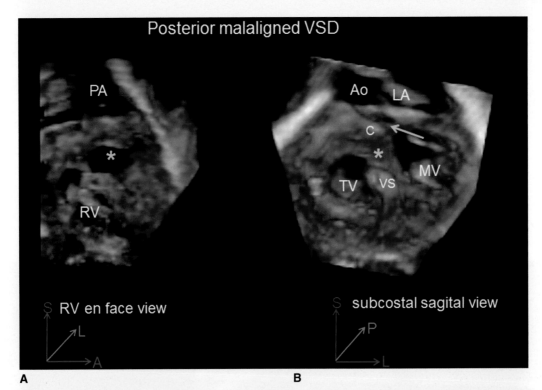

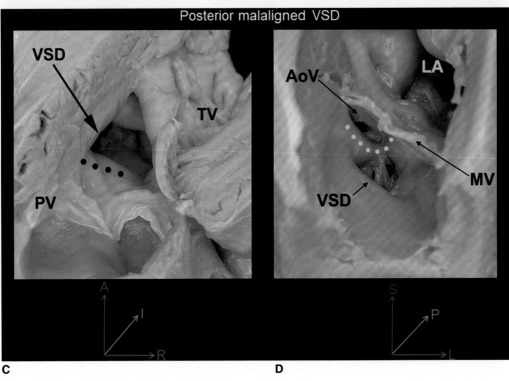

Figure 13-14. Transthoracic 3D echocardiogram of posterior malaligned VSD with interrupted aortic arch complex. A. Right en face view of the VSD (*) acquired from the apical four-chamber view using full-volume 3D acquisition. B. Subcostal sagittal 3D full-volume echocardiogram of the posterior deviation of the conal septum (C) relative to the muscular trabecular septum (VS) resulting in a malaligned VSD (*) and subaortic stenosis (arrow). Malaligned VSD, subaortic stenosis, and interrupted aortic arch often occur together. PA, pulmonary artery. C. Companion pathology specimen to Figure 13-14A of a posterior malalignment VSD. The VSD is seen looking down into the right ventricular outflow tract with the pulmonary valve (PV) in the near field. The hypoplastic outlet septum is deviated posteriorly and seen between the pulmonary valve and VSD. D. Companion pathology specimen to Figure 13-14B, posterior malalignment VSD. This view upward from the LV apex demonstrates the malaligned outlet septum (yellow dots) causing severe subaortic stenosis. Tendinous cords of the TV are seen through the VSD. See accompanying Video 13-18.

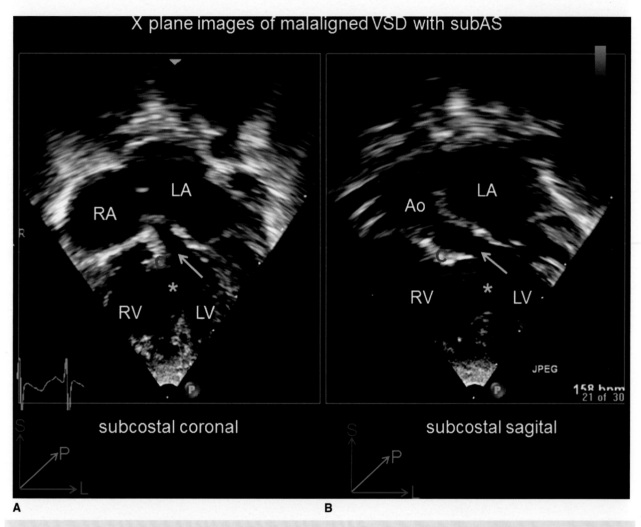

Figure 13-15. Transthoracic X-plane imaging of malaligned VSD. Simultaneous biplane 2D echocardiograms, which demonstrate posteriorly malaligned conus (C) which results in a malaligned VSD (*) and narrow left ventricular outflow tract (*arrow*). A. Subcostal coronal view. B. Sagittal view.

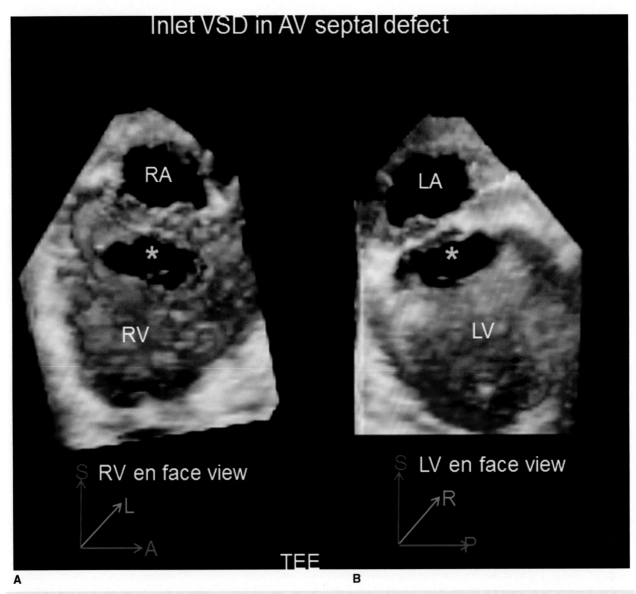

Figure 13-16. Transthoracic 3D echocardiogram of inlet VSD in atrioventricular septal defect. Right side en face view (A) and left side en face view (B) of 3D echocardiograms of inlet VSD in complete atrioventricular septal defect (AV septal defect). Images were obtained from the apical transducer position using 3D full-volume acquisition. The VSD is in the inlet region of the ventricular septum and the superior margin of the defect is the atrioventricular (AV) valves.

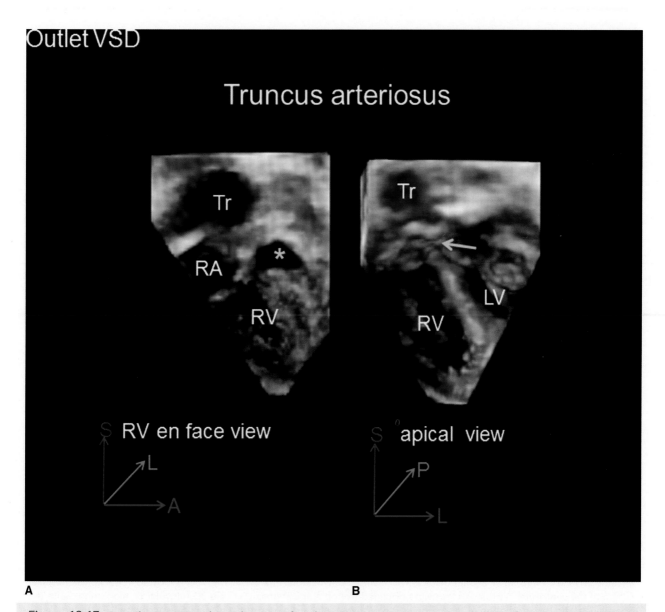

Figure 13-17. Transthoracic 3D echocardiogram of outlet VSD in truncus arteriosus. Right en face view (A) and apical frontal view (B) of outlet VSD (*) in a child with truncus arteriosus (Tr). Images were obtained from the apical position with 3D full-volume acquisition. The VSD is in the outlet region of the septum, the common arterial trunk overrides the defect (*arrow*), and the superior margin of the defect is the truncal valve. See accompanying Video 13-21.

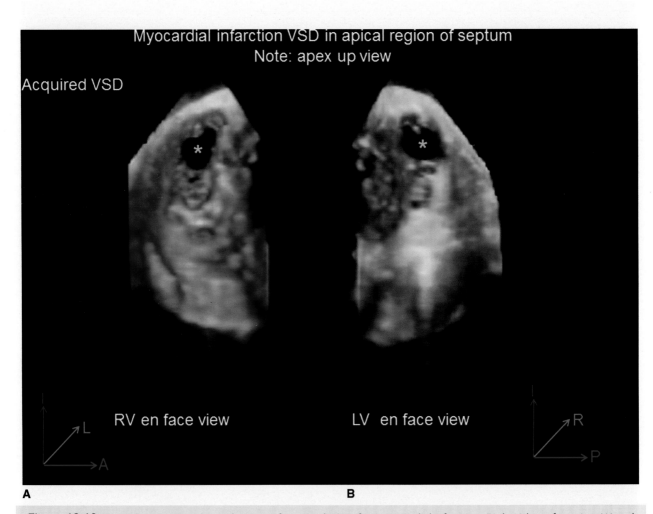

Figure 13-18. Transthoracic 3D echocardiogram of acquired VSD after myocardial infarction. Right side en face view (A) and left side en face view (B) of an acquired apical VSD (*) after a myocardial infarction. The VSD is located in the apical muscular region of the ventricular septum. Images were obtained from the apical position using 3D full-volume acquisition. Note the apex is oriented toward the top of the image as is typical in adult cardiology image display. See accompanying Video 13-22.

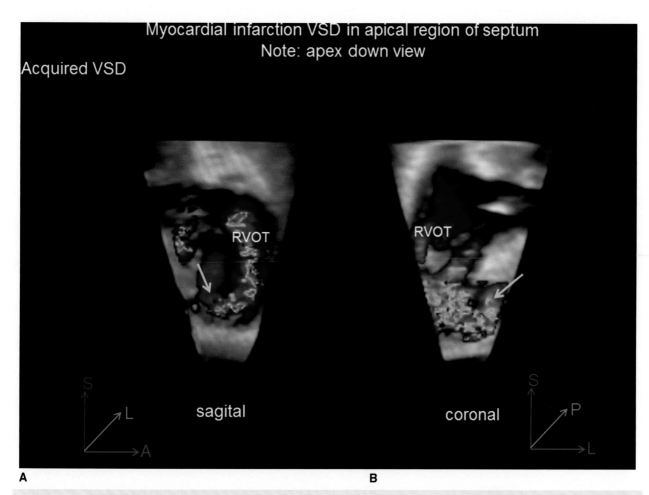

Figure 13-19. Transesophageal 3D echocardiogram of acquired VSD after myocardial infarction. Sagittal view (A) and coronal 3D color Doppler flow maps (B) of the left to right shunt (*arrow*) from a similar case of postinfarction acquired apical VSD. Images were obtained from the deep transgastric position. Note the apex of the heart is oriented at the bottom of the image as is typical in pediatric cardiology. See accompanying Video 13-23.

References

1. Lang RM, Mor-Avi V, Sugeng L, et al. Three-dimensional echocardiography: the benefits of the additional dimension. *J Am Coll Cardiol.* 2006;48:2053–2069.

2. Lang RM, Tsang W, Weinert L, et al. Valvular heart disease: the value of 3-dimensional echocardiography. *J Am Coll Cardiol.* 2011;58:1933–1944.

3. Salustri A, Spitaels S, McGhie J, et al. Transthoracic three dimensional echocardiography in adult patients with congenital heart disease. *J Am Coll Cardiol.* 1995;26:759–767.

4. Seliem MA, Fedec A, Cohen MS, et al. Real-time 3-dimensional echocardiographic imaging of congenital heart disease using matrix-array technology: freehand real-time scanning adds instant morphologic details not well delineated by conventional 2-dimensional imaging. *J Am Soc Echocardiogr.* 2006;19:121–129.

5. Marx GR, Fulton DR, Pandian NG, et al. Delineation of site, relative size and dynamic geometry of atrial septal defects by real-time three-dimensional echocardiography. *J Am Coll Cardiol.* 1995;2:482–490.

6. Magni G, Cao QL, Sugeng L, et al. Volume-rendered, three dimensional echocardiographic determination of the size, shape, and position of atrial septal defects: validation in an in vitro model. *Am Heart J.* 1996;132:376–381.

7. Acar P, Saliba Z, Bonhoeffer P, et al. Influence of atrial sepal defect anatomy in patient selection and assessment of closure with the cardioseal device. *Eur Heart J.* 2000;21:573–581.

8. Van den Bosch AE, Harkel DJT, McGhie JS, et al. Characterization of atrial septal defect assessed by real-time 3-dimensional echocardiography. *J Am Soc Echocardiogr.* 2006;19:815–821.

9. Faletra FF, Ho SY, Auricchio A. Anatomy of right atrial structures by real-time 3D transesophageal echocardiography. *J Am Coll Cardiol Img.* 2010;3:966–975.

10. Pushparajah K, Miller OI, et al. 3D echocardiography of the atrial septum: anatomical features and landmarks for the echocardiographer. *J Am Coll Cardiol Img.* 2010;3:981–984.

11. Saric M, Perk G, Purgess JR, et al. Imaging atrial septal defects by real-time three-dimensional transesophageal echocardiography: step-by-step approach. *J Am Soc Echocardiogr.* 2010;23:1128–1135.

12. Roberson DA, Cui W, Patel D, et al. Three-dimensional transesophageal echocardiography of atrial septal defect: a qualitative and quantitative anatomic study. *J Am Soc Echocardiogr.* 2011;24:600–610.

13. Taniguchi M, Akagi T, Watanabe N, et al. Application of real time three-dimensional transesophageal echocardiography using a matrix array probe for trans-catheter closure of atrial septal defect. *J Am Soc Echocardiogr.* 2009;22:1114–1120.

14. Kardon RE, Cao QL, Masani N, et al. New insights and observations in three-dimensional echocardiographic visualization of ventricular septal defects. *Circulation.* 1998;98:1307–1314.

15. Dall'Agata A, Cromme-Dijkhuis AH, Meijboom FJ, et al. Three dimensional echocardiography enhances the assessment of ventricular septal defect. *Am J Cardiol.* 1999;83:1576–1579.

16. Acar P, Abdel-Massih T, Douste-Blazy MY, et al. Assessment of muscular ventricular septal defect closure by transcatheter or surgical approach: a three-dimensional echocardiographic study. *Eur J Echocardiogr.* 2002;3:185–191.

17. Puri T, Liu Z, Doddamani S, et al. Three-dimensional echocardiography of post myocardial infarction cardiac rupture. *Echocardiography.* 2004;21:279–284.

18. Mehmood F, Miller AP, Nanda NC, et al. Usefulness of live/real time three-dimensional transthoracic echocardiography in the characterization of ventricular septal defects in adults. *Echocardiography.* 2006;23:421–427.

19. Chen FL, Hsiung MC, Nanda N, et al. Real time three dimensional echocardiography in assessing ventricular septal defects: an echocardiographic-surgical correlative study. *Echocardiography.* 2006;23:562–568.

20. van den Bosch AE, Ten Harkel DJ, McGhie JS, et al. Feasibility and accuracy of real-time 3-dimensional echocardiographic assessment of ventricular septal defects. *J Am Soc Echocardiogr.* 2006;19:7–13.

21. Mercer-Rosa L, Seliem MA, Fedec A, et al. Illustration of the additional value of real-time 3-dimensional echocardiography to conventional transthoracic and transesophageal 2-dimensional echocardiography in imaging muscular ventricular septal defects: does this have any impact on individual patient treatment? *J Am Soc Echocardiogr.* 2006;19:1511–1519.

22. Hsu JH, Wu JR, Dai ZK, et al. Real-time three-dimensional echocardiography provides novel and useful anatomic insights of ventricular septal aneurysm. *Int J Cardiol.* 2007;118:326–331.

23. Ishii M, Hashino K, Eto G, et al. Quantitative assessment of severity of ventricular septal defect by three dimensional reconstruction of color Doppler-imaged vena contracta and flow convergence region. *Circulation.* 2001;103:664–669.

24. Rivera JM, Siu SC, Handschumacher MD, et al. Three-dimensional reconstruction of ventricular septal defects: validation studies and in vivo feasibility. *J Am Coll Cardiol.* 1994;23:201–208.

25. Cheng TO, Xie MX, Wang XF, et al. Real-time 3-dimensional echocardiography in assessing atrial and ventricular septal defects: an echocardiographic-surgical correlative study. *Am Heart J.* 2004;148:1091–1095.

PEDIATRIC ASPECTS OF THREE-DIMENSIONAL ECHOCARDIOGRAPHY

14

Girish S. Shirali, John M. Simpson

Complex intracardiac anatomy and spatial relationships are inherent to congenital heart defects (CHDs). This is of great significance in congenital heart disease, where echocardiography is frequently the only imaging modality that is used to define intracardiac anatomy preoperatively. Beginning over 30 years ago and until recently, the clinician's ability to image the heart by echocardiography was limited to two-dimensional (2D) techniques.[1] However, two-dimensional echocardiography (2DE) has fundamental limitations. The very nature of a 2DE slice, which has no thickness, necessitates the use of multiple orthogonal "sweeps." The echocardiographer then mentally reconstructs the anatomy and uses the structure of the report to express this mentally reconstructed vision. This means that the only 3D image of the heart is the "virtual image" that exists in the mind of the echocardiographer, who then translates this vision into words. It is not easy for an observer to understand the images obtained in the course of a sweep: expert interpretation is required. Further, since myocardial motion occurs in three dimensions, 2DE techniques inherently do not lend themselves to accurate quantitation.

Recognition of these limitations of 2DE led to burgeoning research and clinical interest in the modality of three-dimensional echocardiography (3DE). Early reconstructive approaches were based on 2DE image acquisitions that were subsequently stacked and aligned based on phases of the cardiac cycle, in order to recreate a 3DE dataset.[2–4] While these approaches proved to be accurate, the need for time and offline processing equipment imposed fundamental limitations on their clinical applicability. In 1990, von Ramm and Smith[5] published their early results with a matrix array transducer that provided real-time images of the heart in three dimensions. While this was an important breakthrough, this transducer was unable to be steered in the third (elevation) dimension. Over the past decade, dramatic technologic advances have facilitated the ability to perform live 3DE scanning, including the ability to steer the beam in three dimensions and to render the image in real time.[6]

MODIFYING THE CROSS-SECTIONAL PARADIGM: MULTIPLANAR RECONSTRUCTION

One of the advantages of 3DE imaging is that a sonographic volume of data is obtained, which is permanently available for reinterrogation. The size of the volume acquired can be defined by the user, ranging from a relatively small narrow pyramidal shaped volume during a live 3D acquisition to a much larger pyramidal volume obtained over several cardiac cycles. The selection of volume size largely depends on the region of interest that requires to be incorporated within the volume. In some situations, the depth of field provided by a 3D-rendered image may be desirable; however, the alternative is to cut the dataset using a number of planes that can be manually adjusted by the user. Initial inspection of the dataset using this multiplanar approach allows the technical quality of the data to be assessed and artefacts can be readily identified. Planes can be set to cut the dataset in orientations that may be impossible to achieve by 2D echocardiography due to the limitation of an appropriate sonographic window; thus, truly novel cut planes can be displayed.[7] Furthermore, the simultaneous projection of multiple sonographic views, representing different cut planes means that the relative position of different cardiac structures can be appreciated.[8] Careful orientation of a cut plane directly *en face* to a structure means that precise measurements are possible. In practice, atrial and ventricular septal defects (VSDs), for example, can be measured accurately and any irregularity of shape can be clearly appreciated. Multiplanar reformatted imaging is particularly useful for imaging of complex abnormalities of the cardiac connections because individual planes can be moved through the sonographic volume to provide a virtual "walk through" of the heart. Furthermore, in the assessment of atrioventricular valves, the cut planes can be aligned to a single region of interest—such cross-referencing of planes means that precise localization of abnormalities may be achieved.[9,10] An important disadvantage of the multiplanar approach relates to movement of the heart through planes during systole and diastole. Such motion means that cardiac structures may move in and out of the cut plane and may not be displayed throughout the cardiac cycle. The effect of such "through plane" motion can be mitigated by increasing the slice thickness during postprocessing, but this remains a significant issue. In addition to the problem of cardiac motion, a further issue with multiplanar reformatted images is that individual cut planes cannot be rotated to display images in an anatomic format that has been advocated for consistent display of 3D echocardiographic images.[11,12]

CHANGING THE CROSS-SECTIONAL PARADIGM: CROPPING, VIRTUAL DISSECTION

Two-dimensional imaging is inherently cross-sectional. The addition of the third ("elevation") plane to the image transforms the echocardiographer's perspective into one that is similar to that of a surgeon or a pathologist. In this new paradigm, when presented with a 3D image, the echocardiographer must decide to view the structure of interest from specific perspectives. For instance, in order to view the atrioventricular valves en face, choices for viewing perspectives would be either looking down from the atria or looking up from the cardiac apex. In a manner similar to a surgeon or pathologist, the echocardiographer must therefore perform a (virtual) dissection of the heart, cropping off the base and apex of the heart. Similarly, in order to view the ventricular septum en face, the free walls of the heart must be cropped away. Cropping is fundamentally different from the 2D technique of zooming in or magnifying an image. Cropping can be performed after the acquisition, and it does not change line density and spatial or temporal resolution. In order to develop expertise with interpretation of 3D images, the echocardiographer must develop familiarity with these new perspectives and the added anatomic detail that is available using 3DE. The current presentation utilizes pathology specimens to help illustrate these concepts.

NORMAL ANATOMY

Conventional 2DE views and images can be used as a starting point to develop perspectives that are unique to 3DE. Acquisitions from the apical four-chamber window can be cropped and manipulated to provide en-face views of the atrioventricular valves as well as the septal structures (Fig. 14-1 and Video 14-1). The parasternal long-axis view can be rotated to visualize the right heart structures (Fig. 14-2 and Video 14-2). The parasternal short-axis view provides details of mitral valve (MV) anatomy and structure (Fig. 14-3 and Video 14-3). The subcostal long axis (Fig. 14-4 and Video 14-4) provides anatomic details focusing on the right ventricular aspect of the ventricular septum. The subcostal short-axis view (Fig. 14-5 and Video 14-5) can be used to visualize the orifices of the right pulmonary veins. A more advanced 3DE approach focuses on individual cardiac structures such as the tricuspid valve, which can be inspected from both the right atrial and the right ventricular aspects (Fig. 14-6 and Video 14-6).

THE TRICUSPID VALVE

The morphologic features of Ebstein's anomaly of the tricuspid valve are clearly demonstrated using both rendered images (Figs. 14.7–14.10 and Videos 14-7–14-10) and multiplanar reformatting (Fig. 14-11 and Video 14-11).[13,14] Double orifice tricuspid valve is illustrated in Figure 14-12 and Video 14-12.

THE MITRAL VALVE

Congenital malformations of the MV are beautifully illustrated using 3DE.[15–17] The substrate for obstruction to inflow of the left heart may be an obstructive membrane within the left atrium (cor triatriatum, Figs. 14-13 and 14-14 and Videos 14-13 and 14-14). This membrane is located posterosuperior to the base of the left atrial appendage. In contrast, a supramitral ring (Figs. 14-15 and 14-16 and Videos 14-15 and 14-16) is located anteroinferior to the left atrial appendage and may obstruct flow at any level from the hinge to the tips of the MV. The leaflets of the MV may be thick and dysplastic. They may insert onto a single papillary muscle; this leads to a parachute MV, which is best exemplified by contrasting it to the normal attachments of the MV (Fig. 14-17 and Video 14-17). In this malformation, the two mitral leaflets may insert onto either the anterolateral (Fig. 14-18 and Video 14-18) or posteromedial (Fig. 14-19 and Video 14-19) papillary muscle. Mitral leaflets may also insert directly onto papillary muscles without any chordae tendineae and therefore no interchordal spaces (Figs. 14-20 and 14-21 and Videos 14-20 and 14-21). The MV may have two orifices instead of one (Fig. 14-22 and Video 14-22). Rarely, the MV may exhibit Ebstein's malformation. This involves the mural (posterior) mitral leaflet (Fig. 14-23 and Video 14-23).

ATRIOVENTRICULAR SEPTAL DEFECT

The term "atrioventricular septal defect" refers to anomalies that are characterized by a common atrioventricular junction. Morphologic differences between subtypes have important implications for the timing and nature of surgery.[18,19] The components of the partial form of this defect are a primum atrial septal defect (ASD) and a trifoliate left atrioventricular valve, which has a mural leaflet and two bridging leaflets, which are named the superior and inferior bridging leaflet. This form has two atrioventricular (AV) valve orifices (Figs. 14-24–14-30 and Videos 14-24–14-30). The complete form of the defect is characterized by a primum ASD, common AV valve with a single orifice, and a VSD that is roofed by the bridging leaflets of the common AV valve (Figs. 14-31–14-36 and Videos 14-31–14-36). In contrast to AV septal defect, an isolated or true cleft of the MV, directed toward the aorta, is demonstrated in Figures 14-37 and 14-38 and Videos 14-37 and 14-38.

SUBAORTIC AND AORTIC STENOSIS

The substrates leading to subaortic obstruction range from discrete membranes (Figs. 14-39–14-41 and Videos 14-39–14-41) to complex, multilevel muscular tunnels (Fig. 14-42 and Video 14-42).[20] The aortic valve leaflets are thin and lend themselves well to 3D transesophageal imaging (Fig. 14-43 and Video 14-43).[21] Multiplanar reformatting is well suited to understanding the anatomy of the bicuspid aortic valve and the left ventricular outflow tract (Fig. 14-44 and Video 14-44).

TETRALOGY OF FALLOT

3DE views are used to illustrate the classic features of tetralogy of Fallot, including the anterior malalignment-type VSD, located in the "Y" of the septal band, which is best seen in subcostal long-axis views (Figs. 14-45 and 14-46, Videos 14-45 and 14-46). Orthogonal short-axis views (Figs. 14.47 and 14.48, Videos 14.47 and 14.48) illustrate the margins of the VSD and the substrate for subpulmonary stenosis.

d-TRANSPOSITION OF THE GREAT ARTERIES

In its classic and most frequently encountered form, d-transposition of the great arteries is characterized by solitus (usual) arrangement of the viscera and atria, d-loop ventricles, concordant atrioventricular connections, and discordant ventriculoarterial connections. The aorta is connected to the morphologic right ventricle, usually supported by a sleeve of muscle (subaortic conus) that provides for discontinuity between the aortic and tricuspid valves. The pulmonary artery is connected to the morphologic left ventricle (LV), typically with no subpulmonary conus. Issues of importance in d-transposition include VSDs, malalignment of the outlet septum, and the presence and nature of outflow tract obstruction. Figure 14-49 and Video 14-49 illustrate the usual form of d-transposition of the great arteries, with a small perimembranous VSD. Figures 14-50–14-52 and Videos 14-50–14-52 illustrate the application of multiplanar reformatting in d-transposition with a posterior malalignment VSD. This illustrates the utility of 3DE in delineating complex spatial relationships between the VSD and the outflow tracts.

DOUBLE OUTLET RIGHT VENTRICLE

Double outlet right ventricle is a lesion that spans a wide spectrum in terms of outflow tract anatomy and location of the VSD(s). These variations have direct implications for the optimal surgical approach for individual patients. Both rendered images (Figs. 14-53–14-60 and Videos 14-53–14-60) and multiplanar reformatting (Fig. 14-61 and Video 14-61) are useful in evaluating this complex lesion.

TUMORS

Cardiac tumors vary in number, size, shape, and extent, and are well delineated by 3DE.[22,23] Rhabdomyomas may be discrete, involving the aortic valve (Fig. 14-62 and Video 14-62). They may be large, protruding into cardiac chambers; a right atrial rhabdomyoma is illustrated in Figure 14-63 and Video 14-63. Tumors may also be diffuse; a left ventricular fibroma involving most of the free wall is shown in Figure 14-64 and Video 14-64. An atrial myxoma is shown in Figure 14-65 and Video 14-65. The use of multiple planes to understand the extent of a teratoma is shown in Figure 14-66 and Video 14-66.

MISCELLANEOUS LESIONS

The lesions in this section include a persistent left superior vena cava, which connects to the right atrium via the coronary sinus (Fig. 14-67 and Video 14-67). Discordant atrioventricular connections in congenitally corrected transposition, where the right atrium connects to the morphologic LV via the MV and the left atrium connects to the morphologic right ventricle via the tricuspid valve, are illustrated in Figures 14.68 and 14.69 and Videos 14.68 and 14.69.[24] The 3D color flow appearance of a Blalock-Taussig shunt is illustrated in Figure 14-70 and Video 14-70, where, in order to visualize the color flow in the relevant adjacent structures, the grayscale image has been suppressed (the "echocardiographic angiogram," first described by Hlavacek et al.).[25]

CONCLUSIONS

Important technologic advances over the past 5 years have enabled 3DE to emerge as a modality that provides additive value in managing patients with CHD. We anticipate that with continuing improvements in hardware and software, 3DE will become an integral part of a standard echocardiographic examination in the near future.

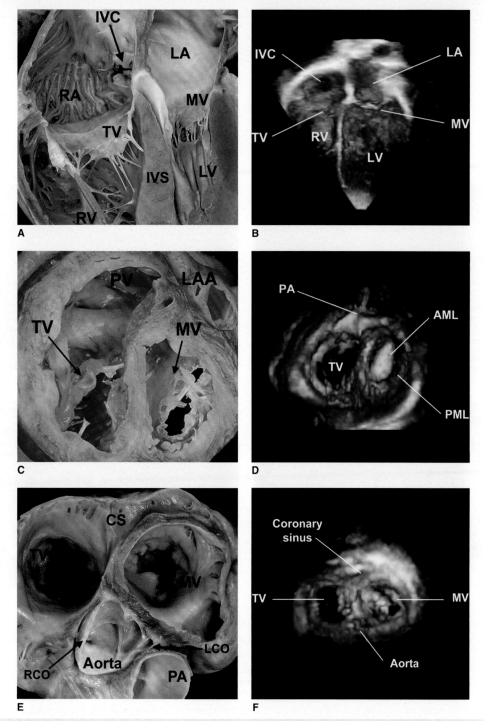

Figure 14-1. A. Apical four-chamber view of the normal heart. This demonstrates normal offset of the atrioventricular valves and the entrance of the inferior vena cava into the right atrium. (IVC, inferior vena cava; LA, left atrium; LV, left ventricle; MV, mitral valve; RA, right atrium; RV, right ventricle; TV, tricuspid valve). B. Live 3DE from an apical four-chamber view. This demonstrates normal offset of the atrioventricular valves and the entrance of the inferior vena cava into the right atrium. (IVC, inferior vena cava; LA, left atrium; LV, left ventricle; MV, mitral valve; RV, right ventricle; TV, tricuspid valve). The companion video (Video 14-1) is an apical four-chamber view, evolving from 2D to 3D imaging. This demonstrates cropping techniques to provide en-face views of the atrioventricular valves and the normal position of the aorta, wedged between the mitral and tricuspid valves. C. Short-axis view of the heart. The heart has been transected in its short axis and is viewed from below. The tricuspid and mitral valves are seen en face. (LAA, left atrial appendage; MV, mitral valve; PV, pulmonary valve; TV, tricuspid valve). D. Apical four-chamber full-volume acquisition. The ventricular apices have been cropped away and the image has been tilted to view the mitral and tricuspid valves from below. (AML, anterior mitral leaflet; PA, pulmonary artery; PML, posterior mitral leaflet; TV, tricuspid valve). E. Aorta wedged between the atrioventricular valves. This atrial view of the base of the heart demonstrates the aorta (Ao) wedged between the two atrioventricular valves. (TV, tricuspid valve; MV, mitral valve; CS, coronary sinus; PA, pulmonary artery; RCO, right coronary orifice; LCO, left coronary orifice). F. Short axis of the heart from an apical full-volume acquisition. The atria have been cropped away and the image has been tilted to view the atrioventricular valves en face, from above downward. The aorta is seen wedged between the mitral and tricuspid valves (MV, mitral valve; TV, tricuspid valve).

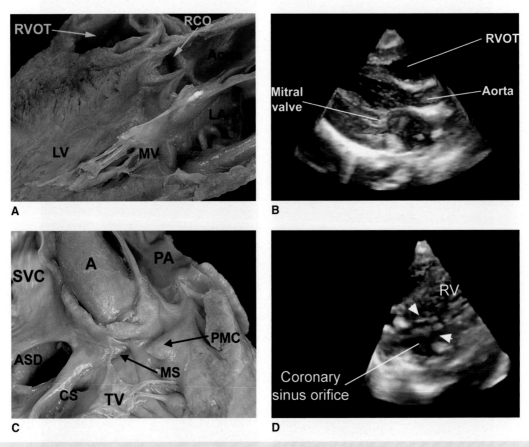

Figure 14-2. A. Parasternal long-axis view of a normal LV. The fibrous continuity between the aortic valve and the mitral valve is seen. The right ventricular outflow tract is seen in cross section. (LA, left atrium; LV, left ventricle; MV, mitral valve; RCO, right coronary orifice; RVOT, right ventricular outflow tract). B. Parasternal long axis live 3DE in a normal heart. Mitral–aortic continuity and the papillary muscles of the MV are well seen. The right ventricular outflow tract is seen in cross section. (RVOT, right ventricular outflow tract). The companion video (Video 14-2) evolves from 2D to 3D imaging to demonstrate the ventricular septum and left heart structures. The image is then rotated to demonstrate the right atrium, tricuspid valve, and right ventricle. C. The right ventricular inflow. The free wall of the right atrium and ventricle, along with the anterior pulmonary artery and a portion of the septal leaflet of the tricuspid valve, has been removed to demonstrate the normal location of the membranous septum. The chordal attachments to the papillary muscle of the conus have been removed; it is seen arising from the septomarginal trabeculation (septal band). Note the secundum ASD. (A, aorta; ASD, atrial septal defect; CS, coronary sinus; MS, membranous septum; PA, pulmonary artery; PMC, papillary muscle of the conus; SVC, superior vena cava; TV, tricuspid valve). D. Parasternal long-axis view of the right heart. This long-axis view has been rotated to demonstrate the right ventricular inflow view: the right atrium, tricuspid valve, and right ventricle. The free walls of the right heart chambers have been cropped off. *Arrowheads* mark the leaflets of the tricuspid valve. The orifice of the coronary sinus is seen. (RV, right ventricle).

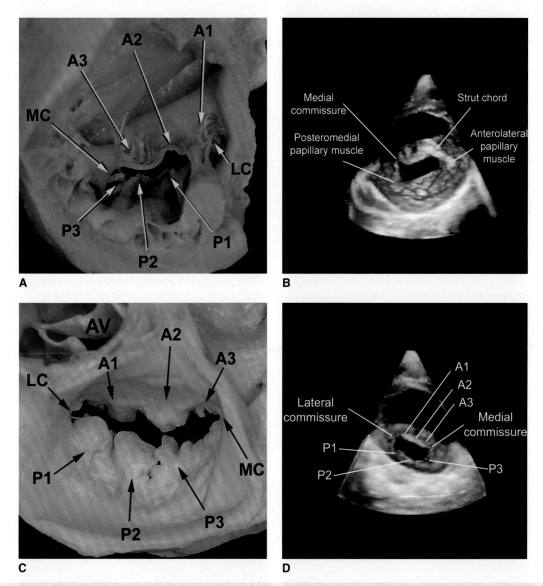

Figure 14-3. A. MV viewed from below. This view of the MV looking up from the apex of the LV demonstrates the medial and lateral commissures, along with the scallops of the anterior mitral leaflet (A1–A3) and the posterior mitral leaflet (P1–P3). (LC, lateral commissure; MC, medial commissure). B. Parasternal short-axis view of the MV. This demonstrates details of mitral leaflet surfaces and chord anatomy, including strut chords that attach to the body of the leaflets (rather than at the tips of the leaflets). The companion video (Video 14-3) evolves from 2D to 3D imaging to demonstrate the MV apparatus as viewed from the LV (*looking up*) and from the left atrium (*looking down*). C. View of the MV from the left atrium demonstrates the medial and lateral commissures. The proximity of the aortic valve to the anterior leaflet of the MV can be appreciated along with the scallops of both the anterior (A1–A3) and posterior (P1–P3) leaflets. (AV, aortic valve; LC, lateral commissure; MC, medial commissure). D. Parasternal short-axis image rotated 180 degrees to view the MV from the left atrium. This view demonstrates the leaflet surfaces, scallops, and commissures of the MV.

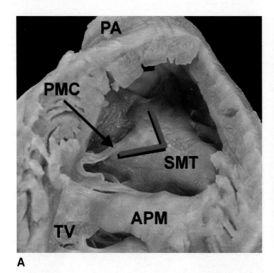
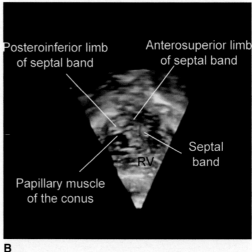

A   B

Figure 14-4. A. Subcostal long-axis view of the right ventricle. The septomarginal trabeculation (septal band) is seen bifurcating into a "Y" (*red lines*). The papillary muscle of the conus inserts into the Y of the septal band. The anterior papillary muscle of the tricuspid valve is seen attaching to the septum. (APM, anterior papillary muscle; PA, pulmonary artery; PMC, papillary muscle of the conus; SMT, septomarginal trabeculation (septal band); TV, tricuspid valve). B. Normal subcostal long-axis view. This provides anatomic details on the pattern of arrangement of muscle bundles in the right ventricular outflow tract. The viewing perspective is from below and rightward. The free wall of the right ventricle has been cropped off. The papillary muscle of the conus is seen attaching between the anterosuperior and posteroinferior limbs of the septal band. (RV, right ventricle). The companion video (Video 14-4) evolves from 2D to 3D imaging to demonstrate the right ventricular aspect of the ventricular septum.

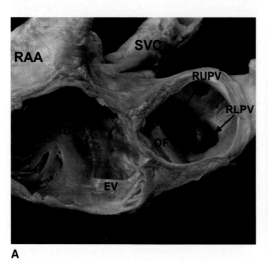
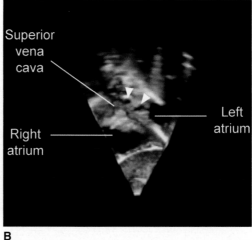

A   B

Figure 14-5. A. Subcostal short-axis view demonstrates the right upper and right lower pulmonary veins. The superior vena cava is seen entering the right atrium (EV, Eustachian valve; OF, foramen ovale; RA, right atrium; RLPV, right lower pulmonary vein; RUPV, right upper pulmonary vein; SVC, superior vena cava; TC, terminal crest). B. Normal subcostal short-axis view. This demonstrates the orifices of the right upper and lower pulmonary veins as they enter the left atrium (*arrowheads*). The companion video (Video 14-5) evolves from 2D to 3D imaging to demonstrate the orifices of both right-sided pulmonary veins as they enter the left atrium.

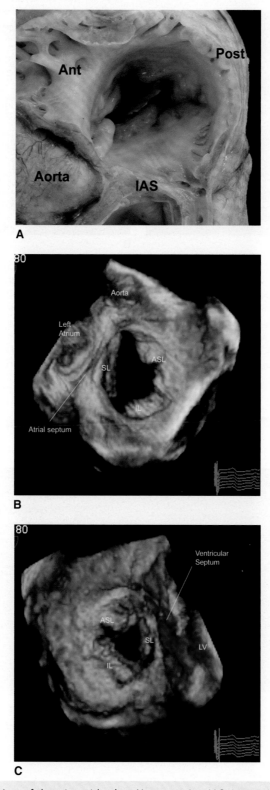

Figure 14-6. A. The right atrial view of the tricuspid valve. (Ant, anterior; IAS, interatrial septum; Post, posterior). B. The tricuspid valve is visualized from the atrial side in this projection. The position of the atrial septum is clearly seen with the aorta in an anterosuperior position. (ASL, anterosuperior leaflet of the tricuspid valve; IL, inferior leaflet of the tricuspid valve; SL, septal leaflet of the tricuspid valve). The companion video (Video 14-6) utilizes a full-volume acquisition of the tricuspid valve using a transesophageal approach. Initially the ventricular and subsequently the atrial aspects of the tricuspid valve are demonstrated. C. The tricuspid valve is visualized from the right ventricular aspect. The three leaflets of the tricuspid valve can be seen including details of the leaflet morphology. (ASL, anterosuperior leaflet of the tricuspid valve; IL, inferior leaflet of the tricuspid valve; SL, septal leaflet of the tricuspid valve; LV, left ventricle).

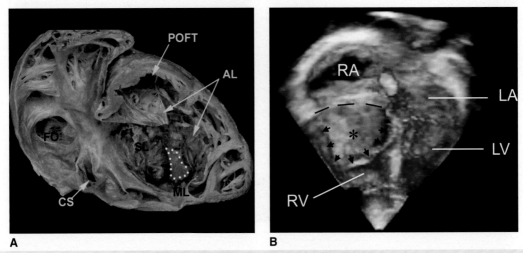

Figure 14-7. A. Ebstein's anomaly. The free wall of the right atrium and right ventricle have been removed to show the marked distortion of the tricuspid valve in this heart with Ebstein's anomaly. The right ventricle is atrialized in the area between the coronary sinus and the septal and mural (posteroinferior) leaflets of the tricuspid valve. The anterior leaflet forms a sail-like structure that partially obstructs the pulmonary outflow tract. The white dots mark the area of noncoaptation of the leaflets of the tricuspid valve. (AL, anterior leaflet; CS, coronary sinus; FO, foramen ovale; ML, mural (posteroinferior) leaflet; POFT, pulmonary outflow tract; SL, septal leaflet). B. Ebstein's anomaly. This apical four-chamber view demonstrates classic features of Ebstein's anomaly. The tricuspid valve leaflets (marked by *arrowheads*) are displaced apically relative to the anatomic annulus (marked by a *dashed line*). The asterisk marks the atrialized right ventricle.

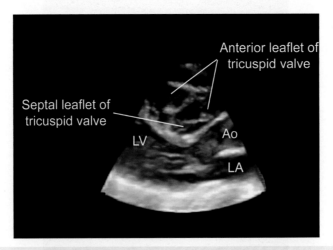

Figure 14-8. Parasternal long-axis view in Ebstein's anomaly demonstrates the rudimentary septal leaflet, the large anterior leaflet, and the gap in coaptation of the leaflets of the tricuspid valve viewed from the right ventricular aspect. See accompanying Video 14-8.

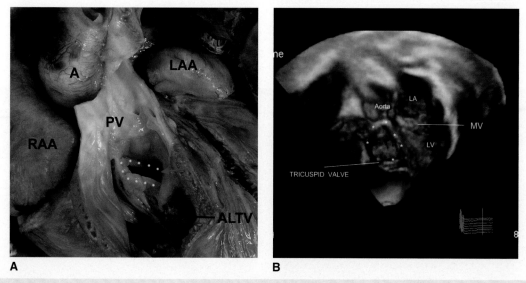

A

B

Figure 14-9. A. Anterior view of the right ventricular outflow tract in a heart with Ebstein's malformation. This shows the stenotic opening (*yellow dots*) formed by the curtain-like anterior leaflet of the tricuspid valve. A portion of the septal leaflet (*red arrow*) also forms a portion of this stenotic opening and lies adjacent to the subpulmonic infundibulum. (A, aorta; ALTV, anterior leaflet of the tricuspid valve; LAA, left atrial appendage; PV, pulmonary valve; RAA, right atrial appendage). B. Rendered 3D view of Ebstein's anomaly of the tricuspid valve demonstrates the abnormal anterosuperior rotation of the tricuspid valve orifice that is seen opening *en face* with a typical "keyhole" appearance. This contrasts with the normal appearance of the tricuspid valve (LA, left atrium; LV, left ventricle; MV, mitral valve). In the corresponding video (Video 14.9), the tricuspid valve can be seen to open and close en face to the crop plane. The orientation and movement of the mitral and aortic valves is normal.

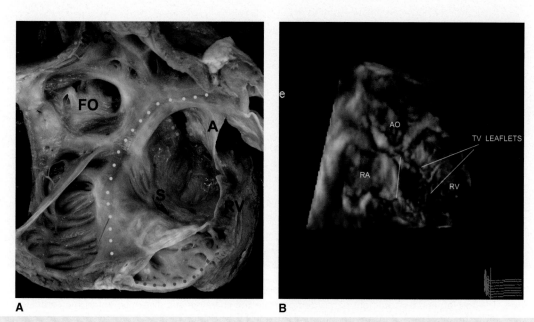

A

B

Figure 14-10. A. Anterior superior view of Ebstein's anomaly. This shows the severity of the malformation with the true tricuspid valve annulus represented with yellow dots. The septal leaflet covers the entire septal surface and the right ventricular apex and partially fuses with the curtain-like anterior leaflet. The orange dots represent the stenotic opening allowing blood to pass from the atrialized right ventricle into the pulmonary outflow. The inferior wall of the right ventricle is thin or atrialized (*red dots*). (A, anterior leaflet; FO, foramen ovale; RV, right ventricle; S, septal leaflet; SVC, superior vena cava). B. Right atrial and right ventricular view of the tricuspid valve leaflets in Ebstein's anomaly. The solid white line marks the normal plane of the tricuspid valve. The superior extension of the tricuspid valve leaflets into the right ventricular outflow tract is illustrated. (Ao, aorta; RA, right atrium; RV, right ventricle; TV, tricuspid valve). The companion video (Video 14-10) demonstrates the tricuspid valve following cropping away of the right ventricular free wall and the lateral wall of the right atrium. The "fan" of tricuspid valve attachments can be clearly seen.

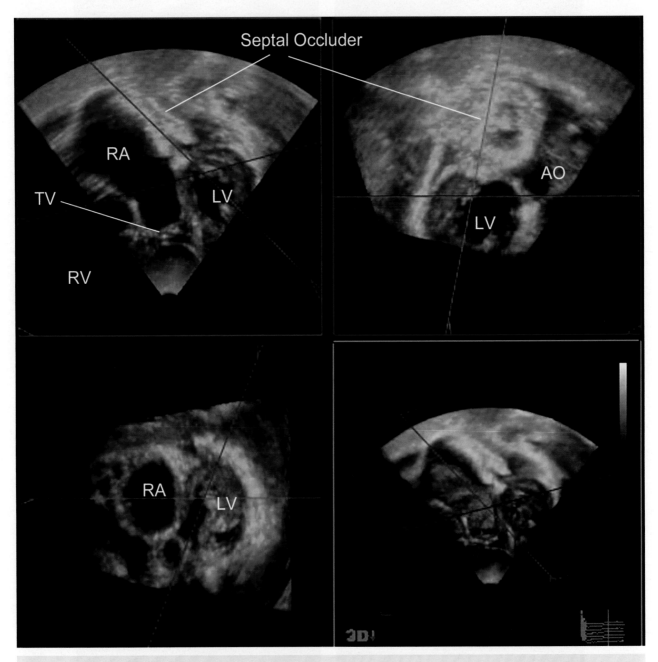

Figure 14-11. Multiplanar reformatted image of Ebstein's anomaly of the tricuspid valve. An atrial septal occluder has been inserted. The top left and bottom right panes demonstrate the characteristic displacement of the septal leaflet of the tricuspid valve. Adjustment of the cut planes permits assessment of the position of the septal occluder to adjacent structures such as the aorta (top right plane). (Ao, aorta; LV, left ventricle; RA, right atrium; RV, right ventricle; TV, tricuspid valve). See accompanying Video 14-11.

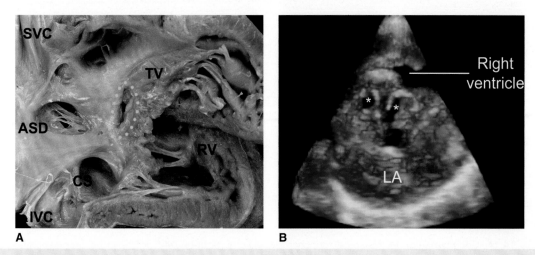

Figure 14-12. **A.** Double orifice tricuspid valve. In this anatomic view of the right ventricle, the free wall has been lifted from the septal component. There is a double orifice tricuspid valve, the second, smaller orifice marked with yellow dots. There is a fenestrated ASD and a dilated coronary sinus secondary to a persistent left superior vena cava. (ASD, atrial septal defect; CS, coronary sinus; IVC, inferior vena cava; RV, right ventricle; SVC, superior vena cava; TV, tricuspid valve). **B.** Double orifice tricuspid valve. This angled parasternal short-axis live 3DE view illustrates double orifice tricuspid valve; the two orifices are marked by asterisks. See Video 14-12.

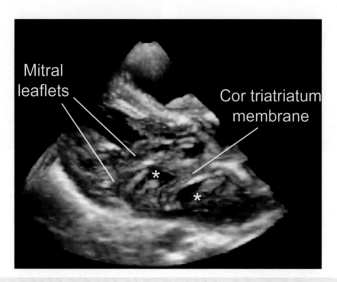

Figure 14-13. Parasternal long-axis image demonstrates cor triatriatum. The membrane separates the left atrium into two chambers, marked by asterisks. See Video 14-13.

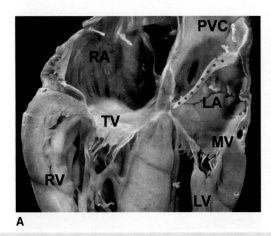

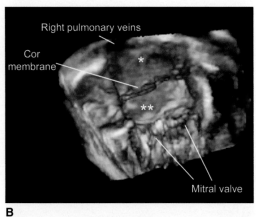

Figure 14-14. A. Cor triatriatum. In this apical four-chamber view, a partition (*red dots*) can be seen separating the left atrium into two compartments. The upper chamber is the pulmonary venous compartment; the lower chamber holds the flap valve of the foramen ovale and abuts on the MV. (LA, left atrium; LV, left ventricle; MV, mitral valve; PVC, pulmonary venous compartment; RA, right atrium; RV, right ventricle; TV, tricuspid valve) (Reproduced with the kind permission of Dr. Robert H. Anderson, London, England). **B.** Apical image demonstrating cor triatriatum. The anterior aspects of the heart have been cropped off to demonstrate the membrane. The pulmonary veins enter the superior chamber (marked by a single *asterisk*), while the inferior chamber (marked by a double *asterisk*) communicates with the MV. See Video 14-14.

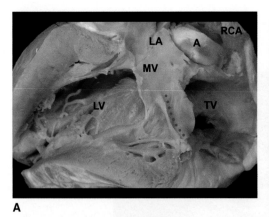

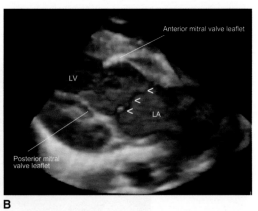

Figure 14-15. A. Supramitral ring. The opened left atrioventricular junction demonstrates a concordant connection between the left atrium and LV with the MV guarding the inlet. The MV is thickened and stenotic with fused chordae tendineae giving it a curtain-like appearance in most areas. At the MV annulus, there is a supramitral ring (*red dots*) that is not circumferential but accentuates the stenosis at the left atrioventricular junction. (A, aorta; LA, left atrium; LV, left ventricle; MV, mitral valve; RCA, right coronary artery, TV, tricuspid valve). **B.** Supramitral membrane (*ring*). This rendered 3D echocardiogram shows a supramitral membrane. The extent of the supramitral membrane (*arrowed*) is appreciated due to the depth of field. (LA, left atrium; LV, left ventricle). See Video 14-15.

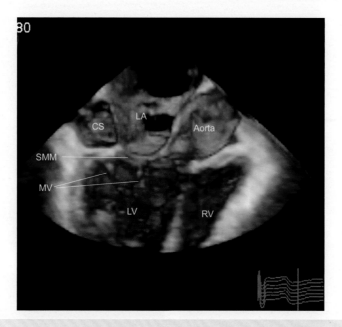

Figure 14-16. Transesophageal 3D echocardiographic view of a supramitral membrane that is immediately above the MV. The coronary sinus is dilated due to a persistent left superior vena cava. (CS, coronary sinus; LA, left atrium; LV, left ventricle; MV, mitral valve; RV, right ventricle; SMM, supramitral membrane). The companion video (Video 14-16) demonstrates fluttering of the aortic valve due to coexistent subaortic stenosis.

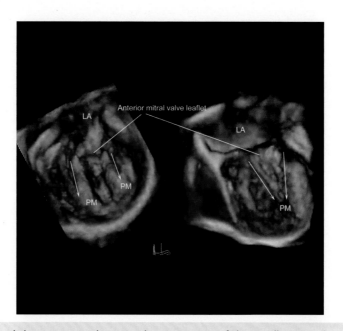

Figure 14-17. The left panel demonstrates the normal arrangement of the papillary muscles and the panel on the right shows a parachute MV characterized by a single papillary muscle. Both rendered images have been cropped along the plane of the anterior MV leaflet. The *arrows* indicate the direction of the chordal attachments to the papillary muscles. (LA, left atrium; PM, papillary muscle). In the companion video (Video 14-17), the left panel demonstrates the normal attachments of the anterior MV leaflet chords to the corresponding papillary muscles. The right panel shows both ends of the anterior leaflet of the MV attaching to a single papillary muscle.

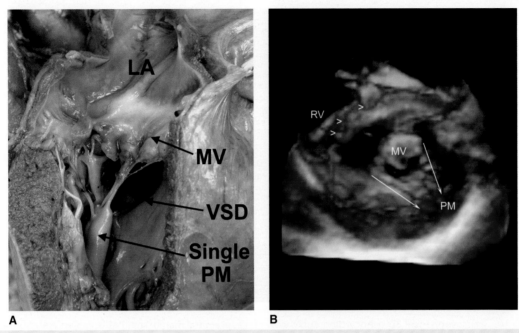

A   **B**

Figure 14-18. A. Parachute MV. The free wall of the LV has been lifted away illustrating a single papillary muscle supporting the MV, consistent with a parachute malformation. The LV was small in this heart with double outlet right ventricle and a VSD. (LA, left atrium: MV, mitral valve; PM, papillary muscle; VSD, ventricular septal defect). B. Rendered 3D view from the left ventricular apex demonstrating a parachute MV. The MV is in an open position and the chords (*arrowed*) attach to a single papillary muscle. The ventricular septum is indicated with *arrowheads* (>). (MV, mitral valve [anterior leaflet]; PM, papillary muscle; RV, right ventricle). See Video 14-18.

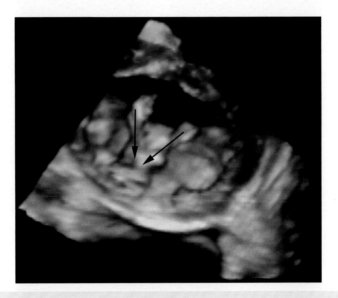

Figure 14-19. Parachute MV and dilated cardiomyopathy. Parasternal short-axis view demonstrates a parachute MV with both leaflets inserting onto a single papillary muscle that is located in the usual position of the posteromedial papillary muscle. This patient also has severe left ventricular dilated cardiomyopathy. See Video 14-19.

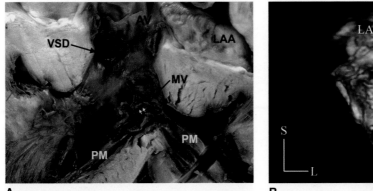

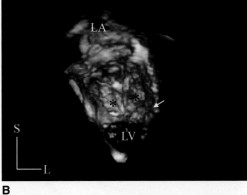

Figure 14-20. A. Dysplastic, stenotic MV. The opened left ventricular outflow tract shows a severely dysplastic MV in fibrous continuity with the aortic valve. Note the slit-like (*yellow arrows*) mitral orifice and the thickened valvar tissue. The tendinous cords are fused and attached directly to the tips of the papillary muscles. This heart also has a VSD and a left ventricular diverticulum (*red arrows*). (AV, aortic valve; LAA, left atrial appendage; MV, mitral valve; PM, papillary muscle; VSD, ventricular septal defect). B. Apical four-chamber view demonstrates a severely malformed, stenotic MV with two leaflets (*asterisks*) inserting directly onto a papillary muscle (*arrow*). There are no identifiable chordae tendineae. See Video 14-20.

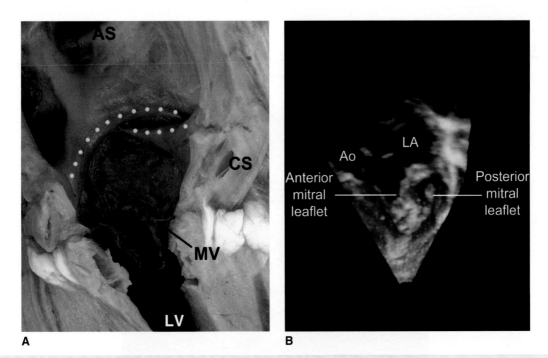

Figure 14-21. A. Dysplastic MV. The left atrioventricular junction has been opened slightly to view the thickened, dysplastic MV. Superior to the valve there is a prominent ridge (*yellow dots*) of tissue adding to the degree of stenosis. (AS, atrial septum; CS, coronary sinus; LV, left ventricle; MV, mitral valve). B. Congenital mitral stenosis. Subcostal view demonstrates a severely malformed, dysplastic MV with no interchordal spaces and multiple diminutive orifices. (Ao, aorta; LA, left atrium). See Video 14.21.

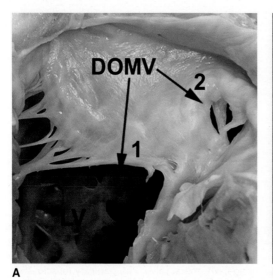
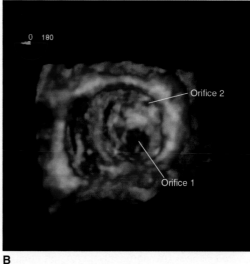

Figure 14-22. A. Double orifice MV. The MV is opened to demonstrate two orifices. Each orifice is numbered (1) and (2); note the thickened edges of the smaller orifice (2). (DOMV, double orifice mitral valve; LV-left ventricle). B. Double orifice MV. Three-dimensional rendered view of a double orifice MV viewed from the LV. There is a smaller, more superior orifice (orifice 2) and a larger more inferior orifice (orifice 1). See Video 14-22.

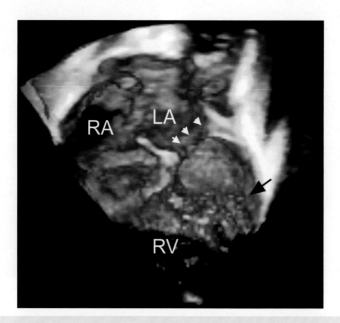

Figure 14-23. Ebstein's anomaly of the MV. Apical four-chamber image demonstrates this rare defect, where the anatomic mitral annulus (*white arrowheads*) is in the normal position, but the hinge of the posterior (mural) mitral leaflet is displaced apically (*black arrow*). (LA, left atrium; RA, right atrium; RV, right ventricle). Valve leaflet excursion and mobility is well appreciated on the companion video (Video 14-23).

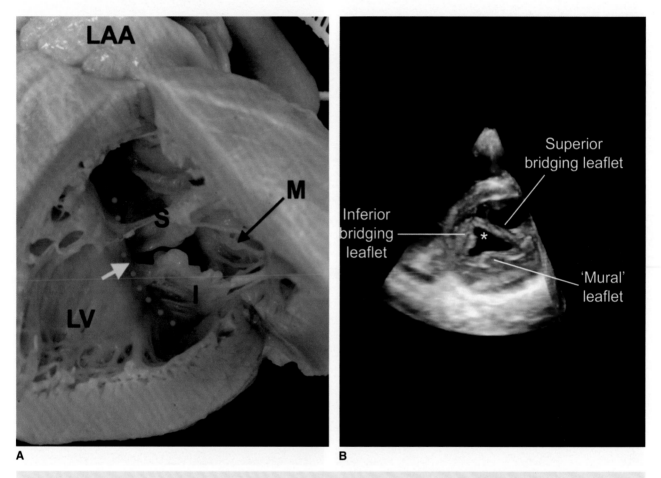

Figure 14-24. A. The free wall of the LV in has been lifted away from the septum to demonstrate the left orifice of the common atrioventricular valve. The zone of apposition between the superior (S) and inferior (I) bridging leaflets is marked with a *yellow arrow*. The leaflets are adherent to the crest of the ventricular septum (*red dots*) (I, inferior bridging leaflet; LAA, left atrial appendage; LV, left ventricle; M, mural leaflet; S, superior bridging leaflet). B. "Cleft" (zone of apposition) viewed in a conventional parasternal short-axis view. This demonstrates the trifoliate left AV valve in the "partial" form of atrioventricular septal defect. Here, the zone of apposition ("cleft," marked by an *asterisk*) between the superior and inferior bridging leaflets is clearly seen extending from the hinge to the tips of the AV valve. See Video 14-24.

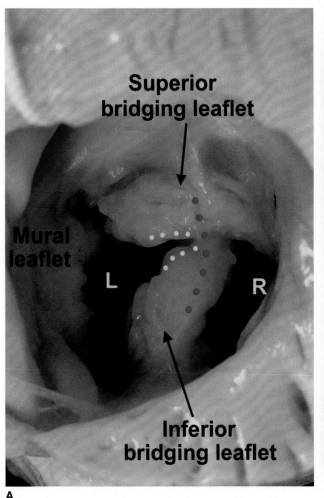

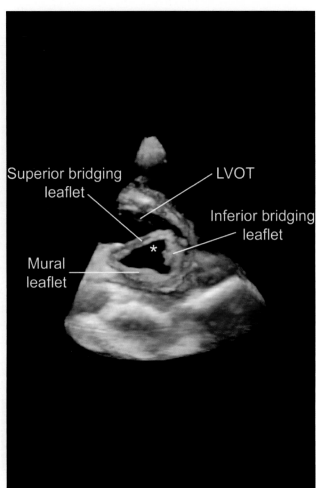

A

B

Figure 14-25. **A.** Trifoliate left atrioventricular valve from above. This short-axis view through the common atrium illustrates a common atrioventricular valve with separate right (R) and left (L) orifices. The leftward components of the superior and inferior bridging leaflets, together with the mural leaflet, comprise the trifoliate left atrioventricular valve. The bridging leaflets are adherent to one another and to the crest of the ventricular septum (*red dots*). The *yellow dots* mark the zone of apposition between the superior and inferior bridging leaflets. **B.** Trifoliate left atrioventricular valve and zone of apposition from above. Parasternal short-axis acquisition that has been rotated to view the left AV valve from above looking down. This demonstrates the classic 3D appearance of a trifoliate left atrioventricular valve. An *asterisk* marks the zone of apposition between the superior and inferior bridging leaflets ("cleft"). LVOT, left ventricular outflow tract. See Video 14-25.

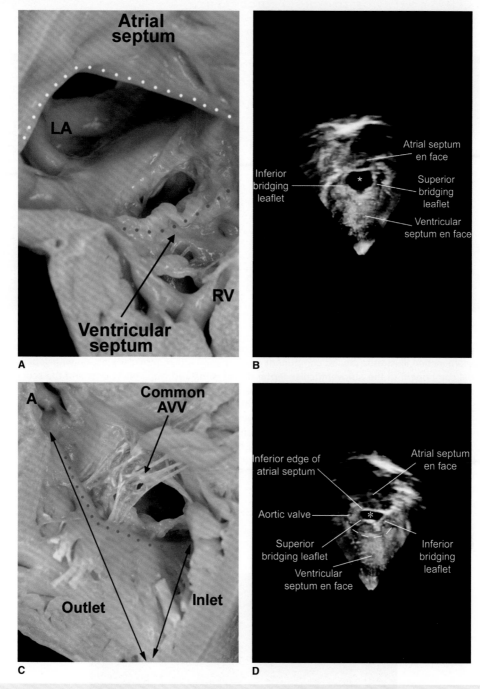

Figure 14-26. A. Partial atrioventricular septal defect, viewed from right to left. En-face view of the septal structures demonstrates the relationships of the bridging leaflets across the slightly scooped out ventricular septum. The bridging leaflets are adherent to the crest of the septum (*red dots*) with no shunting of blood taking place at the ventricular level. The crescent shaped inferior edge of the atrial septum forms the superior edge of a primum ASD (*white dots*) that is larger in its anteroposterior dimension than in its superoinferior dimension. B. Partial atrioventricular septal defect, viewed from right to left in this apical acquisition. In order to view the atrial and ventricular septums en face, the free walls of the right heart chambers have been cropped off. This view shows the crescentic inferior edge of the atrial septum. An *asterisk* marks the primum ASD, which is bordered below by the superior and inferior bridging leaflets. This defect is larger in its anteroposterior dimension than in its superoinferior dimension. Chordal attachments from the bridging leaflets to the ventricular septum have obliterated the potential for ventricular-level shunting. The companion video (Video 14-26) evolves from 2D to 3D imaging to demonstrate en-face views of the septal structures and the ASD. C. Partial atrioventricular septal defect, viewed from left to right. The left ventricular aspect of this heart shows the bridging leaflets adherent along the entire crest of the ventricular septum (*red dots*). Left ventricular inlet—outlet disproportion, with a shorter inlet and longer outlet, is the same as that seen in the complete type of atrioventricular septal defect. (A, aorta; AVV, atrioventricular valve). D. Partial atrioventricular septal defect, viewed from left to right. The free walls of the left heart chambers have been cropped off. This view shows the scooped out edge of the ventricular septum (*white dashed line*), and the crescentic inferior edge of the atrial septum. An *asterisk* marks the primum ASD, which is bordered below by the superior and inferior bridging leaflets. Note the anterior ("sprung") position of the aorta, with the "goose-neck" deformity of the left ventricular outflow tract.

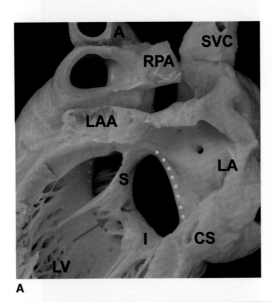
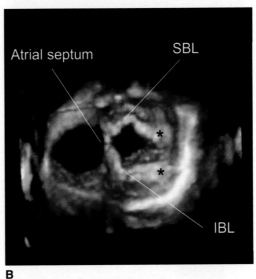

Figure 14-27. **A.** Orientation of the zone of apposition in a "partial" atrioventricular septal defect. This long-axis view of the left atrioventricular junction illustrates the left component of a common atrioventricular junction with separate right and left orifices. The atrial component of the atrioventricular septal defect is marked with *yellow dots* and the scooped out crest of the ventricular septum with *red dots*. The superior (S) and inferior (I) bridging leaflets are adherent to the one another and to the crest of the interventricular septum, forming separate right and left orifices. The zone of apposition (*red arrow*) between the bridging leaflets is clearly seen and points directly at the ventricular septum. (A, aorta; CS, coronary sinus; LA, left atrium; LAA, left atrial appendage; LV, left ventricle; RPA, right pulmonary artery; SVC, superior vena cava). **B.** Partial atrioventricular septal defect viewed from the apex. In this full-volume acquisition, the apices of the ventricles have been cropped off, and the image has been tilted to view the heart from below upward. This demonstrates the zone of apposition or "cleft" between the superior and inferior bridging leaflets. *Asterisks* mark the two left-sided papillary muscles. (IBL, inferior bridging leaflet; SBL, superior bridging leaflet). See Video 14-27.

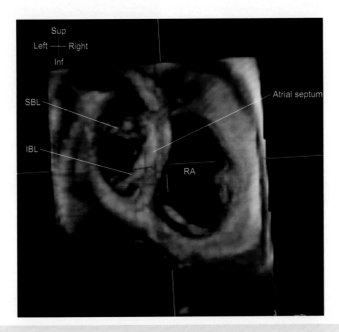

Figure 14-28. Atrioventricular septal defect viewed from the atrial aspect. This demonstrates the superior and inferior bridging leaflets of the left atrioventricular valve with the valve in an open position. (Inf, inferior; IBL, inferior bridging leaflet; RA, right atrium; Sup, superior; SBL, superior bridging leaflet). See Video 14-28.

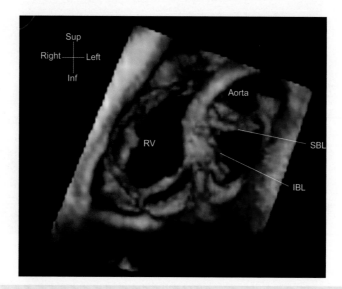

Figure 14-29. A 3D rendered view of atrioventricular septal defect viewed from the ventricles. The superior and inferior bridging leaflets are imaged as well as the relationship of the aorta to the superior bridging leaflet. The zone of apposition between the bridging leaflets is orientated toward the ventricular septum. (Inf, inferior; IBL, inferior bridging leaflet; RV, right ventricle; Sup, superior; SBL, superior bridging leaflet). See Video 14-29.

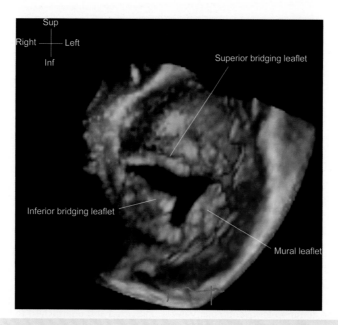

Figure 14-30. Atrioventricular septal defect viewed from the ventricular aspect. This demonstrates the morphology of the left atrioventricular valve, which has been displayed with the valve open. The companion video (Video 14-30) demonstrates the zone of apposition between the superior and inferior bridging leaflets. (Inf, inferior; sup, superior). See Video 14-30.

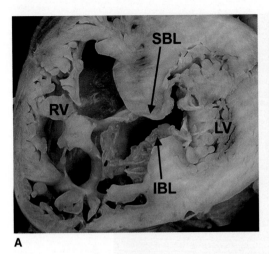

A

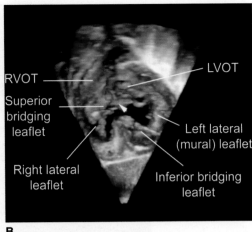

B

Figure 14-31. A. Common atrioventricular valve, Rastelli type A. This short-axis view of the common atrioventricular valve demonstrates the right and left portions of the valve along with the superior and inferior bridging leaflets as they traverse the ventricular portion of the atrioventricular septal defect. (IBL, inferior bridging leaflet; LV, left ventricle; RV, right ventricle; SBL, superior bridging leaflet). B. Common atrioventricular valve, Rastelli type A. Subcostal short-axis view demonstrates the morphology of the common atrioventricular valve. The superior bridging leaflet is divided and attaches to the crest of the septum, shown by an *arrow*. (LVOT, left ventricular outflow tract; RVOT, right ventricular outflow tract). The companion video (Video 14-31) is a subcostal short-axis view that evolves from 2D to 3D imaging to demonstrate the morphology of the common atrioventricular valve.

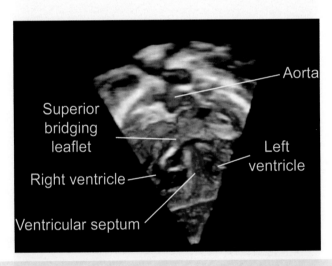

Figure 14-32. Complete atrioventricular septal defect, Rastelli type C. Subcostal short-axis view demonstrates that the superior bridging leaflet of the common atrioventricular valve is undivided and unattached to the septum. Note the position of the aorta, which is sprung anteriorly. See Video 14-32.

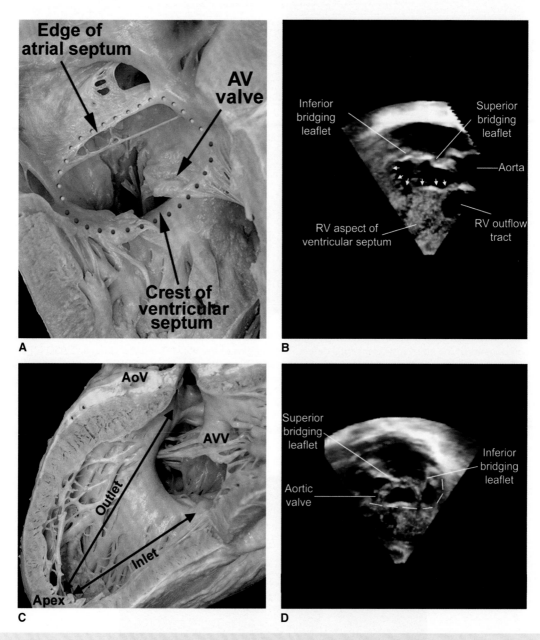

Figure 14-33. A. Right ventricular aspect of complete atrioventricular septal defect. The free walls of the right heart have been retracted. The crescent shaped free edge of the atrial septum (*yellow dots*) and the scooped out edge of the ventricular septum (*red dots*) are easily appreciated in this view of the right ventricular aspect of the atrioventricular septal defect. The bridging leaflets of the common atrioventricular valve can be appreciated extending over the ventricular septum (AV, atrioventricular). B. Right ventricular aspect of complete atrioventricular septal defect. Apical view of the septum en face, viewed from right to left. The free walls of the right heart chambers have been cropped off. It shows the scooped out edge of the ventricular septum (marked by *arrows*) and the extension of the VSD below both the superior and inferior bridging leaflets of the common AV valve. Note that the VSD is larger in its anterior–posterior dimension than in its superior–inferior dimension. The companion video (Video 14-33) evolves from 2D to 3D imaging, demonstrating en-face views of the right and left surfaces of the septal structures and septal defects. C. Left ventricular aspect of complete atrioventricular septal defect. Note the scooped appearance of the crest of the ventricular septum. The VSD is large, extending below both bridging leaflets of the common atrioventricular valve. The left ventricular inlet (distance between the atrioventricular valve and the apex) is shorter than the outlet (the distance between the apex and the AV). (AoV, aortic valve; AVV, atrioventricular valve). D. Left ventricular aspect of complete atrioventricular septal defect. Apical view of the septum en face, viewed from left to right, after cropping off the free walls of the left heart chambers. It shows the scooped out edge of the ventricular septum (*white dashed line*) and the extension of the VSD below both the superior and inferior bridging leaflets of the common AV valve. The aortic valve is "sprung" anteriorly.

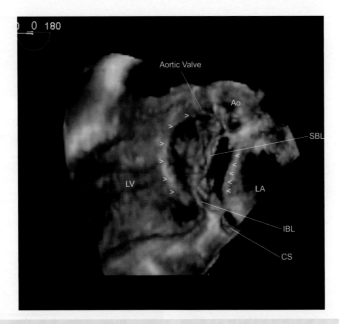

Figure 14-34. View from the left lateral aspect of the ventricular and atrial septal structures. This demonstrates the ventricular and atrial components of the atrioventricular septal defect. The margins of the VSD (>) and the "primum" ASD (<) are marked. (Ao, aorta; CS, coronary sinus; IBL, inferior bridging leaflet; LA, left atrium; LV, left ventricle; SBL, superior bridging leaflet). See Video 14-34.

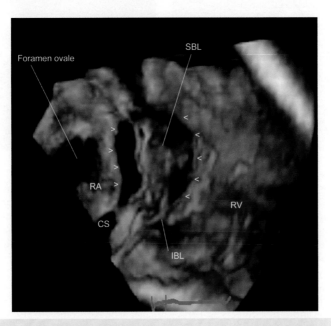

Figure 14-35. A 3D rendered view of atrioventricular septal defect when viewed from the right side of the septal structures. The margins of the ventricular component (<) and atrial margins (>) of the defect are marked. (CS, coronary sinus; IBL, inferior bridging leaflet; RA, right atrium; RV, right ventricle; SBL, superior bridging leaflet). See Video 14-35.

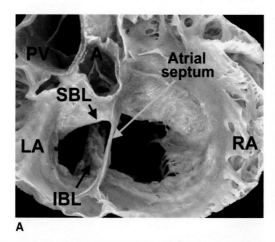
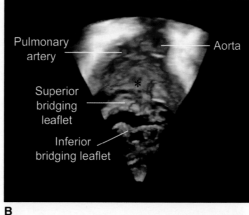

Figure 14-36. A. Unbalanced, right ventricle dominant atrioventricular septal defect. This simulated, short-axis echocardiographic view of the base of the heart illustrates a common atrioventricular valve that has a dominant right-sided component. The lower edge of the atrial septum has been left intact and the crest of the ventricular septum (*red dots*) can be seen deep to it. The superior and inferior bridging leaflets are separate as they cross the septum. Because of the common atrioventricular valve, the aorta is sprung from its usual wedged position between the atrioventricular valves. (A, aorta; IBL, inferior bridging leaflet; LA, left atrium; PV, pulmonary valve; RA-right atrium, SBL, superior bridging leaflet). B. Unbalanced, right ventricle dominant atrioventricular septal defect. This subcostal en-face view of the common atrioventricular valve reveals that that it is exclusively committed to the right ventricle. Both the large aorta and small pulmonary artery arise from the right ventricle. An *asterisk* marks the prominent subaortic conus. See Video 14-36.

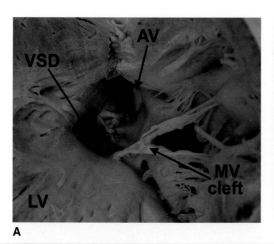
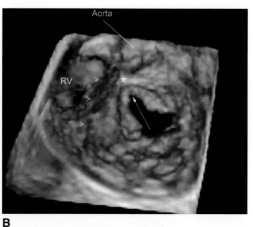

Figure 14-37. A. The free wall of the LV has been lifted from the septal component to demonstrate a true cleft in the MV. Note that the cleft points toward the left ventricular outflow tract and the aortic valve. This is in contrast to atrioventricular septal defect, where the zone of apposition points to the septum. There is a repaired perimembranous VSD (AV, aortic valve; LV, left ventricle; MV, mitral valve). B. Ventricular aspect of true cleft in MV. 3D echocardiographic projection of a true cleft in the MV visualized from the left ventricular aspect. The position of the ventricular septum is marked by *arrowheads* (>). Note that the direction of the cleft is toward the aorta (marked by *arrow*) in contrast to the zone of apposition of leaflets in an atrioventricular septal defect. Furthermore, the true cleft in this example stops short of the aorta (marked by *asterisk*) and the morphology of the tricuspid valve is normal (RV, right ventricle). The companion video demonstrates the trifoliate nature of the cleft MV with the features noted above which distinguish this from an atrioventricular septal defect.

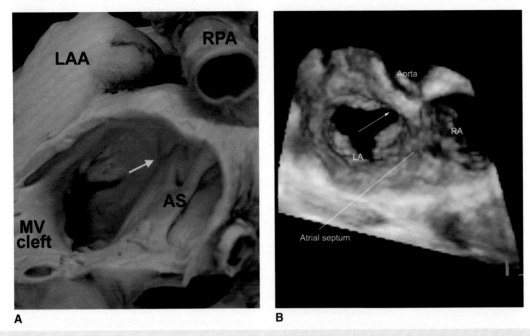

A   B

Figure 14-38. A. This left atrial view illustrates a true cleft of the MV. The plane of the ventricular septum is marked with red dots. The cleft (*yellow arrow*) points away from the septum and toward the aorta and the left ventricular outlet. (AS, atrial septum; LAA, left atrial appendage; MV, mitral valve; RPA, right pulmonary artery). B. Atrial aspect of true cleft in MV. A 3D echocardiographic projection of a true cleft in the MV visualized from the left atrial aspect. The *arrow* depicts the direction of the cleft toward the aortic valve. The three leaflets of the cleft MV can be appreciated (LA, left atrium; RA, right atrium). Similar findings are shown in the companion video (Video 14-38).

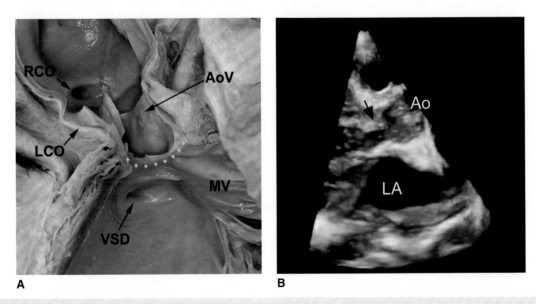

A   B

Figure 14-39. A. Subaortic membrane. The left ventricular outflow tract is opened revealing a discrete, fibrous ring (*yellow dots*) in the subaortic area. The fibrous ring is circumferential, extending over the area where there is aortic–MV fibrous continuity. The aortic valve is slightly thickened but had a normal circumference when viewed from above. There is a VSD. (AoV, aortic valve; LCO, left coronary orifice; MV, mitral valve; RCO, right coronary orifice; VSD, ventricular septal defect). B. Parasternal long-axis view demonstrates a prominent discrete subaortic membrane (*arrow*) in close proximity to the aortic valve leaflets. The companion video (Video 14-39), evolving from 2D to 3DE, demonstrates different viewing perspectives to help visualize the subaortic membrane in its entirety. See Video 14-39.

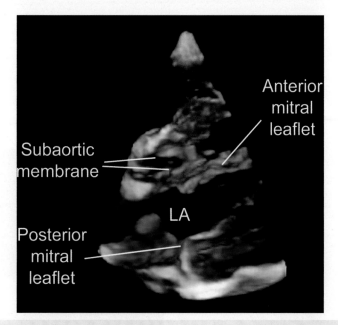

Figure 14-40. View of the leftward aspect of a subaortic membrane (equivalent of the right anterior oblique angiographic projection). This image was reconstructed from a parasternal long-axis image. It demonstrates a discrete circumferential subaortic membrane. See Video 14-40.

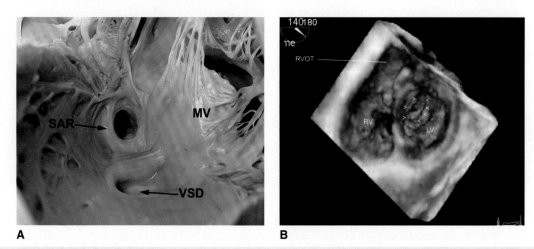

A   B

Figure 14-41. **A.** Subaortic membrane. Looking from the apex of the LV into the MV and subaortic outflow, there is a distinct subaortic ring causing severe subaortic stenosis. The ring is circumferential and crosses the area where the aortic and mitral valves are in fibrous continuity (MV, mitral valve; SAR, subaortic ring; VSD, ventricular septal defect). **B.** Circumferential subaortic ring. Three-dimensional rendered view from the LV. The circumferential subaortic stenosis can be clearly visualized (*arrows*) (LV, left ventricle; RV, right ventricle; RVOT, right ventricular outflow tract). See Video 14-41.

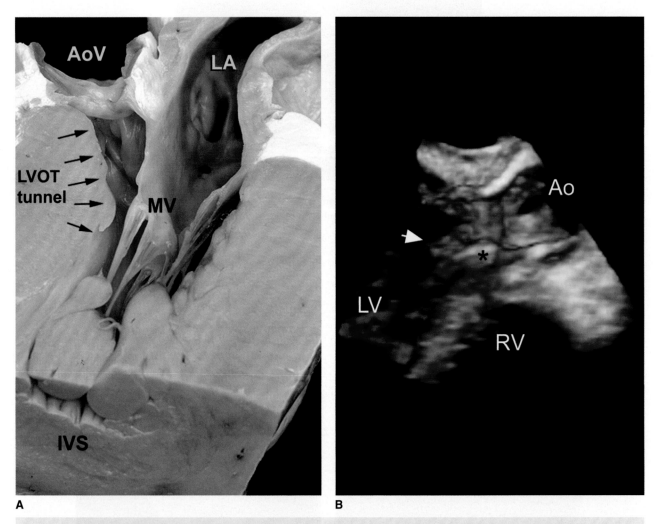

Figure 14-42. A. Tunnel subaortic stenosis. This long-axis view of a heart with hypertrophic cardiomyopathy is viewed from the apex. The thick interventricular septum can be appreciated, especially in the area of the left ventricular outflow tract where it causes a subaortic tunnel (AoV, aortic valve; IVS, interventricular septum; LA, left atrium; LVOT, left ventricular outflow tract; MV, mitral valve). B. Tunnel subaortic stenosis. Transesophageal echocardiogram demonstrates a complex substrate for subaortic stenosis. The left ventricular outflow tract is diffusely narrow. Two levels of obstruction are seen: the *asterisk* marks a long, muscular tunnel, and the *arrowhead* points to a localized discrete shelf located lower in the outflow tract. See Video 14-42.

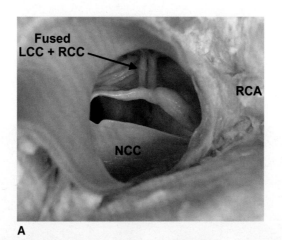

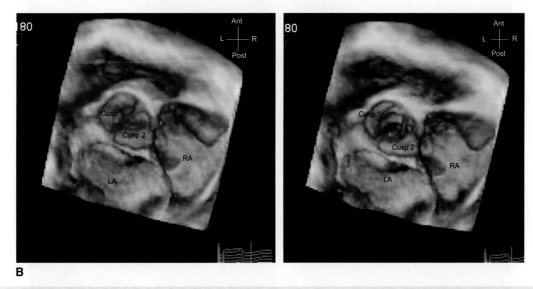

Figure 14-43. **A.** This bicuspid aortic valve is composed of right and left coronary cusps that are fused with thickened free edges of both cusps. The noncoronary cusp does not appear thickened. (LCC, NCC, and RCC: left, non, and right coronary cusp, respectively). **B.** Rendered view of a bicuspid aortic valve in the closed position (*left panel*) and open position (*right panel*) visualized from the ascending aorta. The aortic valve cusps are in a relatively anteroposterior orientation. (Cusp 1, anterior cusp of aortic valve; Cusp 2, posterior cusp of aortic valve; LA, left atrium; RA, right atrium). The companion video (Video 14-43) demonstrates a bicuspid aortic valve when viewed from the ascending aorta. The fluttering of the aortic valve cusps is due to associated subaortic stenosis.

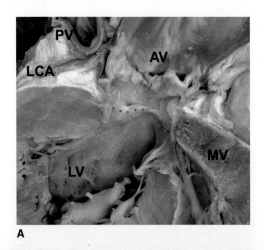

A

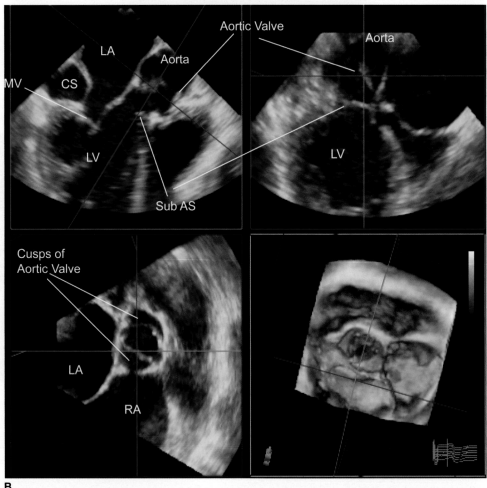

B

Figure 14-44. A. Subaortic membrane and bicuspid aortic valve. This close up view of the aortic outflow from the LV shows a subaortic ridge or membrane (*red dots*) causing severe stenosis. The aortic valve is thickened and bicuspid. (AV, aortic valve; LCA, left coronary artery; LV, left ventricle; MV, mitral valve; PV, pulmonary valve). B. Multiplanar reformatted image of a bicuspid aortic valve with associated subaortic stenosis. Alignment of the blue crop planes through the aortic valve (upper left and right panes) means that a precise cross section of the aortic valve can be obtained (bottom left pane) confirming the bicuspid nature of the valve. The associated subaortic stenosis is visualized in the upper left and upper right panes. (CS, coronary sinus; LA, left atrium; LV, left ventricle; MV, mitral valve; RA, right atrium; Sub AS, subaortic stenosis). In the companion video (Video 14-44), both the bicuspid aortic valve and the anatomy of subaortic stenosis are evident. In the bottom right pane, the subaortic membrane can be visualized through the aortic valve.

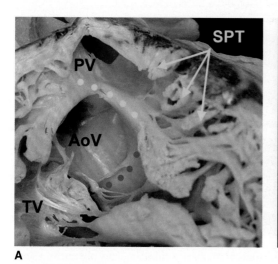

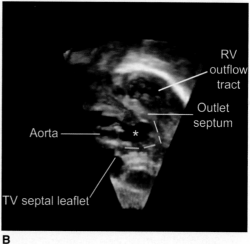

A

B

Figure 14-45. **A.** Tetralogy of Fallot. The long segment muscular nature of subpulmonary stenosis is easily seen with prominent septoparietal trabeculations along the free wall that contribute to the obstruction in this heart with tetralogy of Fallot. The outlet septum (*yellow dots*) is malaligned anteriorly. The aortic valve overrides the ventricular septum. *Red dots* mark the posteroinferior edge of the VSD (AoV, aortic valve; PV, pulmonary valve; SPT, septoparietal trabeculations; TV, tricuspid valve). **B.** Tetralogy of Fallot, subcostal long-axis view. This live 3DE image demonstrates anterior malalignment of the outlet septum. The anterosuperior and posteroinferior limbs of the septal band are marked by white and blue dashed lines, respectively. The asterisk marks the large VSD between the limbs of the septal band. The outlet septum is malaligned anteriorly; it has fused with the anterosuperior limb of the septal band. This leads to stenosis of the subpulmonary outflow tract. See Video 14-45.

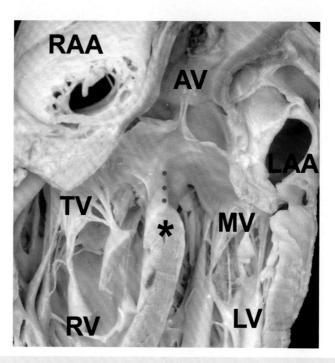

Figure 14-46. This simulated four-chamber echocardiographic view nicely demonstrates the overriding aorta in a heart with tetralogy of Fallot. The aortic valve is committed approximately 50% to the right and LV s. It lies directly over the crest of the ventricular septum (*asterisk*). *Red dots* mark the lower border of the VSD (AV, aortic valve; LAA, left atrial appendage; LV, left ventricle; MV, mitral valve; RAA, right atrial appendage; RV, right ventricle; TV, tricuspid valve). The companion video (Video 14-46) is a subcostal long-axis view that evolves from 2D to 3DE imaging, demonstrating novel viewing perspectives to delineate the anatomy of tetralogy of Fallot. See Video 14-46.

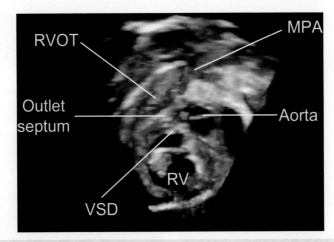

Figure 14-47. Subcostal short-axis view demonstrates the substrate and nature of subpulmonary obstruction, anterior malalignment of the outlet septum and the overriding aorta (MPA, main pulmonary artery; RVOT, right ventricular outflow tract; VSD, ventricular septal defect). See Video 14-47.

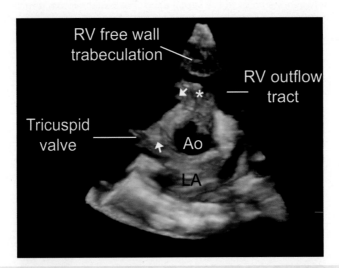

Figure 14-48. Parasternal short-axis view demonstrates the margins of the VSD (*arrows*). The defect extends to the tricuspid valve; as a result, the tricuspid and aortic valves are in continuity through the defect, which classifies this as a perimembranous VSD. The *asterisk* marks the anteriorly malaligned outlet septum. Note the severity of subpulmonary stenosis at the tip of the outlet septum. See Video 14-48.

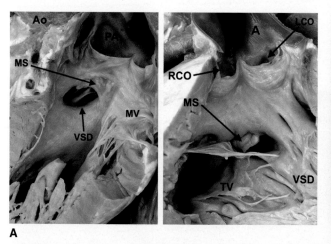
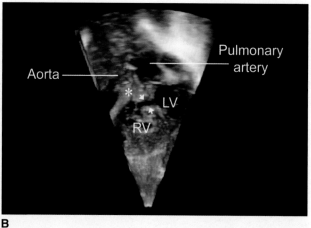

Figure 14-49. A. d-Transposition of the great arteries with a perimembranous VSD. The left panel shows the left ventricular view with the pulmonary artery exiting the morphologically LV and the fibrous continuity between the pulmonary and mitral valves. The perimembranous VSD is easily visualized with a prominent remnant of the membranous septum. The right panel shows the right ventricular view of the same heart with the tricuspid valve guarding the inlet and the aorta in the outlet. Note the muscular infundibulum separating these two valves. The right and left coronary arteries are seen exiting the aorta. There is a perimembranous VSD with a prominent remnant of the membranous septum (Ao, aorta; LCO, left coronary orifice; MV, mitral valve; MS, membranous septum; PA, pulmonary artery; RCO, right coronary orifice; TV, tricuspid valve; VSD, ventricular septal defect). **B.** Subcostal long-axis view in d-Transposition of the great arteries with a perimembranous VSD. This demonstrates connection of the aorta to the right ventricle and the pulmonary artery to the LV. The subaortic conus is marked by an *asterisk*. *Arrowheads* mark a small membranous VSD. The outflow tracts are widely patent. The outlet septum, which is also marked by the upper *arrowhead*, does not show any evidence of malalignment. The companion video (Video 14-49) evolves from 2D to 3D imaging, demonstrating how live 3D imaging, coupled with gentle tilting and rotation of the image, helps illustrate salient anatomic features.

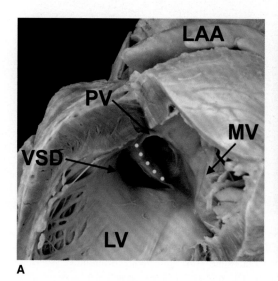
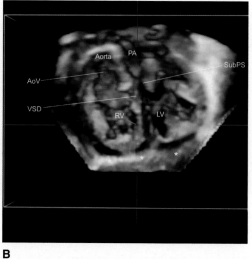

Figure 14-50. A. Transposition with subpulmonary stenosis. The free wall of the morphologically LV has been lifted away from the septal component to illustrate the VSD and the posteriorly malaligned outlet septum (*yellow dots*). The malalignment of the outlet septum causes subpulmonic stenosis in this heart with transposition. (LAA, left atrial appendage; LV, left ventricle; MV, mitral valve; PV, pulmonary valve; VSD, ventricular septal defect). **B.** Rendered subcostal 3D echocardiographic view of transposition of the great arteries with VSD and subpulmonic stenosis. This demonstrates the muscular substrate of the subpulmonic stenosis and the position of the VSD (AoV, aortic valve; LV, left ventricle; PA, pulmonary artery; RV, right ventricle; subPS, subpulmonic stenosis; VSD, ventricular septal defect). See Video 14-50.

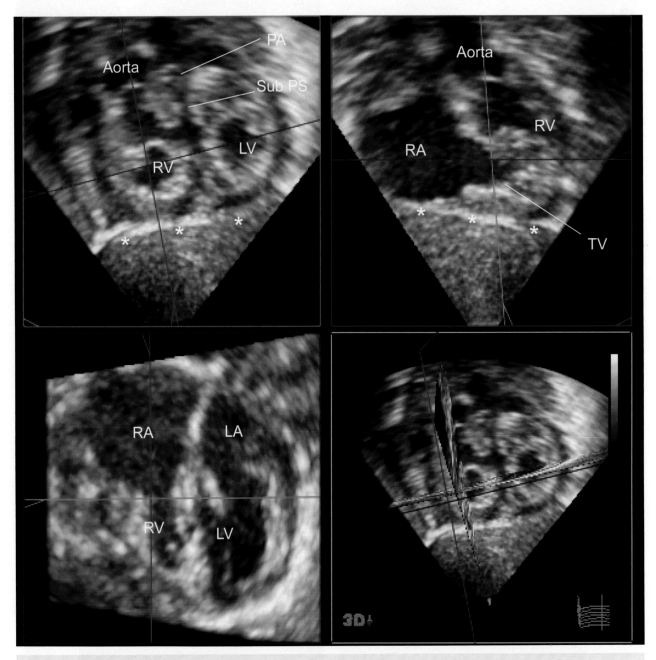

Figure 14-51. Multiplanar reformatted image of transposition of the great arteries with VSD and subpulmonic stenosis. The top left pane demonstrates the aorta arising from the right ventricle and the stenosis below the pulmonary valve. The red cut plane has been aligned to the aorta to demonstrate the subaortic region (**top right** pane). The relative size of the left and right ventricles is shown in the bottom left pane (LA, left atrium; LV, left ventricle; PA, pulmonary artery; RA, right atrium; RV, right ventricle; sub PS, subpulmonic stenosis). See Video 14-51.

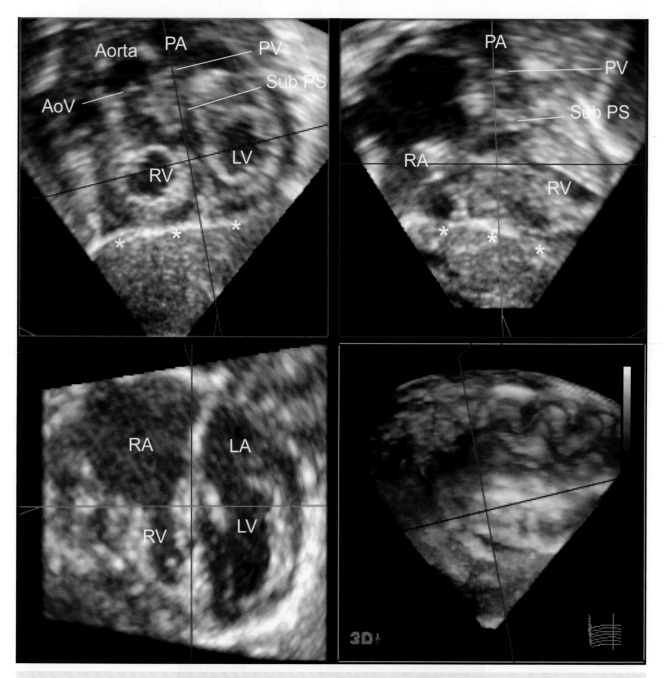

Figure 14-52. Multiplanar reformatted image of transposition of the great arteries with VSD and subpulmonic stenosis. The top left pane demonstrates the muscular subpulmonic stenosis. The red cutting plane has been placed through the subpulmonary region to show the anatomy of the subpulmonic stenosis (top right pane) (LA, left atrium; LV, left ventricle; PA, pulmonary artery; PV, pulmonary valve; RA, right atrium; RV, right ventricle; sub PS, subpulmonic stenosis). See Video 14-52.

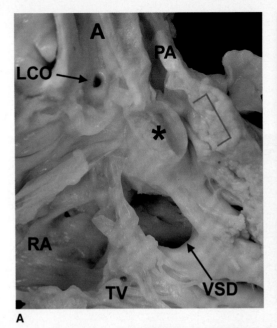
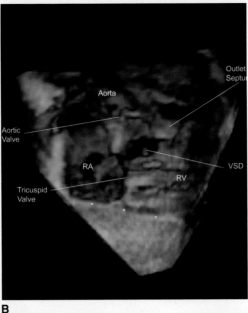

A

B

Figure 14-53. A. Double outlet right ventricle with subaortic VSD. This specimen is consistent with the tetralogy of Fallot variant. The great arteries are normally related, with the aorta posterior and rightward of the pulmonary valve. A muscular infundibulum supports both arterial valves. The VSD is subaortic in location. There is anterior malalignment of the outlet septum (*asterisk*) causing subpulmonic, infundibular stenosis (*red bracket*). (A, aorta; LCO, left coronary artery; PA, pulmonary artery; RA, right atrium; TV, tricuspid valve; VSD, ventricular septal defect). B. Double outlet right ventricle: rendered 3D echocardiographic view of a subaortic VSD and adjacent structures. The projection has been obtained by cropping away the free wall of the right ventricle and the lateral wall of the right atrium. The *asterisks* (*) mark the position of the diaphragm (RA, right atrium; RV, right ventricle; VSD, ventricular septal defect). See Video 14-53.

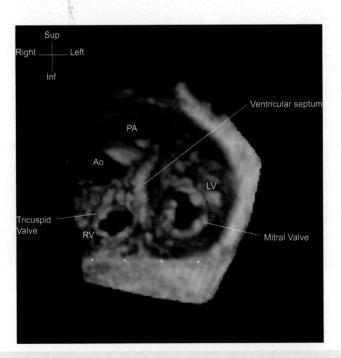

Figure 14-54. Rendered 3D echocardiographic view of double outlet right ventricle viewed from the ventricular aspect. The relationship of the atrioventricular valves and the great arteries is visualized. The position of the ventricular septum is indicated. The diaphragmatic surface is indicated by *asterisks* (*) (Ao, aorta; Inf, inferior; LV, left ventricle; PA, pulmonary artery; RV, right ventricle; Sup, superior). See Video 14-54.

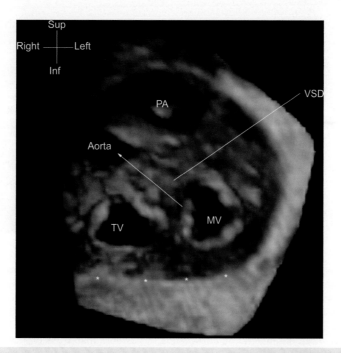

Figure 14-55. Rendered 3D echocardiographic view of double outlet right ventricle with a subaortic VSD, viewed from the ventricular aspect. The cut plane passes through the VSD to confirm the relative position of the atrioventricular valves, great arteries and VSD. The *arrow* demonstrates potential for surgical "routing" from the LV to the aorta. The position of the diaphragm is shown by the *asterisks* (*) (MV, mitral valve; PA, pulmonary artery; TV, tricuspid valve; VSD, ventricular septal defect). See Video 14-55.

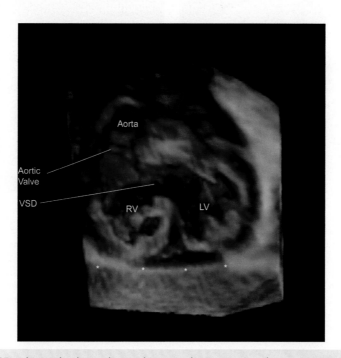

Figure 14-56. Rendered 3D subcostal echocardiographic view demonstrating the aorta arising from the right ventricle as well as the position of the VSD. The diaphragm is marked by *asterisks* (*) (LV, left ventricle; RV, right ventricle; VSD, ventricular septal defect). See Video 14-56.

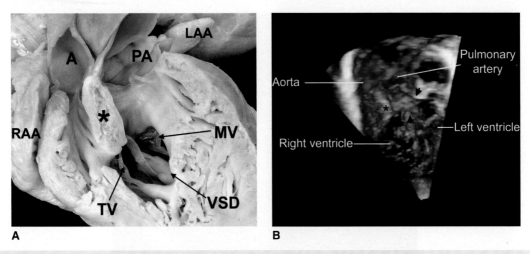

A

B

Figure 14-57. A. Taussig-Bing–type double outlet right ventricle. This anatomic view of the right ventricle clearly shows the double outlet with the aorta to the right of the pulmonary artery and both outlets supported by a complete muscular infundibulum. The outlet septum (*asterisk*) is quite prominent and there is a large, subpulmonic VSD (A, aorta; LAA, left atrial appendage; MV, mitral valve; PA, pulmonary artery; RAA, right atrial appendage; RV, right ventricle; TV, tricuspid valve; VSD, ventricular septal defect). B. Taussig-Bing–type double outlet right ventricle. Subcostal view demonstrates a large subpulmonary VSD, the margins of which are marked by *arrowheads*. An *asterisk* marks the prominent muscular conus between the large subpulmonary outflow tract and the smaller subaortic outflow tract. Surgery for this defect would typically involve placement of a surgical baffle between the tip of the muscular conus (*asterisk*) and the crest of the ventricular septum (*lower arrowhead*), combined with an arterial switch operation. See Video 14-57.

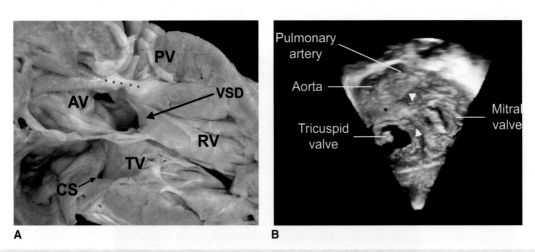

A

B

Figure 14-58. A. Doubly committed subarterial VSD in double outlet right ventricle. The free wall of the right ventricle has been lifted off the septum to demonstrate the tricuspid valve (inlet) and the double outlet. The aortic and pulmonary valves are in fibrous continuity (*red dots*) and the VSD is doubly committed (AV, aortic valve; CS, coronary sinus; PV, pulmonary valve; RV, right ventricle; TV, tricuspid valve; VSD, ventricular septal defect). B. Subcostal view demonstrates double outlet right ventricle with continuity between the aortic and pulmonary valves. In contrast to the specimen demonstrated in Figure 14-58A, both arterial valves are supported by a prominent muscular conus (*asterisk*) that separates them from the atrioventricular valves. *Arrowheads* mark the margins of the VSD. See Video 14-58.

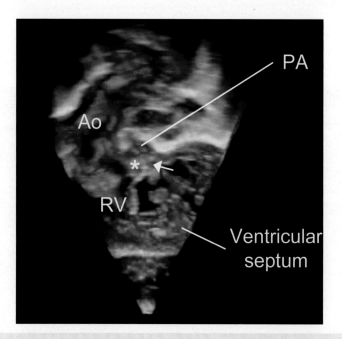

Figure 14-59. Subcostal short-axis view demonstrates a large anterior aorta and a small posterior pulmonary artery. The outlet septum (marked by an *asterisk*) is malaligned posteriorly into the subpulmonary outflow tract. The anteroseptal commissure of the tricuspid valve (marked by an *arrow*) is seen extending into the subpulmonary outflow tract. See Video 14-59.

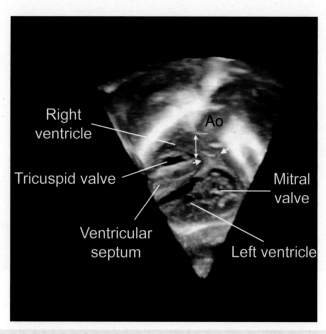

Figure 14-60. Subcostal long-axis view demonstrates dextrocardia and superoinferior ventricles. The LV is located inferior to the right ventricle. *Arrowheads* mark the margins of the VSD, which is subaortic. The two-headed *arrow* indicates the plane of planned placement of a surgical baffle to direct flow from the LV to the aorta. See Video 14-60.

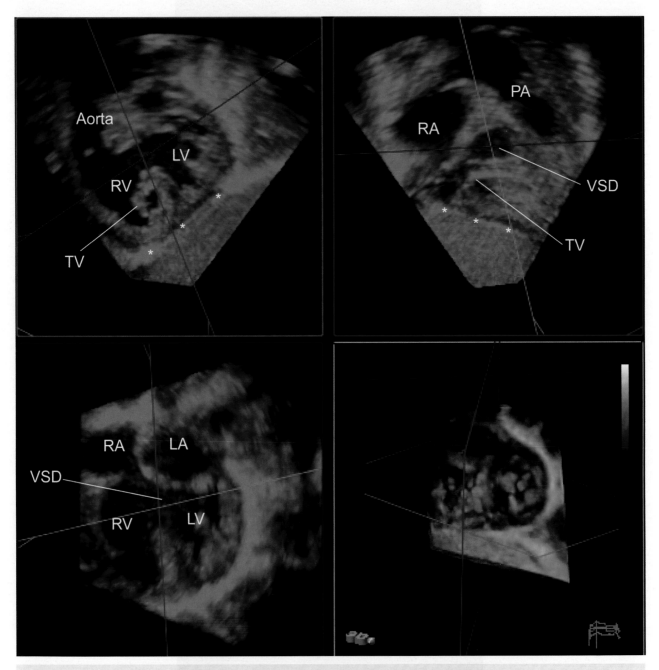

Figure 14-61. Multiplanar reformatted images of double outlet right ventricle. The top left pane demonstrates the aorta arising from the right ventricle as well as the position of the VSD. The top right pane outlines the VSD by appropriate alignment of the red crop planes. Its relationship to the tricuspid valve and pulmonary artery is also appreciated. The bottom left pane outlines the size of the right and LVs as well as the VSD. The diaphragmatic surface is marked by *asterisks* (*) for reference. (LV, left ventricle; PA, pulmonary artery; RA, right atrium; RV, right ventricle; TV, tricuspid valve; VSD, ventricular septal defect). See Video 14-61.

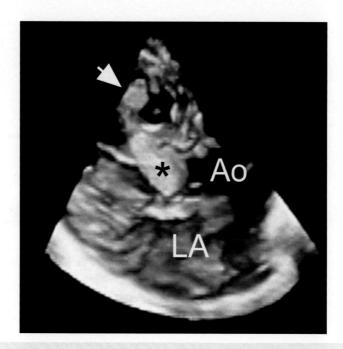

Figure 14-62. **Tumor adjacent to the aortic valve.** Parasternal long-axis view demonstrates a tumor (marked by an *asterisk*) in the left ventricular outflow tract immediately below the right coronary cusp of the aortic valve. A separate tumor (marked by an *arrow*) is seen on the right ventricular aspect of the ventricular septum. The presence of multiple cardiac tumors is suggestive of rhabdomyomas and tuberous sclerosis. See Video 14-62.

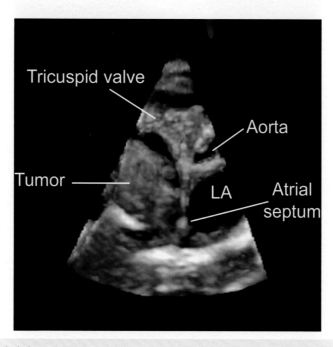

Figure 14-63. **Right atrial rhabdomyoma.** Parasternal short-axis view demonstrates a large tumor occupying much of the cavity of the right atrium. The tumor has a bilobed appearance. It is remote from the tricuspid valve. See Video 14-63.

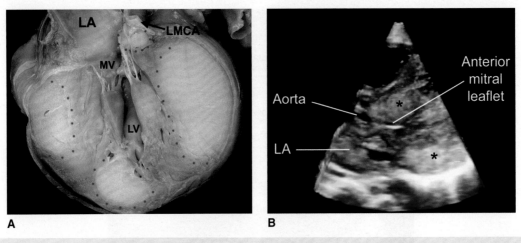

A   B

Figure 14-64. A. This view of the left atrium and LV shows multiple intracardiac tumors that are outlined by red dots, these along the anterior and posterior walls, at the apex and in the area where the MV and aorta are in fibrous continuity. (LA, left atrium; LV, left ventricle; LMCA, left main coronary artery; MV, mitral valve). B. Diffuse left ventricular tumor. Parasternal long-axis view has been rotated 180 degrees into a right anterior oblique projection to demonstrate a large diffuse mass (marked by *asterisks*) that has infiltrated the inferior and lateral walls of the LV (LA, left atrium). See Video 14-64.

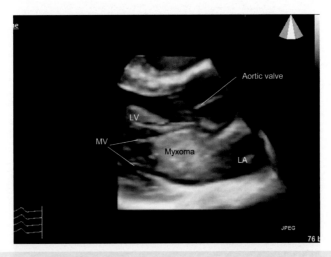

Figure 14-65. Parasternal long-axis view of atrial myxoma. (LA, left atrium; LV, left ventricle; MV, mitral valve). The companion video (Video 14-65) demonstrates motion of the tumor with the cardiac cycle. See Video 14-65.

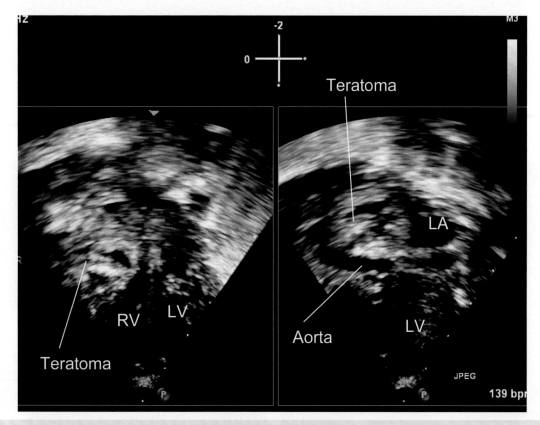

Figure 14-66. Neonatal cardiac teratoma visualized using cross-plane imaging. The left pane shows the apical four-chamber acquisition plane and the right pane shows the orthogonal view. The image on the right demonstrates how the teratoma envelops the ascending aorta. (LA, left atrium; LV, left ventricle; RV, right ventricle). See Video 14-66.

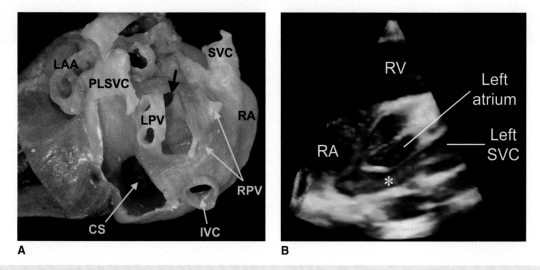

Figure 14-67. A. Left superior vena cava draining to the coronary sinus. In this posterior view, both the left atrium and the persistent left superior vena cava have been windowed. The persistent left superior vena cava extends between the left atrial appendage and the left pulmonary veins to the crux of the heart where it drains to the coronary sinus. The foramen ovale is patent (*black arrow*) (CS, coronary sinus; IVC, inferior vena cava; LAA, left atrial appendage; LPV, left pulmonary veins; PLSVC, persistent left superior vena cava; RA, right atrium; RPV, right pulmonary veins; SVC, superior vena cava). B. Left superior vena cava draining to the coronary sinus. This parasternal short-axis view angled leftward demonstrates the left superior vena cava draining into the coronary sinus, which is marked by an asterisk. See Video 14-67.

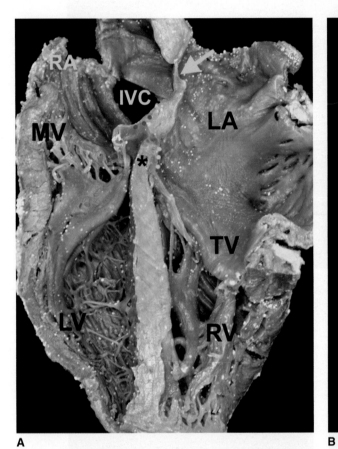

A

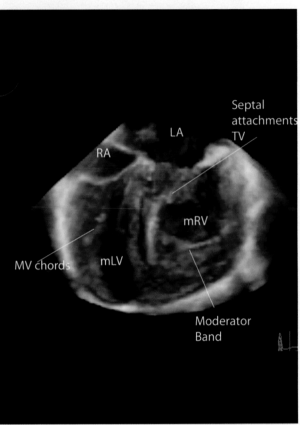

B

Figure 14-68. A. Discordant atrioventricular connections with congenitally corrected transposition. In this simulated four-chamber echocardiographic view, the morphologically right atrium is connected to the (right-sided) morphologically LV and the morphologically left atrium is connected to the (left-sided) morphologically right ventricle. Note the reversed offset of the atrioventricular valves, with the tricuspid valve inserting lower on the interventricular septum (*asterisk*) than the MV. The atrial septum (*yellow arrow*) is intact (IVC-inferior vena cava; LA, left atrium; LV, left ventricle; MV, mitral valve; RA, right atrium; RV, right ventricle; TV, tricuspid valve). B. Rendered three-dimensional echocardiogram demonstrates discordant atrioventricular connections. The left atrium connects to the morphologic right ventricle as evidenced by the moderator band and the septal attachments of the tricuspid valve. The right atrium connects to a smooth walled morphologic LV. The MV chords only have attachment to the free wall of the LV. (LA, left atrium; MV, mitral valve; mRV, morphologic right ventricle; mLV, morphologic left ventricle; RA, right atrium; TV, tricuspid valve). See Video 14-68.

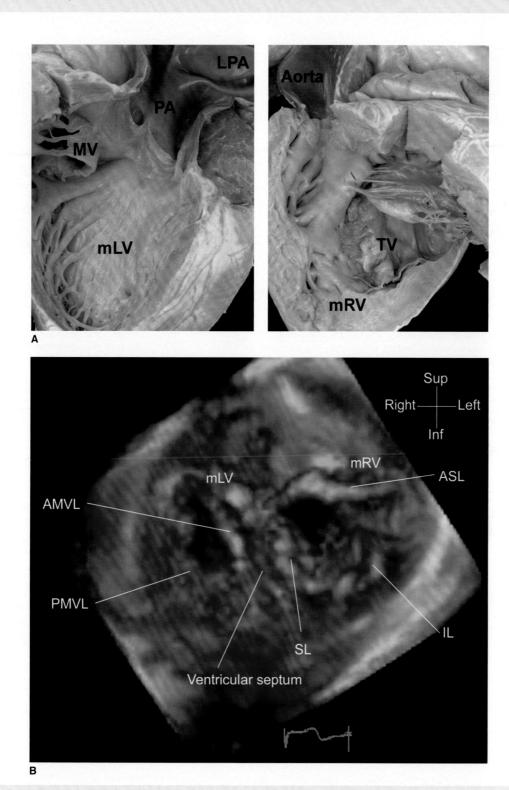

Figure 14-69. **A.** Discordant atrioventricular connections. The left panel demonstrates the morphologically LV on the right side of the heart. Its septal surface is relatively smooth, with a finely trabeculated apical component. The MV guards the inlet and is in fibrous continuity with the pulmonary valve. The right panel demonstrates the morphologically right ventricle on the left side of the heart. Its septal surface is coarsely trabeculated. The tricuspid valve guards the inlet, and there is muscle separating the atrioventricular valve from the arterial valve, in this case, the aorta. There is an Ebstein's malformation of the tricuspid valve (LPA, left pulmonary artery; mLV, morphologic left ventricle; MV, mitral valve; PA, pulmonary artery; TV, tricuspid valve). **B.** Discordant atrioventricular connections viewed from the ventricular apex. The left-sided atrioventricular valve is the trileaflet tricuspid valve and the right-sided atrioventricular valve is the bileaflet MV (AMVL, anterior mitral valve leaflet; ASL, anterosuperior leaflet of the tricuspid valve; IL, inferior leaflet of the tricuspid valve; mRV, morphologic right ventricle; mLV, morphologic left ventricle; PMVL, posterior mitral valve leaflet; SL, septal leaflet of the tricuspid valve). See Video 14-69.

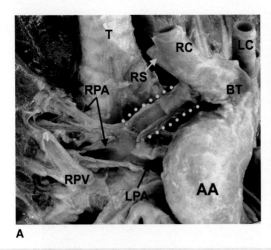

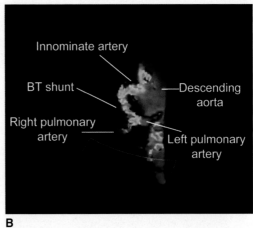

Figure 14-70. **A.** Blalock-Taussig shunt. This anterior view demonstrates a modified Blalock-Taussig shunt (*yellow dots*). It extends from the brachiocephalic trunk to the right pulmonary artery. A few blue sutures are visible at the anastomosis (AA, ascending aorta; BT, brachiocephalic trunk; LC, left common carotid artery; LPA, left pulmonary artery; RC, right common carotid; RPA, right pulmonary artery; RS, right subclavian artery; T, trachea). **B.** Blalock-Taussig shunt. This is a demonstration of 3D color flow in a Blalock-Taussig shunt from the suprasternal notch. In order to visualize the color flow in the relevant adjacent structures, the grayscale image has been suppressed. See Video 14-70.

References

1. Tajik AJ, Seward JB, Hagler DJ, et al. Two-dimensional real-time ultrasonic imaging of the heart and great vessels. Technique, image orientation, structure identification, and validation. *Mayo Clin Proc.* 1978;53(5):271–303.

2. Ariet M, Geiser EA, Lupkiewicz SM, et al. Evaluation of a three-dimensional reconstruction to compute left ventricular volume and mass. *Am J Cardiol.* 1984;54(3):415–420.

3. Linker DT, Moritz WE, Pearlman AS. A new three-dimensional echocardiographic method of right ventricular volume measurement: in vitro validation. *J Am Coll Cardiol.* 1986;8(1):101–106.

4. Matsumoto M, Matsuo H, Kitabatake A, et al. Three-dimensional echocardiograms and two-dimensional echocardiographic images at desired planes by a computerized system. *Ultrasound Med Biol.* 1977;3(2–3):163–178.

5. Von Ramm OT, Smith SW. Real time volumetric ultrasound imaging system. *J Digit Imaging.* 1990;3:261–266.

6. Salgo IS. Three-dimensional echocardiographic technology. *Cardiol Clin.* 2007;25(2):231–239.

7. Buck T, Thiele KE. Basic principles and practical application. In: Buck T, Franke A, Monaghan M, eds. *Three dimensional echocardiography.* Berlin, Germany: Springer; 2011:21–53.

8. Bharucha T, Roman KS, Anderson RH, et al. Impact of multiplanar review of three-dimensional echocardiographic data on management of congenital heart disease. *Ann Thorac Surg.* 2008;86:875–881.

9. Beraud AS, Schnittger I, Miller DC, et al. Multiplanar reconstruction of three-dimensional transthoracic echocardiography improves the presurgical assessment of mitral prolapse. *J Am Soc Echocardiogr.* 2009;22:907–913.

10. Kuppahally SS, Paloma A, Craig Miller D, et al. Multiplanar visualization in 3D transthoracic echocardiography for precise delineation of mitral valve pathology. *Echocardiography.* 2008;25:84–87.

11. Simpson JM, Miller O. Three-dimensional echocardiography in congenital heart disease. *Arch Cardiovasc Dis.* 2011;104:45–56.

12. Simpson J, Miller O, Bell A, et al. Image orientation for three-dimensional echocardiography of congenital heart disease. *Int J Cardiovasc Imaging.* 2012;28:743–753.

13. Vettukattil JJ, Bharucha T, Anderson RH. Defining Ebstein's malformation using three-dimensional echocardiography. *Interact Cardiovasc Thorac Surg.* 2007;6(6):685–690.

14. Muraru D, Badano LP, Sarais C, et al. Evaluation of tricuspid valve morphology and function by transthoracic three-dimensional echocardiography. *Curr Cardiol Rep.* 2011;13(3):242–249 [Review].

15. Espinola-Zavaleta N, Vargas-Barron J, Keirns C, et al. Three-dimensional echocardiography in congenital malformations of the mitral valve. *J Am Soc Echocardiogr.* 2002;15(5):468–472.

16. Vogel M, Simpson JM, Anderson D. Live three-dimensional echocardiography of cor triatriatum in a child. *BMJ Case Rep.* 2009:bcr2007140269.

17. Valverde I, Rawlins D, Austin C, et al. Three-dimensional echocardiography in the management of parachute mitral valve. *Eur Heart J Cardiovasc Imaging.* 2012;13(5):446.

18. Seliem MA, Fedec A, Szwast A, et al. Atrioventricular valve morphology and dynamics in congenital heart disease as imaged with real-time 3-dimensional matrix-array echocardiography: comparison with 2-dimensional imaging and surgical findings. *J Am Soc Echocardiogr.* 2007;20(7):869–876.

19. Hlavacek AM, Crawford FA Jr, Chessa KS, et al. Real-time three-dimensional echocardiography is useful in the evaluation of patients with atrioventricular septal defects. *Echocardiography.* 2006;23:225–231.

20. Bharucha T, Ho SY, Vettukattil JJ. Multiplanar review analysis of three-dimensional echocardiographic datasets gives new insights into the morphology of subaortic stenosis. *Eur J Echocardiogr.* 2008;9(5):614–620.

21. Altiok E, Koos R, Schröder J, et al. Comparison of two-dimensional and three-dimensional imaging techniques for measurement of aortic annulus diameters before transcatheter aortic valve implantation. *Heart.* 2011;97(19):1578–1584.

22. Tolstrup K, Shiota T, Gurudevan S, et al. Left atrial myxomas: correlation of two-dimensional and live three-dimensional transesophageal echocardiography with the clinical and pathologic findings. *J Am Soc Echocardiogr.* 2011;24(6):618–624.

23. Reddy VK, Faulkner M, Bandarupalli N, et al. Incremental value of live/real time three-dimensional transthoracic echocardiography in the assessment of right ventricular masses. *Echocardiography.* 2009;26(5):598–609.

24. Aguiar-Souto P, Labrandero de Lera C, Deiros Bronte L, et al. Congenitally corrected transposition of the great arteries: three-dimensional echocardiography diagnosis. *Neth Heart J.* 2010;18(7-8):384.

25. Hlavacek A, Lucas J, Baker H, et al. Feasibility and utility of three-dimensional color flow echocardiography of the aortic arch: the "echocardiographic angiogram." *Echocardiography.* 2006;23(10):860–864.

Jeanne M. DeCara, Roberto M. Lang

Cardiac masses constitute a small subset of cardiovascular disease. In fact, most cardiac neoplasms are discovered incidentally on cardiac imaging or at autopsy. As a result, determining the etiology of a cardiac mass with confidence can prove challenging and can sometimes only be achieved after surgical resection. However, improvements in echocardiography, including real time three-dimensional (3D) echocardiography, and the evolution of advanced technology such as cardiac magnetic resonance imaging and cardiac computed tomography (CT) have enhanced the cardiologist's ability to better refine the differential diagnosis of a cardiac mass. Of all of the cardiac imaging modalities, echocardiography is the most commonly utilized because of its portability, low cost, lack of radiation exposure, or need for contrast dye. For this reason, cardiac masses are most likely to be first identified antemortem by echocardiography. This chapter briefly outlines some general considerations in the evaluation of a cardiac mass using both 2D and 3D echocardiography.

TUMOR CLASSIFICATION AND FREQUENCY

Cardiac masses can be classified as primary or secondary, benign or malignant, or by their location: atrial, ventricular, or valvular. Tables 15-1–15-3 show the relative frequencies of primary benign, primary malignant and metastatic neoplasms.[1] However, for practical purposes, the differential diagnosis of a cardiac mass is perhaps best fine-tuned when considering the location of a mass because some masses have distinct predilections for specific intracardiac sites.

ATRIAL MASSES

Myxomas are the most common benign tumors of the heart accounting for nearly half of such neoplasms.[2] Although right atrial and atypical locations such as the atrial appendage or ventricular myocardium have been reported, myxomas are classically located in the left atrium attached to the interatrial septum (Fig. 15-1). Myxomas may be broad-based and sessile or attached to the heart via a pedicle. These tend to be sporadic solitary tumors, though multiple myxomas are not uncommon when associated with familial syndromes.[2] Most myxomas are found incidentally on echocardiograms performed for other indications, but vague constitutional symptoms such as fever and malaise may be present. When large, myxomas may cause obstruction to ventricular filling, and syncope or heart failure symptoms may ensue. The friable surface of the tumor and possibly adherent thrombus have been postulated etiologies of the embolic events that may sometimes be seen in patients with myxomas. For patients who have had an embolic event and are found to have a right atrial myxoma, careful examination for a patent foramen ovale must be undertaken since this may be a conduit for further paradoxical embolism. Myxomas have a recurrence rate of approximately 1% to 3% if sporadic and greater in cases of multiple lesions as is seen in familial syndromes.[3,4] Recurrences are either the result of incomplete resection or additional foci that had been undiscovered on initial evaluation. Therefore, a thorough examination intraoperatively is imperative to minimize the chance of recurrence. Distinguishing atrial myxomas from thrombi (Figs. 15-2–15-5) can be challenging. Helpful clues are the presence of pathologic conditions associated with stasis, often coupled with spontaneous echo contrast, and the presence of indwelling catheters or pacemaker/defibrillator leads to which clot may be adherent.

The most common malignant atrial masses are sarcomas. These masses are quite large. Unlike myxomas, they have a predilection for the right atrium.[9–12] Because of their size, they are more often associated with symptoms arising from obstruction to right heart filling. Metastatic disease is often present at the time of diagnosis. Their large size and invasive nature may preclude surgical resection. Unfortunately, these masses are associated with rapidly progressive disease and a poor prognosis.

VALVULAR MASSES

The most common benign valvular mass is a papillary fibroelastoma (Figs. 15-6–15-9). These small masses are most commonly located on the aortic valve, followed closely by the mitral valve. Attachments to the tricuspid and pulmonic have been reported but are far less common. These masses may initially be mistaken for vegetations (Figs. 15-10 and 15-11). As with vegetations, embolic events may occur in affected individuals and are often the impetus for surgical resection. However, unlike vegetations, these tumors are typically round and, although nonencapsulated, are well circumscribed. Additionally, they classically have a shimmering appearance attributed to their frond-like surface (Fig. 15–8). Cropping and manipulation of 3D echocardiographic images may aid in the detection of a discrete stalk, which may not be immediately apparent on 2D echocardiography, particularly when the site of attachment is along the subvalvular apparatus where a nonorthogonal or tangential view of the endocardial surface may be challenging. The presence of a stalk and the solitary nature of these tumors help to distinguish them from Libman-Sacks endocarditis, while their more bulky nature contrasts with the fibrolinear nature of Lambl's excrescence. Caseous mitral annular calcification (Fig. 15-12) may also appear mass-like but is unusually bright and tends to be located along the commissural aspect of the annulus as opposed to the midannulus.

VENTRICULAR MASSES

Ventricular masses are among the hardest to define on echocardiography. In children, rhabdomyomas and fibromas are most common, and, although benign, they may be associated with conduction abnormalities, arrhythmias, and sudden death. Ventricular locations for primary malignant tumors are quite uncommon in adults. Ventricular masses in adults are more frequently metastatic lesions or thrombi (Figs. 15-13–15-15). The distinction between tumor and thrombus is aided by clinical context and associated conditions such as wall motion abnormalities or left ventricular dysfunction. Often the reflective properties of a mass help to discern the type of neoplasm present. For instance, fibromas tend to be hyperreflective on echocardiography. Other tumors such as hemangiomas are highly vascular tumors and may show evidence of perfusion on contrast echocardiography. Indeed, the presence of perfusion within a mass on contrast echocardiography has been reported to help differentiate tumor from thrombus, though it must be noted that this is not an FDA-approved indication of echocardiographic contrast agents.[14] Ventricular masses found in the right heart may be approachable for biopsy. In this setting, 3D echocardiography can provide critical guidance of the bioptome (Fig. 15-15).

ROLE OF 3D ECHOCARDIOGRAPHY

Three-dimensional echocardiography offers the advantage of allowing a volumetric acquisition of the heart encompassing the entire mass. This is helpful in several ways. For example, assessment of the mass is not limited to the finite orthogonal planes offered by 2D echocardiography. The volumetric dataset may be cropped and manipulated not only by the sonographer at the time of data acquisition but also offline by the echocardiographer at the time of interpretation. One example in which these features of 3D echocardiography are particularly valuable is in the evaluation of mass size.[15] The diameter of vegetations, thrombi, and tumors has important implications for patient prognosis, particularly as it relates to embolic potential. Because masses often have irregular shapes, assessment of mass size from a 3D volumetric dataset has an advantage over the planar images of 2D echocardiography. Compared to real-time 3D echocardiography, 2D transthoracic echocardiography has been to shown to underestimate the diameter of cardiac masses by as much 24.6%; 19.8% by 2D transesophageal echocardiography.[16]

Because cardiac masses are uncommon entities, data on the sensitivity and specificity of echocardiography for their detection are limited to relatively small case series. In one series of 149 patients, the sensitivity of 2D transthoracic echocardiography for the detection of a pathologically confirmed tumor was 93.3%, with a minimal detectable tumor size of 0.5 to 1.0 cm². Two-dimensional transesophageal echocardiography had a sensitivity of 96.8%.[10] There are few data on diagnostic accuracy of 3D echocardiography for the detection of masses, perhaps because rather than being utilized as an isolated diagnostic imaging technique, it is usually employed as an adjunct to 2D echocardiography in order to garner additional information about the location, size, means and point of attachment, and potential approach for surgical resection of a mass. This was highlighted in one series where 3D transesophageal echocardiography provided incremental information over 2D echocardiography in preoperative assessment for 37% of the patients studied and was estimated to be able to do so in approximately 18% of all intracardiac masses.[17]

SUMMARY

Cardiac masses are relatively rare within the spectrum of cardiovascular disease and are often first identified using 2D echocardiography. Their location, morphology, and site of attachment are key features that help to refine the diagnostic possibilities. By virtue of its ability to capture a mass in a volumetric dataset, real time 3D echocardiography offers incremental value in the diagnostic evaluation of a cardiac mass and aides in defining potential approaches for surgical resection.

TABLE 15-1 • Primary *Benign* Neoplasms of the Heart (1976–1993)*

Tumor[†]	Total	Surgical	Autopsy	Age ≤15 Years at Diagnosis
Myxoma	114	102	12	4
Rhabdomyoma	20	6	14	20
Fibroma	20	18	2	13
Hemangioma	17	10	7	2
Atrioventricular nodal	10	0	10	2
Granular cell	4	0	4	0
Lipoma	2	2	0	0
Paraganglioma	2	2	0	0
Myocytic hamartoma	2	2	0	0
Histiocytoid cardiomyopathy	2	0	2	2
Inflammatory pseudotumor	2	2	0	1
Fibrous histiocytoma	1	0	1	0
Epithelioid hemangioendothelioma	1	1	0	0
Bronchogenic cyst	1	1	0	0
Teratoma	1	0	1	1
Totals	**199**	**146 (73%)**	**53 (27%)**	**45 (23%)**

*Modified from Burke A, Virmani R. *Atlas of tumor pathology. Tumors of the heart and great vessels.* Washington, DC: Armed Forces Institute of Pathology; 1996:231.
[†]Excludes papillary fibroelastoma and lipomatous hypertrophy of the atrial septum.

TABLE 15-2 • Primary *Malignant* Tumors of the Heart (1976–1993)*

Tumor	Total	Surgical	Autopsy	Age ≤15 Years at Diagnosis
Sarcoma	137 (95%)	116	21	11 (8%)
Angio	33	22	11	1
Unclassified	33	30	3	3
Fibrous histiocytoma	16	16	0	1
Osteo	13	13	0	0
Leiomyo	12	11	1	1
Fibro	9	9	0	1
Myxo	8	8	0	1
Rhabdomyo	6	2	4	3
Synovial	4	4	0	0
Lipo	2	0	2	0
Schwannoma	1	1	0	0
Lymphoma	7 (5%)	1	6	0
Totals	**144 (100%)**	**117 (81%)**	**27 (19%)**	**11 (8%)**

*Modified from Burke A, Virmani R. *Atlas of tumor pathology. Tumors of the heart and great vessels.* Washington, DC: Armed Forces Institute of Pathology; 1996:231.

TABLE 15-3 • Metastatic Neoplasms in the Heart at Necropsy— Order of Frequency of Cancers Encountered*

Primary Tumor	Total Autopsies	Metastases to Heart
1. Lung	1,037	180 (17%)
2. Breast	685	70 (10%)
3. Lymphoma	392	67 (17%)
4. Leukemia	202	66 (33%)
5. Esophagus	294	37 (13%)
6. Uterus	451	36 (8%)
7. Melanoma	69	32 (46%)
8. Stomach	603	28 (5%)
9. Sarcoma	159	24 (15%)
10. Coral cavity and tongue	235	22 (9%)
11. Colon and rectum	440	22 (5%)
12. Kidney	114	12 (11%)
13. Thyroid gland	97	9 (9%)
14. Larynx	100	9 (9%)
15. Germ cell	21	8 (38%)
16. Urinary bladder	128	8 (6%)
17. Liver and biliary tract	325	7 (2%)
18. Prostate gland	171	6 (4%)
19. Pancreas	185	6 (3%)
20. Ovary	188	2 (1%)
21. Nose (interior)	32	1 (3%)
22. Pharynx	67	1 (1%)
23. Miscellaneous	245	0
	6,240	**653 (10%)**

*Modified from Burke and Virmani (who combined studies of McAllister HA and Fenoglia JJ Jr). *Tumors of the cardiovascular system atlas of tumor pathology.* Washington, DC: Armed Forces Institute of Pathology; 1978: 111–119; and Mukai K, Shinkai T, Tominaga K, Shiomosato Y. The incidence of secondary tumors of the heart and pericardium: a 10 year study. *Jpn J Clin Oncol.* 1988;18:195–201.

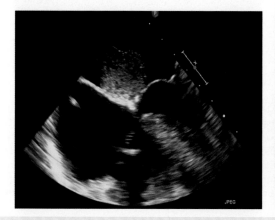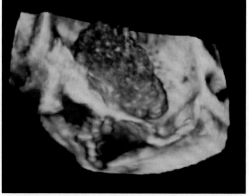

Figure 15-1. **Left atrial myxoma.** As seen here, most myxomas are attached to the interatrial septum in the region of the fossa ovalis. Left atrial locations predominate, but 20% of myxomas are found in the right atrium. Although in this example, the myxoma is sessile, these masses are frequently pedunculated. Three-dimensional echocardiography can be used to determine the presence of a pedicle and its site of attachment (Videos 15-4A,B).

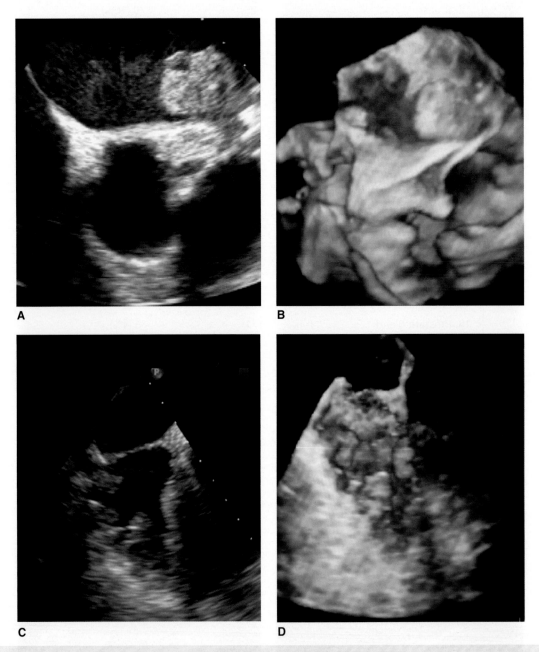

Figure 15-2. **Left atrial appendage thrombus on 2D and 3D transesophageal echocardiogram.** Left atrial myxomas are distinguished from left atrial thrombi primarily based on their location and clinical context. Atrial thrombi are most often found within the atrial appendage in the setting of atrial fibrillation[5] or in the left atrium proper as is more common in the setting of mitral stenosis. An important hint to the diagnosis of thrombus as opposed to myxoma is the presence of spontaneous echo contrast as seen in (A) and (B). Although the left atrial appendage thrombus in the upper panels is large and protrudes into the left atrium, they are more commonly well-circumscribed small echodensities located in the tip of the appendage as seen in (C) and (D) (Video 15-5). They must be distinguished from pectinate muscles, which are linear projections from the wall of the appendage into the body of the atrial appendage.[6]

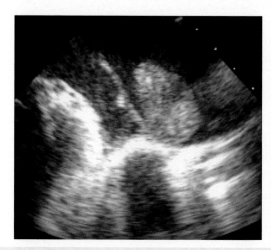
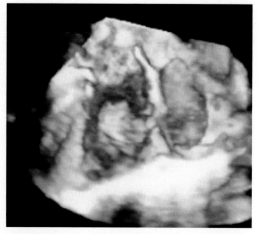

Figure 15-3. Pulmonary vein thrombus. Although atypical locations for myxomas have been reported, a pulmonary vein location would be quite rare. A mass found in this location is more often a tumor coming from the lung. Alternatively, as in this case, a pulmonary vein mass may represent a thrombus following a pulmonary vein ablation (Video 15-6).

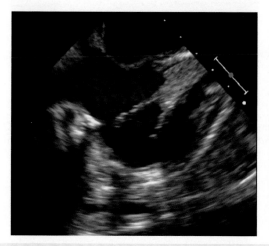
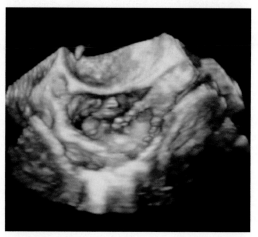

Figure 15-4. Catheter-associated thrombus. A myxoma would be in the differential diagnosis of a benign right atrial mass; however, catheter-associated thrombi are far more commonly encountered. In some cases, the mass may not be on the catheter itself but on the opposing right atrial wall where catheter-associated trauma has become the nidus for thrombus formation[7,8] (Videos 15-7A,B).

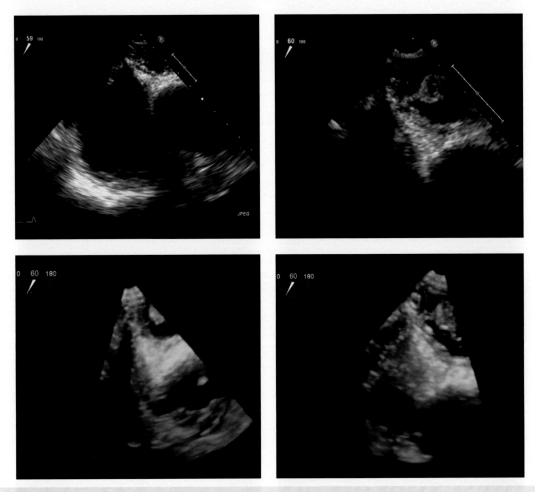

Figure 15-5. Thrombus in transit across the interatrial septum: transthoracic echocardiogram. In these 2D and 3D images, a thrombus is seen within the right atrium and crossing the interatrial septum to the left atrium through the foramen ovale (Videos 15-8A,B).

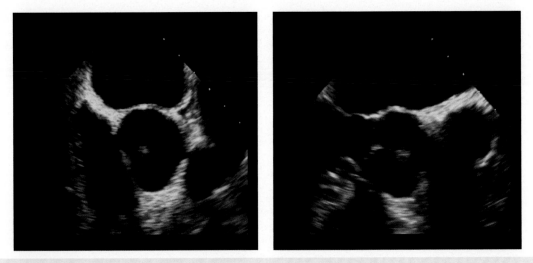

Figure 15-6. Aortic valve papillary fibroelastoma. Papillary fibroelastomas are the most common valvular masses. These nonneoplastic lesions arise from the endocardial surface and are most commonly found attached via a stalk on the aortic valve. The mitral valve is the next most commonly involved valve followed by the tricuspid and pulmonic valves, respectively.

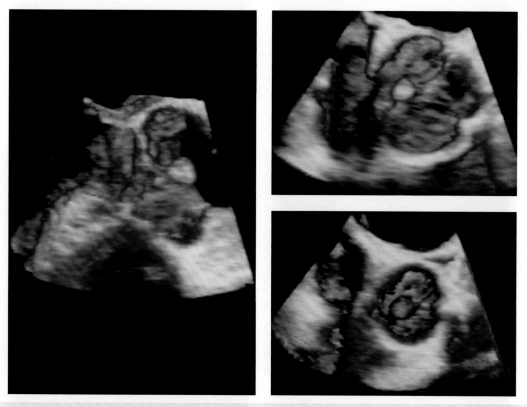

Figure 15-7. Aortic valve papillary fibroelastoma: zoomed 3D transesophageal echocardiogram. In this patient, the aortic valve papillary fibroelastoma on the noncoronary cusp of the aortic valve is well visualized (Video 15-10).

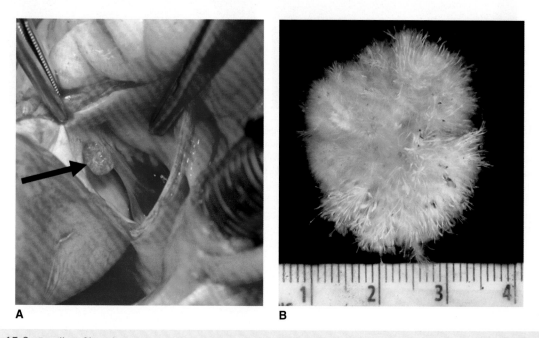

A   **B**

Figure 15-8. Papillary fibroelastoma: gross inspection (A) and pathologic specimen (B). Fibroelastomas are associated with embolic events, which are more common when they are >1 cm in size and highly mobile.[13] It has been postulated that material embolizes from multiple fronds on the surface of the mass. These fronds give fibroelastomas an irregular villous surface that has often compared to a sea anemone as can be appreciated on gross inspection during surgery (A) and on gross pathologic specimen (B).

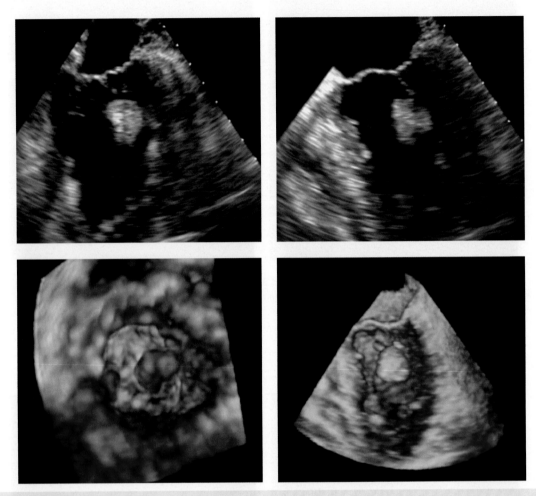

Figure 15-9. Papillary fibroelastoma on the mitral valve apparatus. Atypical locations for papillary fibroelastomas include the mitral valve leaflets, subvalvular apparatus, and endocardium. In this setting, atypical myxoma, Libman-Sacks endocarditis, or infective endocarditis should be considered in the differential diagnosis. The clinical scenario and lesion appearance are helpful to narrow the diagnosis. For instance, Libman-Sacks lesions are often described as sessile kissing lesions along the line of valve leaflet coaptation and may be associated with rheumatologic disorders such as systemic lupus, while the absence of bacteremia or fungemia argues against infective endocarditis. In addition, it is uncommon for a vegetation to be seen on the subvalvular apparatus in isolation. See also the shimmering gelatinous surface characteristic of papillary fibroelastomas in Videos 15-13A,B.

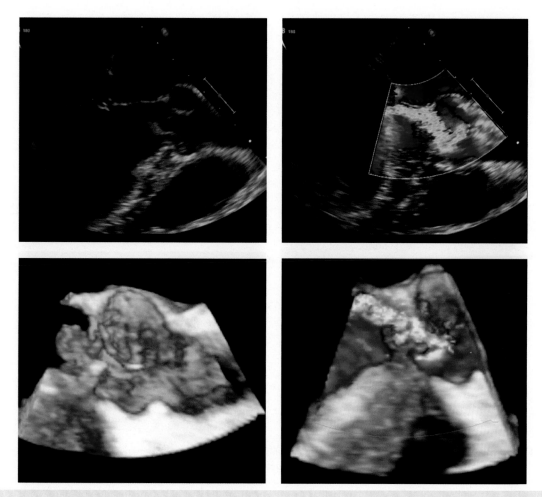

Figure 15-10. Aortic valve vegetation: 2D (upper panels) and 3D (lower panels) transesophageal echocardiograms. In the long-axis view of the aortic valve, an irregularly shaped echodensity is seen attached to the aortic valve. Unlike a papillary fibroelastoma, which tends not to disrupt valvular integrity, this vegetation has destroyed the valve's architecture. Consequently, there is significant eccentrically directed aortic insufficiency (Video 15-12).

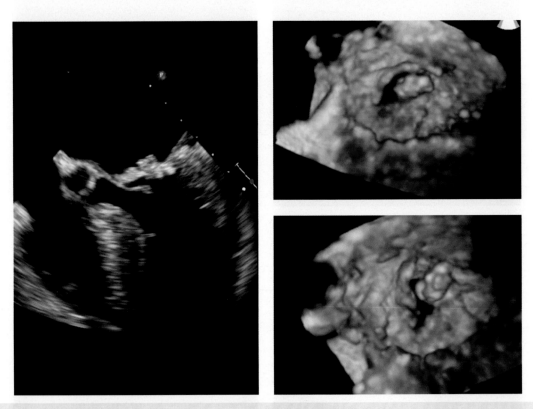

Figure 15-11. Mitral valve vegetation. Unlike the papillary fibroelastomas seen in Figures 15-8 and 15-9, this mass has no clear stalk and is not well circumscribed. A 2D transesophageal echocardiogram reveals an irregularly shaped echodensity along the mitral valve plane. A 3D transesophageal echocardiogram allows the image to be oriented in order to provide a bird's eye view of the mitral valve plane, demonstrating that the echodensity is attached to the anterior mitral valve leaflet. As in this case, most mitral and tricuspid valve vegetations tend to be located along the atrial surface of the valve (Video 15-14).

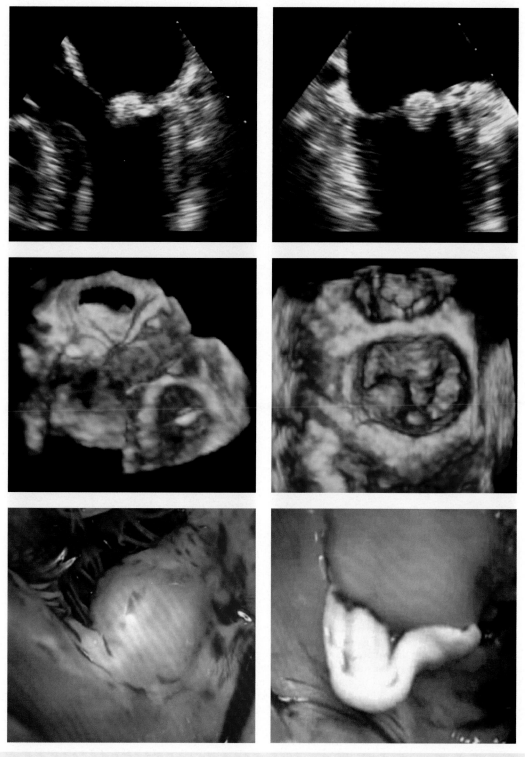

Figure 15-12. Caseous calcification of the mitral annulus. A 2D transesophageal echocardiogram reveals a bright, well-circumscribed but nonpedunculated mass along the mitral valve plane. The round, smooth surface and lack of a pedicle argue against the diagnosis of papillary fibroelastoma. The hyperreflective nature contrasts with the more fleshy nature of vegetations that tend to have an echodensity similar to the myocardium. On 3D transesophageal echocardiogram, this mass appears to affect only the posterior annulus near the lateral commissure. This was confirmed at surgery where the fairly smooth-surfaced mass was found along the posterior mitral annulus. Further probing prompted the extrusion of a milky white material with the consistency of toothpaste, consistent with caseous mitral annular calcification (Videos 15-15A,B).

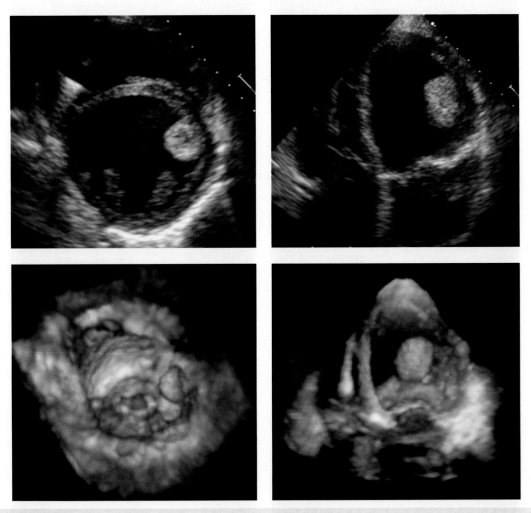

Figure 15-13. **Left ventricular thrombus.** This mass appears quite similar to the papillary fibroelastoma in Figure 15-9. The main distinguishing feature however is not appreciated on this static image. In real time, the mass in this figure is associated with left ventricular dysfunction. This makes thrombus much more likely than papillary fibroelastoma or even atypical myxoma, which are not associated with nor cause wall motion abnormalities. Manipulation of the 3D transthoracic images demonstrates that this lesion is sessile and nonpedunculated, which would be atypical for a fibroelastoma (Videos 15-16A,B).

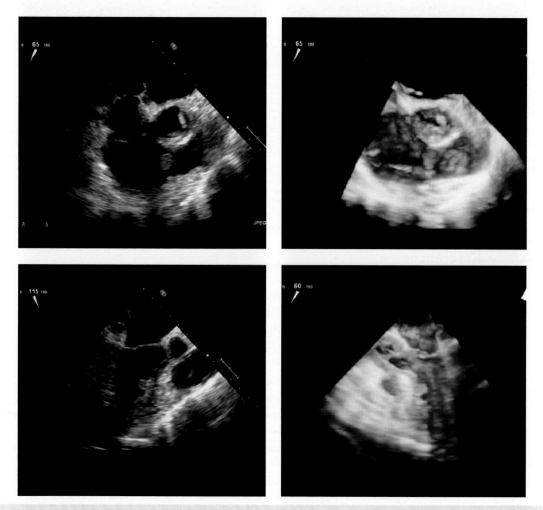

Figure 15-14. **Metastatic melanoma.** Both 2D and 3D echocardiograms show two round well-delineated masses along the right ventricular and left ventricular surfaces of the interventricular septum. Although thrombi are in the differential diagnosis for these masses given coexisting malignancy, there are no regional wall motion abnormalities and no spontaneous echo contrast to suggest stasis. The patient declined biopsy (Videos 15-17A,B).

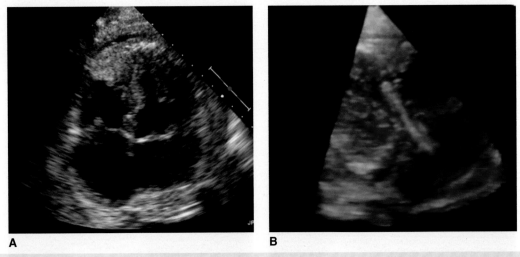

A B

Figure 15-15. Metastatic squamous cell carcinoma. On the 2D transthoracic echocardiogram apical four-chamber view in (A), the right ventricular apex is completely filled with an echodense material. This patient had known tonsillar carcinoma and also had had a pulmonary embolism. The patient agreed to a biopsy of the mass during which 3D echocardiography was utilized to guide the bioptome, as shown in the RV inflow view in (B). The pathologic diagnosis confirmed metastatic malignancy (Videos 15-18A,B).

References

1. Roberts WC. Primary and secondary neoplasms of the heart. *Am J Cardiol* 1997;80(5):671–682.

2. Reynen K. Cardiac myxomas. *N Engl J Med.* 1995;333(24):1610–1617.

3. Waller DA, Ettles DF, Saunders NR, et al. Recurrent cardiac myxoma: the surgical implications of two distinct groups of patients. *Thorac Cardiovasc Surg.* 1989;37(4):226–230.

4. McCarthy PM, Piehler JM, Schaff HV, et al. The significance of multiple, recurrent, and "complex" cardiac myxomas. *J Thorac Cardiovasc Surg.* 1986;91(3):389–396.

5. Klein AL, Grimm RA, Murray RD, et al. Use of transesophageal echocardiography to guide cardioversion in patients with atrial fibrillation. *N Engl J Med.* 2001;344(19):1411–1420.

6. Orsinelli DA, Pearson AC. Usefulness of multiplane transesophageal echocardiography in differentiating left atrial appendage thrombus from pectinate muscles. *Am Heart J.* 1996;131(3):622–623.

7. Fuchs S, Pollak A, Gilon D. Central venous catheter mechanical irritation of the right atrial free wall: a cause for thrombus formation. *Cardiology.* 1999;91(3):169–172.

8. Gilon D, Schechter D, Rein AJ, et al. Right atrial thrombi are related to indwelling central venous catheter position: insights into time course and possible mechanism of formation. *Am Heart J.* 1998;135(3):457–462.

9. Putnam JB Jr, Sweeney MS, Colon R, et al. Primary cardiac sarcomas. *Ann Thorac Surg.* 1991;51(6):906–910.

10. Meng Q, Lai H, Lima J, et al. Echocardiographic and pathologic characteristics of primary cardiac tumors: a study of 149 cases. *Int J Cardiol.* 2002;84(1):69–75.

11. Burke AP, Cowan D, Virmani R. Primary sarcomas of the heart. *Cancer.* 1992;69(2):387–395.

12. Bear PA, Moodie DS. Malignant primary cardiac tumors. The Cleveland Clinic experience, 1956 to 1986. *Chest.* 1987;92(5):860–862.

13. Sun JP, Asher CR, Yang XS, et al. Clinical and echocardiographic characteristics of papillary fibroelastomas: a retrospective and prospective study in 162 patients. *Circulation.* 2001;103(22):2687–2693.

14. Kirkpatrick JN, Wong T, Bednarz JE, et al. Differential diagnosis of cardiac masses using contrast echocardiographic perfusion imaging. *J Am Coll Cardiol.* 2004;43(8):1412–1419.

15. Nanda NC, Abd-El Rahman SM, Khatri G, et al. Incremental value of three-dimensional echocardiography over transesophageal multiplane two-dimensional echocardiography in quantitative and qualitative assessment of cardiac masses and defects. *Echocardiography.* 1995;12(6):619–628.

16. Asch FM, Bieganski SP, Panza JA, et al. Real-time 3-dimensional echocardiography evaluation of intracardiac masses. *Echocardiography.* 2006;23(3):218–224.

17. Muller S, Feuchtner G, Bonatti J, et al. Value of transesophageal 3D echocardiography as an adjunct to conventional 2D imaging in preoperative evaluation of cardiac masses. *Echocardiography.* 2008;25(6):624–631.

Note: Page numbers in *italics* denote figures; those followed by "t" denote tables.